PLAY IN CLINICAL PRACTICE

Play in Clinical Practice

Evidence-Based Approaches

edited by
SANDRA W. RUSS
LARISSA N. NIEC

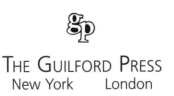

THE GUILFORD PRESS
New York   London

© 2011 The Guilford Press
A Division of Guilford Publications, Inc.
72 Spring Street, New York, NY 10012
www.guilford.com

Printed in the United States of America

This book is printed on acid-free paper.

Last digit is print number: 9 8 7 6 5 4 3 2 1

Library of Congress Cataloging-in-Publication Data is available
from the Publisher.

ISBN 978-1-60918-046-1

To Nathaniel,
who understood the importance of play,

and to all the children
who have taught us about play

About the Editors

Sandra W. Russ, PhD, a child clinical psychologist, is Professor of Psychology at Case Western Reserve University, where she teaches courses in Child and Family Intervention and Psychology of Creativity. She has served as president of the Society for Personality Assessment; the Society of Clinical Child and Adolescent Psychology (American Psychological Association [APA] Division 53); and the Society for the Psychology of Aesthetics, Creativity and the Arts (APA Division 10). Dr. Russ's research program has focused on pretend play, creativity, and adaptive functioning in children. She developed the Affect in Play Scale, which assesses pretend play in children, and she and her students are developing a play facilitation intervention. She is the author of *Affect and Creativity: The Role of Affect and Play in the Creative Process* (1993) and *Play in Child Development and Psychotherapy: Toward Empathically Supported Practice* (2004).

Larissa N. Niec, PhD, is Professor of Psychology in the Clinical Psychology Doctoral Program at Central Michigan University and Director of the University's Parent–Child Interaction Therapy Clinic. She conducts basic and applied research on play, child maltreatment, and parent–child interaction therapy. The overarching goal of her research program is to reduce barriers to evidence-based treatment for children and families. Currently, Dr. Niec is involved in national efforts to increase the effectiveness of treatment dissemination to community therapists. Her first novel, *Shorn,* was published in 2008.

Contributors

Emily Abbenante, MA, Department of Psychology, Central Michigan University, Mt. Pleasant, Michigan

Sarah E. Baker, PhD, Pediatric Prevention Research Center, Wayne State University School of Medicine, Detroit, Michigan

Sandra J. Bishop-Josef, PhD, Edward Zigler Center in Child Development and Social Policy, Child Study Center, Yale School of Medicine, New Haven, Connecticut

Elizabeth Brestan-Knight, PhD, Department of Psychology, Auburn University, Auburn, Alabama

Kristin M. Briggs, EdD, NJ Cares Institute, School of Osteopathic Medicine, University of Medicine and Dentistry of New Jersey, Stratford, New Jersey

Rhea M. Chase, PhD, Center for Child and Family Health, University of North Carolina at Chapel Hill, Chapel Hill, North Carolina

Candice Chow, MA, Center for Anxiety and Related Disorders, Boston University, Boston, Massachusetts

Gina B. Christopher, MA, Baylor College of Medicine, Houston, Texas

Meena Dasari, PhD, Metropolitan Center for Cognitive Behavioral Therapy, New York, New York

Esther Deblinger, PhD, NJ Cares Institute, School of Osteopathic Medicine, University of Medicine and Dentistry of New Jersey, Stratford, New Jersey

Julie Fiorelli, BA, Department of Psychology, Case Western Reserve University, Cleveland, Ohio

Cheryl Gering, MA, Department of Psychology, Central Michigan University, Mt. Pleasant, Michigan

Suzanne Gorovoy, MA, Department of Psychology, Case Western Reserve University, Cleveland, Ohio

Amanda C. Gulsrud, PhD, UCLA Semel Institute for Neuroscience and Human Behavior, Los Angeles, California

Linh Huynh, MA, UCLA Semel Institute for Neuroscience and Human Behavior, Los Angeles, California

Jason F. Jent, PhD, Miller School of Medicine, University of Miami, Miami, Florida

Connie Kasari, PhD, UCLA Semel Institute for Neuroscience and Human Behavior, Los Angeles, California

Astrida Seja Kaugars, PhD, Department of Psychology, Marquette University, Milwaukee, Wisconsin

Sue M. Knell, PhD, Spectrum Psychological Associates, Mayfield Village, Ohio

Barbara Lewis, PhD, Department of Communication Sciences, Case Western Reserve University, Cleveland, Ohio

Michael J. Manos, PhD, Center for Pediatric Behavioral Health, Cleveland Clinic, Cleveland, Ohio

May Matson, MA, Department of Psychology, University of Texas at Austin, Austin, Texas

Larissa N. Niec, PhD, Department of Psychology, Central Michigan University, Mt. Pleasant, Michigan

Maia Noeder, MA, Department of Psychology, Case Western Reserve University, Cleveland, Ohio

Beth L. Pearson, PhD, Children's Health Council, Palo Alto, California

Jessica Pian, BS, Center for Anxiety and Related Disorders, Boston University, Boston, Massachusetts

Donna B. Pincus, PhD, Center for Anxiety and Related Disorders, Boston University, Boston, Massachusetts

Melissa K. Runyon, PhD, NJ Cares Institute, School of Osteopathic Medicine, University of Medicine and Dentistry of New Jersey, Stratford, New Jersey

Sandra W. Russ, PhD, Department of Psychology, Case Western Reserve University, Cleveland, Ohio

Christie A. Salamone, PhD, Columbus Psychological Associates, Columbus, Georgia

Elizabeth J. Short, PhD, Department of Psychology, Case Western Reserve University, Cleveland, Ohio

Sara Cain Spannagel, MA, Department of Psychology, Case Western Reserve University, Cleveland, Ohio

Deborah J. Tharinger, PhD, Department of Educational Psychology, University of Texas, Austin, Austin, Texas

Courtney L. Weiner, MA, Center for Anxiety and Related Disorders, Boston University, Boston, Massachusetts

Edward F. Zigler, PhD, Edward Zigler Center in Child Development and Social Policy, Child Study Center, Yale School of Medicine, New Haven, Connecticut

Preface

Play is important for children. Mental health professionals have known this for decades. Research has supported the importance of play in child development for decades as well. Play was first used in therapy by psychoanalytic therapists in the 1930s but soon became part of nondirective client-centered therapies. Recently, play has been integrated into cognitive-behavioral approaches with children. One of the unique characteristics of play is that the processes that occur in play have important functions in child development. The use of play in therapy fits with a developmental perspective in working with children.

Play has many functions. In daily life, children communicate through play; express emotions and worries in play; and develop many abilities through play. In therapy, with adult guidance, the play process can be used to bring about change in a variety of ways.

A plethora of clinical literature presents a rich clinical base for the effectiveness of play in therapy to bring about change. However, as the field moves toward empirically supported practice, it is imperative that an empirical base be developed for the use of play in therapy. For play to continue to be used in therapy, we must learn when and how play is effective and for which child populations. Also, we need to know what types of play and techniques are helpful under which specific circumstances. Ideally, these studies will inform us about why play helps. There are many theories about how play aids the child, but empirical support for various theoretical explanations will help identify the mechanisms of change and inform future practice.

The aim of this book is to contribute to the growing base of empirical support for the use of play in therapy. The research findings presented in this book also have implications for the use of play in prevention and intervention programs.

A large body of basic research supports the important role of play in child development. Play influences cognitive, emotional, and interpersonal development and has been linked to areas of adaptive functioning such as creativity, coping, emotional understanding, and affect regulation. The findings from this basic research have important implications for the development of assessment and intervention programs for emotionally disturbed children and prevention programs in early childhood.

Within the area of applied research, a number of evidence-based interventions for children exist that include play as a key component of treatment. These treatments are often outside the realm of traditional play therapy and include, for example, behavioral and cognitive-behavioral interventions such as parent–child interaction therapy, trauma-focused cognitive-behavioral therapy, and cognitive-behavioral play therapy.

These two important areas of play research—basic and applied—remain largely unintegrated. There is a growing need for translational work that links the basic developmental research in play with the applied work in assessment, intervention, and prevention. This book provides a bridge between the literatures.

Part I focuses on the research on play and child development. Chapter 1, by Russ, Fiorelli, and Spannagel, presents an overview of cognitive and affective processes in play and their role in adaptive functioning in children. Chapter 2, by Jent, Niec, and Baker, reviews play and interpersonal functioning. Both chapters discuss implications of the child development research on play for the use of play in therapy.

Part II presents evidence-based play assessment approaches. Chapter 3, by Kaugars, presents an overview of play assessment measures and empirical support. Chapter 4, by Breslan-Knight and Salamone, focuses on the assessment of parent–child interaction through a structured play-based assessment. Chapter 5, by Tharinger, Christopher, and Matson, focuses on the use of play in the increasingly popular therapeutic assessment approach.

Part III presents evidence-based intervention approaches that integrate play as an important component. Chapter 6, by Niec, Gering, and Abbenante, reviews the empirical support for parent–child interaction therapy, in which play is a key component. Chapter 7, by Briggs, Runyon, and Deblinger, reviews play in trauma-focused cognitive-behavioral treatment. Next, Kasari, Huynh, and Gulsrud (Chapter 8) review the play intervention research with children with autism. Pincus, Chase, Chow, Weiner, and Pian (Chapter 9) review the use of play in cognitive-behavioral therapy for anxiety disorders. In Chapter 10, Knell and Dasari present cognitive-behavioral play therapy, an integrated treatment approach. Finally, Short, Noeder, Gorovoy, Manos, and Lewis (Chapter 11) present research on play in assessment and treatment with children with special needs and with attention-deficit/hyperactivity disorder, Asperger syndrome, and language disabilities.

Part IV focuses on play intervention and prevention programs in school settings. Bishop-Josef and Zigler (Chapter 12) give an overview of the history and research in Head Start programs with preschool children and discuss the role of play in the curricula. Russ and Pearson (Chapter 13) review the focused play intervention studies in primarily elementary school settings and implications for future programs in the schools.

Finally, in Chapter 14, Russ and Niec offer some thoughts and conclusions that emerge from the chapters. Implications for integrating play into therapy, prevention programs, and research are discussed.

We are fortunate to have such outstanding authors who are experts in the field contributing to this volume. These expert clinicians and researchers present the current knowledge base of research in the play area as it pertains to intervention and prevention. We hope that this book will provide a base for future research and practice with play.

ACKNOWLEDGMENTS

We want to express appreciation to Rochelle Serwator, our editor at The Guilford Press, for her excellent guidance in shaping this book. Her understanding of the child area and consistent support was essential in the development of this project.

We also want to thank the leading group of scholars and researchers who contributed to this book.

Sandra W. Russ also wants to thank her husband, Tom Brugger, for his constant love and support.

Contents

PART I
Play in Child Development

1

Cognitive and Affective Processes in Play

Sandra W. Russ, Julie Fiorelli,
and Sarah Cain Spannagel

Play is a universal phenomenon for children around the world. Is play just another way of having fun? Or is play—and the many forms of play—serving a larger purpose? Research evidence suggests that a larger purpose is being served, that of adaptive functioning. The child development literature finds many associations among play, especially pretend play, and areas of adaptive functioning for children such as creative problem solving, coping ability, and perspective taking. Cognitive and affective processes that emerge in pretend play are key processes in many of these adaptive behavioral correlates of play. This chapter focuses on cognitive and affective processes in pretend play and implications for the use of play in therapy. (Interpersonal processes are reviewed in Chapter 2).

WHAT IS PLAY?

Krasnor and Pepler (1980) developed a model of play that involves four components: nonliterality, positive affect, intrinsic motivation, and flexibility. They believed that "pure play" involves all four components to varying degrees. In their model, we can see the presence of both cognitive and affective processes. Flexibility and the use of symbolism and pretend are important aspects of cognitive functioning. Positive affect and intrinsic motivation—doing something for the love of doing it—are important affective processes. The processes that occur in pretend play are important in both child development and child psychotherapy.

Pretend play involves the use of fantasy and make-believe and the use of symbolism. Fein (1987) stated that pretend play is a symbolic behavior in which "one thing is playfully treated as if it were something else" (p. 282). Fein also thought that pretense is charged with feelings and emotional intensity, so that affect is intertwined with pretend play.

Hirsh-Pasek and Golinkoff (2003) concluded that around the age 2, children begin to discover pretend play. For example, they can pretend to talk on a telephone. Pretend play becomes more evident by the third and fourth year. Children are able to think symbolically, use objects to represent different things, and consider worlds outside their own. Play follows developmental stages in which a child moves from reacting to characteristics of objects, to exploring objects, to symbolically using objects (Belsky & Most, 1981).

Krasnor and Pepler (1980) articulated three perspectives on the role of play in child development. First, play reflects the developmental level of the child and can be used as a diagnostic tool. Second, play provides an opportunity to practice skills. Third, play is a causal agent in developmental change. Child therapists are in a unique position to use play to help bring about developmental change.

COGNITIVE AND AFFECTIVE PROCESSES IN PLAY

What kind of processes occur in pretend play? Russ (2004) identified a number of cognitive and affective processes in play that emerged in the clinical and research literature. This framework for conceptualizing the processes in play was based on the theory and research in child development and psychotherapy.

Fantasy is an integral part of pretend play (Klinger, 1971). Piaget (1945/1967) conceptualized fantasy as "interiorized play," while J. Singer (1981) viewed play as the "externalization" of fantasy. Sherrod and Singer (1979) identified processes involved in both fantasy and pretend play activities: the ability to form images, skill in storing and retrieving stored images, possessing a store of images, skill in recombining and integrating these images as a source of internal stimulation and divorcing them from reality, and reinforcement for skillful recombining of images.

They believed that the last two processes were unique to fantasy and play activities.

After reviewing the literature, Russ (2004) identified the following cognitive processes as occurring in play:

- *Fantasy/make-believe.* The ability to engage in "as-if" play behavior. Pretending to be in a different time and space. Role-playing different characters.
- *Symbolism.* The ability to transform ordinary objects (blocks, Legos) into representations of other objects (e.g., a block becomes a telephone).
- *Organization.* The ability to tell a story with a logical time sequence, plot, and indications of cause and effect. Narratives can vary in elaboration of detail and complexity.
- *Divergent thinking.* The ability to generate a number of different ideas, story themes, and symbols.

Affective processes identified by Russ were:

- *Expression of emotion.* The ability to express affect states in a pretend play situation. Both positive and negative emotions are expressed. For example, the doll expresses aggression by angrily yelling at another doll "I don't like you."
- *Expression of affect themes.* The ability to express affect images and content themes in play. For example, the child builds a fortress with guns to prepare for battle. This is aggressive ideation, even though no fighting has occurred.
- *Enjoyment of play.* The ability to "get lost" in the play experience and to experience pleasure and joy.
- *Cognitive integration, emotion regulation, and modulation of affect.* The ability to process emotion and to integrate affect into a cognitive context.

Because both cognitive and affective processes occur in play, often simultaneously, we can learn about cognitive–affective interaction (Singer & Singer, 1990). This is especially important in order to develop play therapy interventions. Slade and Wolf (1994) stated that the cognitive and affective functions of play are intertwined: "Just as the development of cognitive structures may play an important role in the resolution of emotional conflict, so emotional consolidation may provide an impetus to cognitive advances and integration" (p. xv).

In order to study these cognitive and affective processes in play, we need to be able to measure them. Much of the early research on play measured cognitive processes. Rubin, Fein, and Vandenberg referred to this phenomenon as the "cognification" of play (1983). There has been increasing study of affect in play. Russ developed the Affect in Play Scale (APS) in the late 1980s in order to study affective processes and a number of studies have since been carried out with this measure (Russ, 1987, 1993, 2004). The APS consists of a 5-minute task with puppets and blocks in which the child is instructed to play any way he or she likes. The play is videotaped and coded for amount of affect themes and expressions in the play narrative, variety of affect themes, imagination, organization of the story, and enjoyment of the play. What follows is a review of the play and adaptive functioning literature. Some of these studies used the APS.

PRETEND PLAY AND ADAPTIVE FUNCTIONING

Both cognitive and affective processes in pretend play relate to many areas of adaptive functioning in children. In a meta-analysis of 46 play studies, Fisher (1992) found the largest effect sizes for relationships between play and divergent thinking and for perspective taking (effect sizes = 0.387 and 0.392, respectively). Fisher concluded that research supported the thesis that play results in improvement in children's development.

Creativity

Divergent thinking and perspective taking are important ingredients in creativity. A large body of research links pretend play and creativity. In general, children who have better pretend play skills are more creative, independent of intelligence. This finding is relevant to child therapy because the ability to problem-solve in innovative ways can generalize to everyday problems in living. Ruth Richards's concept of "everyday creativity" stresses the importance of creative problem solving in daily life (1990).

A number of cognitive processes have been found to be involved in and unique to creative problem solving. Two major cognitive processes are divergent thinking and transformation abilities, identified by Guilford (1968). *Divergent thinking* is the generation of a variety of ideas. This kind of thinking goes off in different directions, in contrast to *convergent thinking* which focuses in on a specific solution. Divergent thinking involves following associations and having a breadth of attention to internal cues (Kogan, 1983). Wallach (1970) stated that divergent thinking is dependent on the flow of ideas and "fluidity in generating cognitive units" (p. 1240). Divergent thinking has been found to be relatively independent of intelligence (Runco, 1991). *Transformation ability* is the capacity to break out of a set or a fixed way of thinking and to see a new solution or new configuration of a pattern. Flexibility of thought is involved in this ability to follow different paths in problem solving.

Other cognitive processes that are important but not unique to creative thinking are insight and synthesizing abilities (Sternberg, 1988), sensitivity to problems and problem finding (Runco, 1994), having a wide breadth of knowledge (Barron & Harrington, 1981), and evaluative ability (Guilford, 1950).

Affective processes are also involved in creativity. Joy and love of the work is important and can result in the "flow" state (Csikszentmihalyi, 1990) in which the person "gets lost" in the task. Openness to affect-laden images and memories is involved in artistic production as well as in divergent thinking itself. The ability to be open to affect in fantasy and not repress has been associated with creativity. A positive emotional state has also been related to creativity. For a review of the research and theoretical literature on cognitive and affective processes involved in creativity, see Russ (1993, 2004).

It makes theoretical sense that pretend play would relate to creativity because so many of the cognitive and affective processes involved in creativity occur in play. Much of the research has focused on the play and divergent thinking relationship. Theoretically, play should be related to divergent thinking because in play children generate a variety of ideas and recombine ideas and symbols. Singer and Singer (1990) think of play as actual practice with divergent thinking. Russ (1993) has stressed the importance of affect in divergent thinking. The involvement of emotion in play should increase access to emotional memories and broaden the associative network. In addition, Fein (1987) proposed that children use play to develop and manipulate an affective symbol system. Fein conceptualized this affective symbol system as representing real or imagined experience at a general level. These affective units constitute affect-binding representational templates that store information about affect-laden events. The units are "manipulated, interpreted, coordinated and elaborated in a way that makes affective sense to the players" (p. 292). These affective units are a key part of pretend play and of creative thinking. Fein thought that activities that involved divergent thinking, like daydreaming, pretend play, and drawing, activated the affective symbol system. Fein concluded that creative processes could not be studied independently of an affective symbol system.

A large number of studies have found a relationship between play and divergent thinking (Johnson, 1976; Pepler & Ross, 1981; Singer & Rummo, 1973). Russ and Grossman-McKee (1990) found that both cognitive and affective processes in play related to divergent thinking, independent of intelligence. Lieberman (1977) found a relationship between playfulness and joy and divergent thinking in kindergarten children. Both positive and negative affect in play relates to divergent thinking. Russ and Schafer (2006) found a relationship between negative affect in fantasy play and divergent thinking. Children who could express negative themes in play, such as aggression or fear, generated more uses for objects and more original uses for objects than children who expressed less negative affect. Kaugars and Russ (2009) also found a relationship between affect expression in pretend play and divergent thinking in preschool children. In a recent study, pretend play ability and divergent thinking related to storytelling ability (Dillon & Russ, 2010), suggesting that processes involved in both play and divergent thinking could be involved in real-world creativity.

In a longitudinal study, Russ, Robins, and Christiano (1999) found that imagination and organization of fantasy in play in first and second graders was associated with divergent thinking in the fifth and sixth grades. As in many other studies, this relationship was independent of intelligence. The relationship between play and divergent thinking was stable over a 4-year period.

Much of the research on play and divergent thinking has been correlational and can not imply a causal relationship. However, there have been some experimental studies in the literature. In two important studies, play facilitated divergent thinking in preschool children (Dansky & Silverman, 1973; Dansky, 1980). These two studies are important in that they show a direct effect of play on divergent thinking. Smith and Whitney (1987) have criticized many play and divergent thinking studies because of experimenter bias. However, a number of studies did control for experimenter bias and found facilitative effects for play (Dansky, 1999).

Pretend play has also been found to facilitate insight in problem-solving tasks. Vandenberg (1980), in a review of insight and pretend play studies, concluded that all of these studies had the consistent finding that play facilitated insightful tool use and enhanced motivated task activity. Vandenberg pointed to the similarity between play and creativity. In both play and creativity, one is creating novelty from the commonplace and has a disregard for the familiar.

Russ (2004) concluded that, over time, engaging in pretend play helps the child become more creative in the following ways:

1. Practice with the free flow of associations that is part of divergent thinking.
2. Practice with symbol substitution, recombining of ideas, and manipulation of object representations. These processes are part of transformation ability and insight ability.
3. Express and experience positive affect. Positive affect is important in creativity. In addition, positive affect in play could be the precurser of the passion and joy that people take in the creative act. Children who can get lost in play could also get lost in the creative act. Getting lost in play could be the child's form of the "flow" state identified by Csikszentmihalyi (1990) as experienced during creative activities.
4. Express and think about affect themes and images. Learn to code and manipulate the affective symbols that Fein proposed. Emotion-laden content is permitted to surface and be expressed through play. Over time, the child develops access to a variety of memories, associations, and affective and nonaffective cognition. This broad repertoire of associations helps with creative problem solving.

The research findings that have established a relationship between play and creativity are relevant to the area of play therapy. Play is involved in creative problem solving. Children who engage in pretend play and who can express emotion in play are able to think flexibly, generate alternatives to problems, and come up with novel solutions. This ability generalizes to solving problems in daily living and to coping with stress.

Coping

Play has also been found to relate to coping ability. Coping refers to efforts to manage stress (Lazarus & Folkman. 1984). The link between play and divergent thinking probably partially accounts for the play and coping connection. Good divergent thinkers should be able to think of alternative solutions to real-life problems. There is some empirical support for this concept. Russ (1988) found a relationship between divergent thinking and teachers' ratings of coping in fifth-grade boys. Similarly, Carson, Bittner, Cameson, Brown, and Meyer (1994) found a significant relationship between figural divergent thinking and teacher's ratings of coping. Russ et al. (1999) found a relationship between divergent thinking and quality of coping responses in a self-report scale. So there is some evidence that the ability to generate different solutions to problems is a factor in daily coping.

Much of the research that has investigated the relationship between play and coping has been done with the APS as the measure of children's play. These studies have used different coping measures and were carried out by different researchers. For example, in a study of 7- to 9-year-old children undergoing an invasive dental procedure, Christiano and Russ (1996) found a positive relationship between play and coping and a negative relationship between play and distress. Children who were "good" players on the APS (in that they expressed affect and imagination in their play) implemented a greater number and variety of coping strategies and reported less distress during the dental procedure than did children who expressed less affect and fantasy in play. In a longitudinal study, Russ et al. (1999) found that play ability significantly predicted self-reported coping over a 4-year period.

Adjustment

Play and adjustment is an area very relevant to play therapy. Although there is less research in this area than in the creativity area, some studies do suggest a relationship with adjustment or aspects of adjustment. Certainly the research on play and coping just reviewed relates to adjustment. Children who have more coping strategies available to them should be better adjusted in general.

In a recent study by Burck (2010), play ability on the APS was positively related to parents' rating of adaptive functioning. Singer and Singer (1990) concluded that imaginative play related to academic adjustment and flexibility of thought. They also found that preschoolers who engaged in make-believe play were better adjusted across different situations. In a study of urban children from 4 to 5 years of age, Rosenberg (1984) found that quality of fantasy play for children playing in dyads was positively related to social competence and ego resilience. Positive themes and relationship themes in the play related to the social competence and ego resilience measures. D'Angelo (1995) also found that ego-resilient children had better play than undercontrolled or overcontrolled children. Grossman-McKee (1989) found that boys who expressed more affect in play had fewer pain complaints than boys with less affect in play. Good players were also less anxious on an anxiety rating scale. The conclusion from this study was that the ability to express affect in play was related to fewer psychosomatic complaints. Several other studies also found a negative relationship between play ability and anxiety (Goldstein, 2002; Christian, 2009).

Another component of adjustment is emotion regulation. Shields and Cicchetti (1988) defined *emotion regulation* as the ability to modulate emotion and engage in an adaptive way with the environment. Berk, Mann, and Ogan (2006) found that a play intervention with preschoolers resulted in increased emotion regulation. Recent research in our research lab by Jessica Dillon (Dillon & Russ, 2010) found a relationship between play ability and parents' ratings of emotion regulation. Also in our lab, Karla Fehr (2009) found a positive relationship between play ability and prosocial behavior and a negative relationship between play and physical aggression in the classroom in preschoolers.

PROCESSING OF EMOTIONS IN PLAY

One of the reasons that play ability relates to areas of adjustment is that children use play to process emotions. Because play is a natural way for emotion to be expressed, it is one of the major ways children learn to deal with emotions. Fein's (1987) concept of manipulation of affect symbols that represent experience and relationships is an important concept. In play, children act out emotion-laden memories and change the scripts in innumerable ways. Children also use play to elevate their mood. Kenealy (1989) reported that 50% of children ages 4–11 used play strategies to feel better when they were depressed. And, as just discussed, children learn to regulate their emotions in play. Mennin, Heimberg, Turk, and Fresco (2002) concluded that an emotion regulation perspective would have as goals of treatment to help individuals (1) become more comfortable with arousing emotional experience; (2) be more able to access and utilize emotional information in adaptive problem solving; and (3) be better able to modulate emotional experience and expression. Play can help children accomplish these goals. Russ (2004) reviewed a number of theoretical frameworks that could explain the role of play in processing emotions.

Of particular importance to child psychotherapy, children utilize play to manage negative emotions. How does this happen in play? What are the cognitive-affective mechanisms that enable anxiety to be reduced? How does play help the child deal with fear, anger, or sadness? Singer and Singer (1990) suggested that play is reinforcing when it permits expression of positive affect and the appropriate control of negative affect. Research by Golomb and Galasso (1995) supports this idea. In a study with preschoolers, they found that when the affective valence of an imagined situation was negative, children would modify the theme to diminish their fear, such as by imagining a "friendly" monster. In a positive affect situation, they concluded that children monitor and regulate affect in play so as not to exceed a certain threshold while still having enough emotional involvement to enjoy the play. Children are making the affect manageable through play.

Singer (1995) referred to Tomkins's (1970) concept of "miniaturization." Play is a way that children "cut down the large things around it to manageable proportions" (p. 191). By creating manageable situations in a pretend, safe setting, negative emotions can be expressed. Singer proposed that children can then increase positive affect and reduce negative affect through play. This conceptualization fits with the idea that play is one way in which children learn to regulate their emotions. Waelder (1933) described the play process as one in which the child repeats an unpleasant experience over and over until it becomes manageable. As he puts it, the child "digests the event." Erikson (1963) thought of the child as mastering traumatic events and conflicts through play.

Psychodynamic theory and treatment focuses on helping the child to reexperience unpleasant emotions in a safe setting through play. The therapist helps the child to reexperience major developmental conflicts or situational traumas in therapy. For many children, this reexperiencing occurs through play. The therapist labels feelings and makes interpretations, guides the play to varying degrees, and helps with the working-through process. Freedheim and Russ (1992) described the slow process of gaining access to conflict-laden content and playing it out until resolution has occurred.

Recent conceptualizations specify mechanisms by which negative affect is managed. Strayhorn (2002) discussed the role of fantasy rehearsal in developing self-control. This can occur in play. Strayhorn stated that fantasy rehearsal helps the child build up habit strength for the handling of conflict situations . A child could reduce fears and anxiety around separation and other issues by acting out adaptive ways of handling the separation and feelings around it in a pretend play situation.

Exposure to negative emotions that the child has been avoiding is central to cognitive-behavioral treatments. Play is one way children can gain exposure in a controlled manner to these emotions and painful memories. Jacobsen and colleagues (2002) found that avoidance coping predicted symptom severity in a posttraumatic stress disorder (PTSD) population of adults who had undergone bone marrow transplants. They utilized a social-cognitive-processing model of trauma recovery (Lepore, Silver, Wortman, & Wayment, 1996) to understand the results. Greater use of avoidance coping such as denial, escape, and avoidance, would give individuals fewer opportunities to process or habituate to the thoughts, images, and memories. There would be less integration of the negative memories. Therapists who work with children with PTSD or with traumatized backgrounds offer many clinical descriptions of the effective use of play to help children integrate traumatic experiences (Gil, 1991; D. Singer, 1993; Terr, 1990).

Using a different framework, Harris (2000) conducted a number of studies and viewed pretend play as helping the child to construct a situation model that is revisable. Children go back and forth between reality and an imagined world. Learning how reality could be different helps children make causal judgments. The play process could help children reduce anxiety by developing a new cognitive appraisal of the situation.

Pennebaker's research on the emotional expression writing paradigm is also relevant to the play area. His studies randomly assign adults to write either about superficial topics or about important personal topics for 15–30 minutes a day for 3–5 days. His studies have found that the emotional writing group's physical and mental health improves (Pennebaker, 2002; Pennebaker & Graybeal, 2001). Mental health measures included drops in rumination and depression and higher grades among students. One of the possible change mechanisms that Pennebaker suggests is that the coherence of the narrative that is constructed produces a transformation of the emotional event. A new meaning to the event is developed. New meanings are also developed in the play situation. Children are expressing emotions and developing narratives. In play therapy, the therapist helps tie the narrative to the child's own life and put the play event into a meaningful context. One implication of Pennebaker's findings is that the coherent narrative in which the emotion is placed is important.

Developing a coherent narrative is central to the structured play techniques used by Gaensbauer and Siegal (1995) with very young children. They use structured play techniques with toddlers who have experienced traumatic techniques. They think that the mechanisms of change when play is used are similar to the mechanisms of change in older children with PTSD. With these young children, the therapists actively structure the play to re-create the traumatic event. Gaensbauer and Siegel (1995) outlined three purposes of structured play reenactment. First, play enables the child to organize fragmented experiences into meaningful narratives. Second, the interpretive work by the therapist helps the child understand the personal meanings of the trauma. Third, the child experiences desensitization to the anxiety and fear and other negative emotions associated with trauma.

Gaensbauer and Siegel (1995) describe how they work with these children. They use toys that are relevant to the trauma for that particular child. For example, if the child had been in a car accident, they would use cars, a hospital room, and so on. Then they ask the child to play out "what happens next." The therapist is very active in acting out the events as well. Parents are often involved in the reenactments too, and are soothing and comforting, as is the therapist. They concluded that these children would "repeatedly return to play vehicles that provide them an opportunity to express their unresolved feelings" (p. 303). They stressed that the key element that enables the child to use the play adaptively, rather than in a repetitive fashion, is the "degree to which the affects can be brought to the surface so that the child can identify them and integrate them in more adaptive ways" (p. 297).

Play Intervention Studies and Anxiety

A few well-done studies have found that focused play interventions reduce anxiety. Although these studies do not investigate mechanisms that underlie the anxiety reduction, they do point the way for research and practice. Phillips (1985) reviewed two studies that used puppet play to reduce anxiety in children facing surgery. Johnson and Stockdale (1975) measured Palmer Sweat Index level before and after surgery. Puppet play in the study involved playing out the surgery. They found less anxiety in the puppet play group before and after surgery. Cassell (1965) also found that anxiety was reduced before surgery for a puppet play group when compared with a no-treatment control. There were no differences after surgery. The treatment group was less disturbed during the cardiac catheterization and was more willing to return to the hospital for further treatment.

An important study by Rae, Worchel, Upchurch, Sanner, and Dainiel (1989) investigated the effects of play on the adjustment of 46 children hospitalized for acute illness. Children were randomly assigned to one of four experimental groups:

1. A therapeutic play condition in which the child was encouraged to play with medical and nonmedical materials. Verbal support, reflection, and interpretation of feelings were expressed by the research assistant.
2. A diversionary play condition in which children were allowed to play with toys, but fantasy play was discouraged. The toys provided did not facilitate fantasy, nor did the research assistant.
3. A verbally oriented support condition in which children were encouraged to talk about feelings and anxieties. The research assistant was directive in bringing up related topics and would ask about procedures.
4. A control condition in which the research assistant had no contact with the child.

All treatment conditions consisted of two 30-minute sessions. The main result was that children in the therapeutic play group showed significantly greater reduction in self-reported hospital-related fears than the children in the other three groups. Because this study had comparison groups that controlled for non-fantasy-based play and also controlled for verbal expression with an understanding adult, one can conclude with more certainty that the fantasy play was the element that helped the child deal with the fears. This study has important implications for many child life programs that are based in hospitals. Child life specialists use play and medical play with hospitalized children to help them cope with medical procedures and the hospital stay.

Focused play interventions have also been effective in reducing separation anxiety in children. In a carefully controlled study, Milos and Reiss (1982) used play interventions for 64 preschoolers who were rated as high separation-anxious by their teachers. The children were randomly assigned to one of four groups. Three play groups were theme-related: the free-play group had appropriate toys; the directed-play group had the scene set with the mother doll bringing the child to school; the modeling group had the experimenter playing out a separation scene. A control group used play with toys irrelevant to separation scenes (blocks, puzzles, crayons). All children received three individual 10-minute play sessions on different days. Quality of play was also rated. The results showed that all three thematic play groups were effective in reducing separation anxiety when compared with the control group. An interesting finding was that, when the free-play and directed-play groups were combined, the quality-of-play ratings were significantly negatively related to a posttest anxiety rating ($r = -.37$). High-quality play was defined as play that showed more separation themes and attempts to resolve the conflicts. It appeared that children who were good players were better able to use the play sessions to master their anxiety. They were able to play out the themes. This finding is consistent with creativity research by Dansky (1980) which found that free play facilitated creativity but only for those children who were able to use make-believe in their play.

Barnett (1984) also looked at separation anxiety and expanded upon the work of Barnett and Storm (1981) in which free play was found to reduce distress in children following a conflict situation. In the 1984 study, a natural stressor was used the first day of school. Seventy-four preschool children were observed separating from their mothers and were rated as anxious or nonanxious. These two groups were further divided into play or no-play conditions. The play condition was a free-play condition. The no-play condition was a story-listening condition. For half of the play session, play was solitary. For the other half, peers were present. The story condition was also split in a similar way. Play was rated by observers and categorized in terms of types of play. Anxiety was measured by the Palmer Sweat Index. The main result was that play significantly reduced anxiety in the high-anxious group. There was no effect for the low-anxious group. For the anxious children, solitary play was best in reducing anxiety. High-anxious children spent more time in fantasy play than did low-anxious children, who showed more functional and manipulative play. Barnett interpreted these findings to mean that play was used to cope with a distressing situation. These findings supported her idea that it was not social play that is essential to conflict resolution, but rather imaginative play qualities that the child introduces into playful behavior. The presence of peers increased anxiety in the high-anxious group.

These play intervention studies suggest that play helps children reduce fears and anxieties and that there is something about play itself that serves as a vehicle for change. These studies suggest that the involvement of fantasy and make-believe is involved in anxiety reduction. Although not directly measured, affect was likely involved in the play as well. In the Milos and Reiss (1982) study, presence of separation themes and attempts to resolve the conflict was related to anxiety reduction. Those are examples of affect themes in play. Results also suggest that children who are already good players are more able to use play opportunities to resolve problems. Teaching children play skills would provide children with a resource for future coping with fears and anxiety.

IMPLICATIONS OF RESEARCH ON PLAY IN CHILD DEVELOPMENT FOR THE USE OF PLAY IN THERAPY

Research findings in the area of play, creativity, coping, processing and regulating emotions, and adjustment have not yet had a direct impact on the use of play in therapy. Many of the cognitive and affective processes that research has shown to relate to play, or to be facilitated by play, are probably being worked with and affected in play therapy, but not in a systematic fashion. As Russ concluded from the empirical literature in 2004, play relates to or facilitates:

1. Problem solving that requires insight ability
2. Flexibility in problem solving
3. Divergent thinking ability
4. Ability to think of alternative coping strategies in coping with daily problems
5. Experiencing positive emotion
6. Ability to think about affect themes (positive and negative)

7. Ability to understand the emotions of others and take the perspective of another (reviewed in Chapter 2)
8. Aspects of general adjustment

In addition, focused play intervention studies with nonclinical populations have found that play reduces fears and anxieties. Research suggests that imagination and fantasy components of play are key. Play intervention is effective for children who already use play to express fantasy and make-believe. Although not investigated in the research, the clinical literature reports that expressing affect in the play is crucial for change to occur.

These research findings are consistent with psychodynamic theoretical and clinical literature that utilizes play to help with internal conflict resolution and traumatic events. Traditional psychodynamic approaches have been targeted for children whose fantasy skills are normally developed and who can use play in therapy to reduce anxiety. These research findings are also consistent with cognitive-behavioral uses of play where playing out fears and anxieties would result in extinction of the fears. Children who could already use fantasy could better imagine scenarios and enable desensitization to occur.

The child development research on play supports the concept that play is related to important areas of adaptive functioning and facilitates development of many cognitive and affective processes. Play ability is a resource for children. Prevention programs that can build play skills would be a worthwhile investment in that they would help children build this internal resource of pretend play. Heckman and Masterov (2007) has made a strong economic argument for the need to invest in children for the benefit of society. Helping children to develop cognitive and affective processes through play would be a wise investment for children and for our society.

REFERENCES

Barnett, I. (1984). Research note: Young children's resolution of distress through play. *Journal of Child Psychology and Psychiatry, 25*, 477–483.

Barnett, I., & Storm, B. (1981). Play, pleasure, and pain: The reduction of anxiety through play. *Leisure Science, 4*, 161–175.

Barron, F., & Harrington, D. (1981). Creativity, intelligence, and personality. In M. Rosenzweig & L. Porter (Eds.), *Annual review of psychology* (Vol. 32, pp. 439–476). Palo Alto, CA: Annual Reviews.

Belsky, J., & Most, J. (1981). From exploration to play: A cross-sectional study of infant free play behavior. *Developmental Psychology, 17*, 630–639.

Berk, L., Mann, T., & Ogan, A. (2006). Make-believe play: Wellspring for development of self-regulation. In D. Singer, R. Golinkoff, & K. Hirsh-Pasek (Eds.), *Play = learning: How play motivates and enhances children's cognitive and social-emotional growth* (pp. 74–100). New York: Oxford University Press.

Burck, A. (2010). *Relationships among play, coping and adjustment in young children.* Unpublished raw data collected for doctoral dissertation, Case Western Reserve University, Cleveland, OH.

Carson, D., Bittner, M., Cameron, B., Brown, D., & Meyer, S. (1994). Creative thinking as a predictor of school-aged children's stress responses and coping abilities. *Creativity Research Journal, 7,* 145–158.

Cassell, S. (1965). Effect of brief puppet therapy upon the emotional response of children undergoing cardiac catheterization. *Journal of Consulting Psychology, 29,* 1–8.

Christian, K. (2009). *Effects of anxious mood on play processes.* Unpublished master's thesis, Case Western Reserve University, Cleveland, OH.

Christiano, B., & Russ, S. (1996). Play as a predictor of coping and distress in children during an invasive dental procedure. *Journal of Clinical Child Psychology, 25,* 130–138.

Csikszentmihalyi, M. (1990). *Flow: The psychology of optimal experience.* Grand Rapids, MI: Harper & Row.

D'Angelo, L. (1995). *Child's play: The relationship between the use of play and adjustment styles.* Unpublished doctoral dissertation, Case Western Reserve University, Cleveland, OH.

Dansky, J. (1980). Make-believe: A mediator of the relationship between play and associative fluency. *Child Development, 51,* 576–579.

Dansky, J. (1999). Play. In M. Runco & S. Pritzker (Eds.), *Encyclopedia of creativity* (pp. 393–408). San Diego: Academic Press.

Dansky, J., & Silverman, F. (1973). Effects of play on associative fluency in pre-school-aged children. *Developmental Psychology, 9,* 38–43.

Dillon J., & Russ, S. W. (2010). *Pretend play, creativity, and emotion regulation in children.* Manuscript submitted for publication.

Erikson, E. (1963). *Childhood and society.* New York: Norton.

Fehr, K. (2009). *Aggression in play, aggression in the classroom, and parenting style.* Unpublished master's thesis, Case Western Reserve University, Cleveland, OH.

Fein, G. (1987). Pretend play: Creativity and consciousness. In P. Gorlitz & J. Wohlwill (Eds.), *Curiosity, imagination, and play* (pp. 281–304). Hillsdale, NJ: Erlbaum.

Fisher, E. (1992). The impact of play on development: A meta-analysis. *Play and Culture, 5,* 159–181.

Freedheim, D., & Russ, S. (1992). Psychotherapy with children. In C. Walker & M. Roberts (Eds.), *Handbook of clinical child psychology* (2nd ed., pp. 765–781). New York: Wiley.

Gaensbauer, T., & Siegel, C. (1995). Therapeutic approaches to posttraumatic stress disorder in infants and toddlers. *Infant Mental Health Journal, 16,* 292–305.

Gil, E. (1991). *The healing power of play.* New York: Guilford Press.

Goldstein, A. (2002). *The effect of affect-laden reading passages on children's emotional expressivity in play.* Unpublished doctoral dissertation, Case Western Reserve University, Cleveland, OH.

Golomb, C., & Galasso, L. (1995). Make believe and reality: Explorations of the imaginary realm. *Developmental Psychology, 31,* 800–810.

Grossman-McKee, A. (1989). The relationship between affective expression in fantasy play and pain complaints in first and second grade children. *Dissertation Abstracts International, 50.*

Guilford, J. P. (1950). Creativity. *American Psychologist, 5,* 444–454.

Guilford, J. P. (1968). *Intelligence, creativity, and their educational implications.* San Diego, CA: Knapp.

Harris, P. (2000). *The work of the imagination.* Oxford, UK: Blackwell.

Heckman, J. J., & Masterov, D. V. (2007). The productivity argument for investing in young children. *Review of Agricultural Economics, 29,* 446–493.

Hirsh-Pasek, K., & Golinkoff, R. M. (2003). *Einstein never used flashcards: How our children really learn—and why they need to play more and memorize less* (rev.). Emmaus, PA: Rodale Press.

Jacobsen, P., Sadler, F., Booth-Jones, M., Soety, E., Weitzner, M., & Fields, K. (2002). Predictors of post trauma stress disorder symptomatology following bone marrow transplantation for cancer. *Journal of Consulting and Clinical Psychology, 76,* 235–240.

Johnson, J. (1976). Relations of divergent thinking and intelligence test scores with social and nonsocial make-believe play of preschool children. *Child Development, 47,* 1200–1203.

Johnson, P., & Stockdale, D. (1975). Effects of puppet therapy on Palmar sweating of hospitalized children. *Johns Hopkins Medical Journal, 137,* 1–5.

Kaugars, A., & Russ, S. (2009). Assessing preschool children's pretend play: Preliminary validation of the Affect of Play Scale—Preschool Version. *Early Education and Development, 20,* 733–755.

Kenealy, P. (1989). Children's strategies for coping with depression. *Behavior Research Therapy, 27,* 27–34.

Klinger, E. (1971). *Structure and functions of fantasy.* New York: Wiley-Interscience.

Kogan, N. (1983). Stylistic variation in childhood and adolescence: Creativity, metaphor, and cognitive styles. In P. Mussen (Ed.), *Handbook of child psychology* (Vol. 3, pp. 631–706). New York: Wiley.

Krasnor, L., & Pepler, D. (1980). The study of children's play: Some suggested future directions. *New Directions for Child Development, 9,* 85–94.

Lazarus, R., & Folkman, S.(1984). *Stress, appraisal, and coping.* New York: Springer.

Lepore, S., Silver, R.,Wortman, C., & Wayment, H. (1996). Social constraints, intrusive thoughts, and depressive symptoms among bereaved mothers. *Journal of Personality and Social Psychology, 70,* 271–282.

Lieberman, J. N. (1977). *Playfulness: Its relationship to imagination and creativity.* New York: Academic Press.

Mennin, D., Heimberg, R., Turk, C., & Fresco, D. (2002). Applying an emotion regulation framework to integrative approaches to generalized anxiety disorder. *Clinical Psychology, 19,* 85–90.

Milos, M., & Reiss, S. (1982). Effects of three play conditions on separation anxiety in young children. *Journal of Consulting and Clinical Psychology, 50,* 389–395.

Pennebaker, J. (2002, January/February). What our words can say about us: Toward a broader language psychology. *APA Monitor,* pp. 8–9.

Pennebaker, J., & Graybeal, A. (2001). Patterns of natural language use: Disclosure, personality, and social integration. *Current Directions in Psychological Science, 10,* 90–93.

Pepler, D., & Ross, H. S. (1981). The effects of play on convergent and divergent problem solving. *Child Development, 52,* 1202–1210.

Phillips, R. (1985). Whistling in the dark?: A review of play therapy research. *Psychotherapy, 22,* 752–760.

Piaget, J. (1967). *Play, dreams, and imitation in childhood.* New York: Norton. (Original work published 1945)

Rae, W., Worchel, R., Upchurch, J., Sanner, J., & Dainiel, C. (1989). The psychosocial impact of play on hospitalized children. *Journal of Pediatric Psychology, 14,* 617–627.

Richards, R. (1990). Everyday creativity, eminent creativity, and health: Afterview for CRT issues on creativity and health. *Creativity Research Journal, 3,* 300–326.

Rosenberg, D. (1984). *The quality and content of preschool fantasy play: Correlates in concurrent social-personality function and early mother–child attachment relationships.* Unpublished doctoral dissertation, University of Minnesota, MN.

Rubin, K., Fein, G., & Vandenberg, B. (1983). Play. In P. Mussen (Ed.), *Handbook of child psychology* (Vol. 4, pp. 693–774). New York: Wiley.

Runco, M. (1991). *Divergent thinking.* Norwood, NJ: Ablex.

Runco, M. (1994). Conclusions concerning problem finding, problem solving and creativity. In. M. A. Runco (Ed.), *Problem finding, problem solving, and creativity* (pp. 272–290). Norwood, NJ: Ablex.

Russ, S. W. (1987). Assessment of cognitive affective interaction in children: Creativity, fantasy, and play research. In J. Butcher & C. Spielberger (Eds.), *Advances in personality assessment* (Vol. 6, pp. 141–155). Hillsdale, NJ: Erlbaum.

Russ, S. W. (1988). Primary process thinking on the Rorschach, divergent thinking, and coping in children. *Journal of Personality Assessment, 52,* 539–548.

Russ, S. W. (1993). *Affect and creativity: The role of affect and play in the creative process.* Hillsdale, NJ: Erlbaum.

Russ, S. W. (2004). *Play in child development and psychotherapy: Toward empirically supported practice.* Mahwah, NJ: Erlbaum.

Russ, S. W., & Grossman-McKee, A. (1990). Affective expression in children's fantasy play, primary process thinking on the Rorschach, and divergent thinking. *Journal of Personality Assessment, 54,* 756–771.

Russ, S. W., & Schafer, E. (2006). Affect in fantasy play, emotion in memories, and divergent thinking. *Creativity Research Journal, 18,* 347–354.

Russ, S. W., Robins, D., & Christiano, B. (1999). Pretend play: Longitudinal prediction of creativity and affect in fantasy in children. *Creativity Research Journal, 12,* 129–139.

Sherrod, L., & Singer, J. (1979). The development of make-believe play. In J. Goldstein (Ed.), *Sports, games, and play* (pp. 1–28). Hillsdale, NJ: Erlbaum.

Shields, A., & Cicchetti, D. (1998). Reactive aggression among maltreated children: The contributions of attention and emotion dysregulation. *Journal of Clinical Child Psychology, 27,* 381–395.

Singer, D. G. (1993). *Playing for their lives.* New York: Free Press.

Singer, D. G., & Rummo, J. (1973). Ideational creativity and behavioral style in kindergarten aged children. *Developmental Psychology, 8,* 154–161.

Singer, D. G., & Singer, J. L. (1990). *The house of make-believe: Children's play and the developing imagination.* Cambridge, MA: Harvard University Press.

Singer, J. L. (1981). *Daydreaming and fantasy.* New York: Oxford University Press.

Singer, J. L. (1995). Imaginative play in childhood: Precursor of subjunctive thoughts, daydreaming, and adult pretending games. In A. Pellegrini (Ed.), *The future of play therapy* (pp. 187–219). Albany: State University of New York Press.

Slade, A., & Wolf, D. (1994). *Children at play.* New York: Oxford University Press.

Smith, P., & Whitney, S. (1987). Play and associative fluency: Experimenter effects may be responsible for positive results. *Developmental Psychology, 23,* 49–53.

Sternberg, R. (1988). A three-facet model of creativity. In R. Sternberg (Ed.), *The nature of creativity* (pp. 125–147). Cambridge, UK: Cambridge University Press.

Strayhorn, J. (2002). Self-control: Toward systematic training programs. *Journal of the American Academy of Child and Adolescent Psychiatry, 41,* 17–27.

Terr, L. (1990). *Too scared to cry: Psychic trauma in childhood.* New York: Harper & Row.

Tomkins, S. (1970). A theory of memory. In J. Antrobus (Ed.), *Cognition and affect* (pp. 59–130). Boston: Little, Brown.

Vandenberg, B. (1980). Play, problem-solving, and creativity. *New Directions for Child Development, 9,* 49–68.

Waelder, R. (1933). Psychoanalytic theory of play. *Psychoanalytic Quarterly, 2,* 208–224.

Wallach, M. (1970). Creativity. In P. Mussen (Ed.), *Carmichael's manual of child psychology* (Vol. 1, pp. 1211–1272). New York: Wiley.

2

Play and Interpersonal Processes

Jason F. Jent, Larissa N. Niec, and Sarah E. Baker

Begin therefore betimes nicely to observe your son's temper; and
that, when he is under least restraint in his play ... see what are
his predominant passions and prevailing inclinations; whether he
be fierce or mild, bold or bashful, compassionate or cruel, open
or reserved, &c. For as these are different in him, so are your
methods to be different, and your authority must hence take
measures to apply itself different ways to him.

—JOHN LOCKE (1693/1890)

Awareness that play reveals something about children's per-
sonalities and social functioning is not recent. For centuries, philoso-
phers, researchers, and clinicians have considered the existence of a link
between play and children's development. Early play literature focused
largely on the origins of play and the categorization of play types (e.g.,
Groos & Baldwin, 1901; Hall, 1907/1995; Lehman & Witty, 1927).
Attention later turned to the study of play processes in normative and
non-normative samples (e.g., Arey, 1941; Despert, 1938; Erikson, 1940),
and to the influence of play in applied settings (Lebo, 1953; Levitt, 1957).
Over time, play research has benefited from improvements in scientific
rigor and developments in statistical analyses that have strengthened
the knowledge base. For example, using standardized play situations,
normed criterion measures, and a variety of empirical designs, researchers have gained a clearer understanding of the relationship between chil-

dren's play and interpersonal development (Butcher & Niec, 2005; Niec & Russ, 2002; Russ, 2004).

Throughout the history of play research, basic and applied studies have emerged as two relatively segregated bodies of literature. The aim of this chapter is to discuss the basic research on children's play and interpersonal processes within a context that facilitates the integration of the basic and applied fields. Specifically, we examine three questions:

1. How does play relate to important interpersonal processes?
2. What cultural factors influence the link between play and interpersonal processes?
3. What relevance does the basic play research have for applied settings?

In order to address these questions, we first briefly review the development of social play and present definitions of the play types that hold particular relevance to interpersonal functioning: pretend play and rough-and-tumble (R&T) play. The interpersonal processes manifested within play are vast and multifaceted. For the purposes of this chapter, we focus on perspective taking, empathy, emotion regulation, and interpersonal schemas. Next, we review cultural influences on play. Finally, we discuss the implications of current research for applied study, such as the development of prevention and intervention programs.

THE DEVELOPMENT OF SOCIAL PLAY

While definitions of play vary widely, most broadly defined, *play* is a flexible activity that evokes positive emotion, is intrinsically motivating, freely chosen, episodic, creative, fluid, and active (Ashiabi, 2007; Dansky, 1999; Fromberg, 1992; Rubin, Fein, & Vandenberg, 1983). The origins of play can be seen as early as the first few months of infancy, when object play is most prevalent. Object play is initially defined by primary circular reactions (Piaget, 1962) in which the infant engages in repetitive motor behaviors focused on the body (e.g., opening and closing fingers; Gardner & Bergen, 2006). At approximately 4 months of age, object play begins to transition from internal objects (i.e., the body) to external objects, including people. As infants' motor and language capacities increase, they display a higher capacity for exploring, manipulating, and making inferences about objects. Through this process, infants begin to develop a better understanding of cause and effect and object properties. For example, infants learn that if they push a button on a pop-up toy, it causes a character to pop up.

Object play is thought to assist children's mastery of emotions and cognitions that are not yet part of their existing schemas (Erikson, 1963/1977; Piaget, 1962). Object play also facilitates the development of shared meanings between individuals and provides a mechanism for social development (Morgenthaler, 2006). Through object play, young children interact in a variety of ways with their parents and peers. For instance, children must define the meaning of objects in play through ongoing dialogue with others in order to sustain and enhance interactions. The quality and length of object play is greater when mothers or peers engage in object play with a child compared to when the child is engaging in object playing alone (Cielinski, Vaughn, Seifer, & Contresas, 1995; Morgenthaler, 2006).

Object play paves the way for the emergence of *pretend play*. Pretend play is defined by the use of fantasy, make-believe, and symbolism (Moore & Russ, 2006). Fein suggests pretend play must meet one of five criteria (Fein, 1981, 1987). These criteria include (1) activities outside the child's typical setting without the normal objects, (2) normal activities that go beyond their typical circumstances, (3) inanimate materials used as animates (e.g., toy tiger becomes animated tiger that is hunting), (4) objects substituted for other objects (e.g., rectangle block is used as a cell phone), and (5) activities not typically expected of a child (e.g., toddler pretends to cook a meal for parents).

Pretend play begins to emerge when children are approximately 1 year old and appears to be a cross-cultural developmental process (Fein, 1981; Gardner & Bergen, 2006). Initially, pretend play is directed internally and is solitary (e.g., child places a play cell phone to her ear; Fein, 1981). Toddlers' use of objects in play continues to be exploratory and manipulative to learn about how objects can be used, but begins to become more symbolic in nature (Fenson, 1986; Gardner & Bergen, 2006). Initially, there is high similarity between a play object and its pretend play function (e.g., using a toy hammer to hit a wooden peg board). As play continues to develop, children also begin to incorporate toys that represent animate objects (e.g., dolls, toy animals, character toys) in their pretend play (Tamis-LeMonda & Bornstein, 1991). For example, a child may take his toy dog for a walk on its leash or play with toy animals in a toy barn.

Pretend play becomes increasingly social as children develop. Reciprocal imitation of pretend play tends to appear between the ages of 15 and 20 months (e.g., two toddlers manipulating cars back and forth next to each other). During this period, toddlers begin to display prosocial behavior such as sharing toys (Hay, Payne, & Chadwick, 2004). Between 20 and 24 months, positive social interactions during pretend play such as laughing, verbalizations, smiling, sharing, and eye contact increase (Gardner & Bergen, 2006). The amount that 2-year-olds engage in pretend play appears to be significantly dependent upon children's language ability (McEwen et al., 2007). Similar themes in pretend play emerge between peers at age 2, but pretend play continues to be parallel rather than interactive. Between 2½ and 3 years old, children develop a better understanding of social roles, and role taking within pretend play increases (Howes, Unger, & Seidner, 1989). Between the ages of 3 and 4 years, the use of objects (e.g., blocks, cars, dolls) as props within pretend play assists with the development of the actual play episodes. As long as the meaning of the objects is shared among players, social pretend play will continue (Morgenthaler, 2006).

Within younger elementary school-age children, pretend play persists in both solitary and group play. However, the need for realistic objects for pretend play decreases (Fenson, 1986). Objects are typically used as props to assist with the progression of the play. During this period, children are able to enact the roles of a range of characters (e.g., family roles, occupational roles, superhero and fictional roles). Children display significant verbal and social reciprocity within their pretend play. Overt pretend play in social situations (e.g., school, playground) peaks around age 5. At that time, the prevalence of other types of play (e.g., physical play, constructive play, games with rules) emerges among peers. While children maintain a high interest in pretend play, this type of play is displayed in somewhat less social settings, such as the child's home or other semiprivate environments (Johnson, 2006).

The prevalence of overt pretend play in elementary school-age children begins to decrease as children get older, but the presence of solitary pretend play persists in private settings (Manning, 2006). During this period, children's solitary pretend play becomes more of an internal process than an external one (Singer & Singer, 2005). That is, older children's pretend play consists of more dynamic scripts, complex plots, and elaboration than younger children's pretend play (Johnson, 2006).

R&T play is different from pretend play in that it does not occur in a solitary setting and may or may not include a fantasy or pretend component. We have included R&T play in this chapter because it relates to children's interpersonal functioning in several domains. Broadly defined, R&T play is social play that includes voluntary play fighting (e.g., wrestling, chasing each other) and is accompanied by positive affect (Burghardt, 2005; Pellegrini, 2006). Developmentally, R&T play emerges in the free play of preschoolers, peaks in the play of elementary school children, and decreases in middle school (Pellegini, 2006). R&T play is seen more frequently in boys than girls throughout childhood, possibly due in part to socialization pressures (Colwell & Lindsey, 2005; Maccoby, 1998; Pellegrini, 2006).

When discussing R&T play, it is important to make clear that it is not the same as aggression. R&T play can be differentiated from real fighting in that it is associated with continued peer affiliation and positive affect (Pellegrini, 1988, 2003). R&T play is often confused with physical aggression because, to the casual observer, the behaviors are similar. For example, it is difficult to distinguish between real wrestling and play wrestling without evaluating children's facial and verbal expressions. R&T play generally includes happiness (e.g., smiles and laughter), whereas aggressive behavior includes anger and sadness (e.g., frowns, furrowed eyebrows; Pellegrini, 2006). When R&T play ends, children typically continue to play together, whereas children generally separate from one another after aggressive acts (Pellegrini, 1988).

PLAY AND INTERPERSONAL PROCESSES

The child's disposition must be early and secretly studied, especially while at *play*....

—JOHN LOCKE (1693/1890)

A meta-analysis of 46 studies measuring the impact of play on a range of child outcomes (e.g., language skill, perspective taking) found that social pretend play related to better language and socioemotional functioning (Fisher, 1992). More recent studies have focused on specific play types and narrower definitions of outcome. In the following section we ask:

1. What can be learned about the way children interact with others by observing their social and pretend play?
2. Do different types of play relate to different aspects of interpersonal functioning?

We address these questions by reviewing some of the recent literature linking play with four interpersonal processes: perspective taking, empathy, emotion regulation, and interpersonal schemas. Each of these processes has implications for children's functioning at school, with peers, and in the family.

Play, Perspective Taking, and Empathy

The ability to understand social interactions from multiple perspectives outside of oneself—*perspective taking*—develops and becomes more sophisticated over time. Understanding others' perspectives contributes to successful interactions. Children who are at risk for problematic peer and family interactions have demonstrated deficits in perspective taking. Specifically, children with conduct problems, children with attention-deficit/hyperactivity disorder (ADHD), and children who have experienced maltreatment have demonstrated problems understanding the points of view of others (Anastassiou-Hadjicharalambous & Warden, 2008; Burack et al., 2006; Marton, Wiener, Rogers, Moore, & Tannock, 2009).

While perspective taking is a necessary component of empathy, empathy includes an emotional experiential component that is not part of perspective taking. Empathy has been conceptualized as "an affective reaction that stems from the apprehension or comprehension of another's emotional state or condition, and that is identical or very similar to what the other person is feeling or would be expected to feel" (Eisenberg & Fabes, 1998, p. 702). Children high in empathy tend to engage in more prosocial behaviors, are viewed as exhibiting less shyness, are perceived as displaying fewer behavior problems (e.g., aggression), and are able to represent the emotional state of others in play better than children low in empathy (e.g., Eisenberg & Fabes, 1998; Findlay, Girardi, & Coplan, 2006; Miller & Jansen op de Haar, 1997; Niec & Russ, 2002; Strayer & Roberts, 2004; Zhou et al., 2002).

The ability to understand and experience others' perspectives is one of the developmental domains most impacted by play (Shirk & Russell, 1996). Pretend play, in particular, provides an ideal medium for children to practice perspective taking and empathy. When children include animate objects or people in their play (e.g., using dolls to play house, playing "school" with friends), they must simultaneously represent multiple perspectives (e.g., parents, teachers, children). Taking on roles within pretend play allows children the opportunity to learn communication skills, problem solving, and empathy (Hughes, 1999). Within collaborative pretend play, the process of representing multiple perspectives appears to help children in the development of theory of mind and schemas of emotions, as well as understanding others' intentions, social roles, and norms (Ashiabi, 2007; Curran, 1999; Jenkins & Astington, 2000; Kavanaugh & Harris, 1999; Leslie, 1987; Nourot, 2006; Rubin & Howe, 1986). In the process of acting out multiple perspectives during pretend play, children may develop sensitivity toward the needs and views of others as they begin to recognize and experience others' emotional states (Ashiabi, 2007; Findlay et al., 2006). The extent to which children can engage in perspective taking also affects their capacity for understanding others' emotions when negotiating play.

The quality of children's pretend play, both solitary and dyadic, has been associated with the ability to understand others' emotions (Cutting & Dunn, 2006; Seja & Russ, 1999; Youngblade & Dunn, 1995). In a study of first- and second-grade children, the quality of the child's solitary fantasy play with puppets significantly related to the child's ability to describe emotional experiences and to understand others' emotions (Seja & Russ, 1999). Young children who engage in more dyadic pretend play with their siblings, particularly older siblings, have been found to display a more advanced understanding of other people's beliefs and feelings than children who less frequently participate in fantasy play (Cutting & Dunn, 2006; Youngblade & Dunn, 1995).

Expressing and experiencing emotions in pretend play may help children to recognize emotions in themselves and in other people. Pretend play provides a socializing atmosphere in which children acquire and practice culturally appropriate emotional communication and regulation (Haight, Black, Ostler, & Sheridan, 2006). Perhaps fostering this type of play may help children to take the perspective of others and adaptively interpret emotions and behaviors in the social environment.

Play and Emotion Regulation

Although emotion regulation has been defined in a variety of ways, it is generally thought to encompass a diverse set of skills rather than a single ability. In a thorough review of emotion regulation and its pervasiveness in varied disciplines of psychology, Gross (1998) defined the construct as "the process by which individuals influence which emotions they have, when they have them, and how they experience and express these emotions" (p. 275). Regulation of emotion involves the ability not only to genuinely experience emotions but also to express them in ways that achieve important goals, such as maintaining important relationships (Bridges, Denham, & Ganiban, 2004).

R&T play and pretend play both have been associated with children's regulation of emotion. R&T play is thought to provide children with the opportunity to practice emotion regulation, as well as perspective taking and emotional expression (Lindsey & Colwell, 2003; Pellegrini & Smith, 1998). This makes sense when one considers the high level of physical contact among children during R&T play and the likely potential for conflict. In a study of elementary school children's R&T play, boys with high levels of aggression and peer rejection were more likely to engage in aggressive acts at the end of R&T play (Pellegrini, 1988). Similar results were found among peer-rejected adolescent boys who were viewed as aggressive. That is, adolescent boys who were perceived by others as aggressive had an increased tendency to use R&T

play to bully others (Pellegrini, 2003). Among peer-rejected and aggressive boys, the frequency of R&T play remains relatively stable, whereas most boys show a decline in R&T play during adolescence.

R&T play appears to serve different functions for different ages. Evidence is mixed regarding the relationship between younger children's R&T play and peer rejection. Some studies have shown that R&T play play in preschool children is related to higher levels of peer rejection (Hart, DeWolf, Wozniak, & Burts, 1992; Ladd & Price, 1987). In other studies, same-sex R&T play was related to positive perceptions of boys' social and emotional competence (Colwell & Lindsey, 2005; Lindsey & Colwell, 2003); however, R&T play between boys and girls was associated with being disliked by peers (Colwell & Lindsey, 2005). A study of elementary school-age children demonstrated that R&T play was positively related to increased cooperative play and social problem-solving skills for socially accepted boys (Pellegrini & Smith, 1998). This suggests that R&T play does not lead to aggression for most boys, but leads to multiple positive social outcomes (Pellegrini, 2006).

Overall, R&T play appears to relate to positive social development when socially accepted children engage in same-sex play of this type. However, R&T play may be contraindicated for peer-rejected and aggressive children, as this type of play may lead to aggressive behavior that remains stable in frequency over time. Given the strong school policies against R&T play and the mixed evidence for the importance of R&T play in promoting children's positive social development, additional research is needed to further delineate under what conditions R&T play leads to healthy interactions between peers.

Although pretend play is different in many ways from R&T play, in pretend play characterized by imaginative engagement with others children may also have opportunities to regulate his or her emotions in adaptive ways (Russ, 2004). Pretend play provides children with a safe arena to explore and practice emotions they have observed in others or have experienced themselves (Haight et al., 2006; Singer, 1995). Emotional expression can be practiced within pretend play without actually experiencing the intensity of the emotion (Moore & Russ, 2006). From the informal "training" that this type of play can provide, children begin to discern meaning from emotional exchanges with others, learn when to apply specific emotions to novel situations, and develop an ability to control emotional expression when the social setting requires it (Singer, 1998; Russ, 2004). For example, emotional regulation is vital in the negotiation of objects and character roles within pretend play. If a child is not given a desired role, this may result in negative affect (e.g., anger, sadness). This experience provides the child the opportunity to practice regulating their affect outside of the play situation or within a character role (Ashiabi, 2007). Through the rehearsal of adaptive emotional expression and regulation within pretend play, children may enhance their ability to utilize similar skills when presented with live interpersonal difficulties (Strayhorn, 2002). In a review of play research, Singer (1998) pointed to the adaptive advantages of pretend play and concluded that it is central in children's ability to regulate their emotions and behavior. In addition, emotion regulation processes in play relate to and facilitate important adaptive functions in children, including creativity, problem solving, coping, and the acquisition of social skills (Russ, 2004).

Managing emotion is critical because it relates to children's level of behavioral adjustment in school and other domains. Children who demonstrate intense displays of emotion and are slow to regulate their emotions are more likely to exhibit disruptive behavior problems than children who more successfully manage their feelings (e.g., Batum & Yagmurlu, 2007; Butcher & Niec, 2005; Eisenberg & Fabes, 2006; Hill, Degnan, Calkins, & Keane, 2006). These children are often less able to cooperate with peers and collaborate in social exchanges, resulting in undesirable outcomes that include higher levels of aggression, withdrawal, and academic disengagement (Fantuzzo, Sekino, & Cohen, 2004).

Research has recently begun to explore pretend play as a possible medium through which children develop the ability to access, organize, and control their emotions. A high level of dyadic pretend play in preschoolers has been associated with a more advanced ability to regulate emotions as rated by mothers and teachers, although this finding was more robust for girls than for boys (Lindsey & Colwell, 2003). Similarly, children in a Head Start program who demonstrated high levels of interactive play with a peer were more competent in their use of emotion regulation skills in the classroom (Fantuzzo et al., 2004). When confronted with conflict, these children engaged in more prosocial behaviors such as sharing and turn taking and displayed fewer temper tantrums than children with lower levels of peer play interaction. It should be noted that in this study, the definition of "interactive" play included but was not limited to pretend/fantasy play and also comprised more general prosocial play behaviors.

Dyadic pretend play with mothers has also been associated with more advanced emotion regulation abilities in young children. Preschoolers who demonstrate a high level of emotional regulation in structured pretend play with their mothers have been rated by their parents as being better able to regulate their emotions in their daily behavior (Galyer & Evans, 2001). This link may indicate that children who engage in emotionally arousing play scenarios develop a variety of viable responses they can keep in their emotional repertoire for later use. Frequency of pretend play with mothers has also been found to correlate with greater emotion regulation ability in children, suggesting that more exposure and practice in regulating emotion facilitates skill generalization from the play to the "real world" (Galyer & Evans, 2001). Some mothers may approach pretense as a teaching opportunity (deliberately or inadvertently) and show their children how and when to express emotion via modeling. The question of whether child–mother pretend play is more significantly associated with emotional regulation ability than child–peer pretend play has not yet been examined.

Both R&T play and social pretend play create situations in which children must regulate their emotions in order to sustain positive interactions with others. The nature of R&T play perhaps makes it more likely to incite aggression in children who have problems with emotion regulation. In contrast, by giving children the opportunity to create, rehearse, and modify emotional situations, pretend play constitutes a socializing experience that may enhance children's ability to regulate emotions. For these reasons, pretend play may be a valuable resource for children coping with anxiety-provoking or otherwise distressing situations (Berk, Mann, & Ogan, 2006; Moore & Russ, 2006).

Play and Interpersonal Schemas

Children's mental models of past interpersonal experiences shape how they view themselves and others. Various terms have been given to these models: interpersonal schemas, internal representations, relational schemas, and internal working models (Baldwin, 1992; Bowlby, 1973; Safran, 1990; Westen, 1991). However, they share in common the concept that repeated behavioral interactions between children and others become represented internally, and children begin to behave dependent upon anticipated responses (Shirk & Russell, 1996; Sroufe, 2000). Interpersonal schemas influence how children approach, negotiate, and sustain interactions with others (Levine & Tuber, 1993).

The content of social pretend play may be driven, in part, by interpersonal schemas (Fromberg, 2002). Scripts for play can be derived from events (e.g., personal experiences, television, and story books) and can express emotions associated with those events (Nourot, 2006). Peers and siblings who have a shared history (e.g., previous interactive play experiences, classroom experiences, historical events, parent–child interactions) may negotiate pretend play with relative ease given previous experiences with patterns of compromise and reciprocity (Howes, Unger,

& Matheson, 1992; Nourot, 2006). In fact, children with a history of shared scripts are likely to prefer to play with one another (Howes & Phillipsen, 1992).

Elements of pretense are added to event scripts and are guided by implicit and explicit prompts while children play (Fromberg, 2002). That is, play is driven by children signaling and responding to one another outside and within pretend play. Children can give explicit directives or prompts by stepping out of the play to make suggestions about roles, objects, and events within the play script. These suggestions are often accompanied by tag questions (e.g., Okay?) to ensure agreement between peers about the flow of the play (Giffin, 1984; Nourot, 2006). Once children agree upon changes in the script, they reenter the play (Fromberg, 2002). Implicit pretend directives about scripts are given within the actual play (Giffin, 1984). Children negotiate within play through the use of a pretend character role, which requires the ability to present others' perspectives (Ariel, 2002). Children must not only represent their own perspectives, but must also represent the perspective of their character role(s) within the play (Nourot, 2006).

Themes manifested in children's play scripts may reveal various dimensions of their interpersonal schemas. Affect tone is one dimension of interpersonal schemas that relates to how children approach and respond to the world (Westen, 1991) and can be measured in children's play (Niec, Yopp, & Russ, 2009). It has been conceptualized as the extent to which an individual expects relationships to be threatening/ destructive or safe/enriching, ranging from predominantly malevolent to predominantly benevolent expectations. Children develop a model of affect tone through early experiences with others, and once formed, the model remains fairly constant over time (Niec & Russ, 2002; Westen et al., 1991). Children are more likely than adults to organize and retrieve social information on the basis of affective valence, with a greater tendency to categorize others as "all good" or "all bad." Those who have trouble regulating their emotions may be particularly prone to experiencing other people in this polarizing fashion, resulting in persistent instability in interpersonal relationships (Westen, 1991). Therefore, affect tone can be a valuable indicator of how well children interact with important people in their lives, including parents and peers. Malevolent affect tone has been associated with a number of negative interpersonal circumstances, including maternal separation, maternal neglect, frequent family moves, and physical and sexual abuse (Downey & Walker, 1989; Freedenfeld, Ornduff, & Kelsey, 1995; Ornduff, Freedenfeld, Kelsey, & Critelli, 1994). Conversely, children with a more benevolent affect tone scored higher on self-report and teacher report measures of empathy and helpfulness (Niec & Russ, 2002).

Children's affect tone may be manifested in the quality and themes of their pretend play. In general, pretend play is characterized by cooperation and communication between playmates (Howes et al., 1992). However, in a study of 80 preschoolers, children whose pretend play included a high proportion of violent themes and reenactments (e.g., killing, inflicting pain) displayed poor emotional regulation skills and socioemotional functioning (Dunn & Hughes, 2001). These children were less positive, more often angry, and engaged in more frequent delinquent behaviors such as bullying and rule breaking in their day-to-day social interactions than children whose pretend play included a lower proportion of violence. Children with more violent play themes also engaged in pretend play significantly less often than children whose pretense did not involve violence. At a 2-year follow up, the children who engaged in violent pretense at age 4 were less likely to give empathic responses for victims and remorseful responses for perpetrators on a measure of moral sensibility at age 6. Pretend play themes contributed to the prediction of later social functioning.

The quality and duration of pretend play is also associated with children's affective state. Children who express frequent negative affect in play (e.g., anger, crying, protesting, whining) tend to engage in less role enactment in pretend play than children who express more positive affect (e.g., smiling, laughing; Dunn & Brown, 1994). Russ and Kaugars (2000) experimentally induced either happy or sad mood in young children and found that negative mood related to more instances of negativity during solitary pretend play. When children enter the context of play with preexisting negative affect, negative themes may also be apparent in the play. Recurrent negative play themes may be an indicator of a malevolent affect tone.

Children who express a range of affect, both within and outside the context of play, develop a repertoire of affective memories that facilitate the development of divergent thinking and complex problem solving (Russ, 2004). However, children who are often angry, have difficulty regulating their emotions, and are unable to read others' emotional signals are at significant risk of experiencing poor peer relationships (Denham et al., 2002). Examining the themes expressed by children in pretend play can provide a window through which their interpersonal schemas may be better understood.

In summary, multiple interrelated interpersonal processes in children's play are associated with social and emotional development. Children's ability to represent the perspective of others is thought to develop through their pretend play with persona objects (e.g., dolls) and others (e.g., playmates, caregivers). Through pretend play, children are provided the opportunity to safely experience personal emotional states and the emotions of others. These experiences may contribute to the development of emotional regulation skills that assist in the negotiation of play, as well as other interactions with peers and adults. Through repeated play patterns and life experiences, children begin to internalize schemas about how they view themselves and the world, and this affects how they approach and respond to interactions. These interpersonal processes are related to more adaptive problem solving, better communication skills, greater prosocial behavior, and fewer internalizing and externalizing behavior problems (e.g., Butcher & Niec, 2005; Findlay et al., 2006; Hughes, 1999; Miller & Jansen op de Haar, 1997).

CULTURAL DIFFERENCES IN PLAY

How do cultural differences impact play and what aspects of culture most contribute to these differences? Pretend play is considered to be a developmental process that occurs across cultures. The use of objects, whether they be toy miniatures or props constructed from materials at hand, appear to support children's participation in pretend play across cultures (Haight, Wang, Fung, Williams, & Mintz, 1999). Similarly, parents and/or family members from diverse cultures have been found to participate in their children's pretend play, suggesting that this is a fundamental social activity (Cote & Bornstein, 2009; Goncu, Mistry, & Mosier, 2000; Haight et al., 1999).

Not all aspects of pretend play are universal, however. The frequency and content of pretend play, as well as the type of caregiver–child interactions within play, appear to vary across cultures (Farver, Kim, & Lee, 1995). In a study that examined the pretend play of five different groups (i.e., Indian, seashore, low-socioeconomic status [SES] urban, high-SES urban, and mixed-SES urban) of Brazilian 4- to 6-year-olds, children from high and mixed SES groups engaged in more pretend play than children in the other groups (Gosso, de Lima Salum e Morais, & Otta, 2007). However, the structure of the pretend play remained similar across groups. Gosso and colleagues suggested that the lower frequency of pretend play among Indian, seashore, and low SES urban children may have been reflective of more simple communication codes within these societies. Also, it may be that child-rearing practices within these groups emphasize concrete and immediate solutions to daily life hassles and practical problems (e.g., the importance of adult work) rather than symbolic thoughts. Alternatively, Indian and seashore cultural groups may place much higher emphasis on exploring and learning about nature than pretend play.

The type and extent of caregiver–child interactions during pretend play also vary among cultures. An investigation of the pretend play of South American Latino immigrant, Japanese immigrant, and European American mother–toddler dyads revealed that differences in children's play were dependent upon maternal interactions (Cote & Bornstein, 2009). That is, Japanese and Latino immigrant children engaged in more exploratory play than symbolic play when they instigated pretend play with their mothers. When mothers initiated pretend play, these children engaged in more symbolic than exploratory play. Mothers from different cultural groups also differed in how they engaged in pretend play with their children. Japanese and Latino immigrant mothers demonstrated (e.g., modeled an action for child) more play with their children than European American mothers, whereas European American mothers solicited (e.g., verbally encouraged the child to participate) more play with their toddlers than the immigrant mothers (Cote & Bornstein, 2009).

Other studies have examined to which extent that caregivers engage in pretend play within specific cultures. In an observational study that examined the pretend play of children within a Mayan village in Mexico, children were observed to spend very little of their time engaging in pretend play, and caregivers were rarely observed reinforcing or acknowledging children's pretend play or play in general (Gaskins, 2000). Within the Mayan culture, economic production is still a family activity and children participate in adult work. It is generally perceived that adult work is the most important family task, and children participate in work duties when able, or at the least they do not interrupt adults' work (Gaskins, 2000). Therefore, caregivers rarely initiate interactions based on their children's social desires. "The Maya believe that the source of development is internal and preprogrammed" (Gaskins, 2000, p. 380). That is, it is believed that children's social development will emerge on its own without significant caregiver–child interactions.

Beyond differences in the frequency of caregiver–child interactions within pretend play, other research has demonstrated differences in the emotional themes and conflict between cultural groups (Farver et al., 1995; Farver & Lee-Shim, 1997). In a series of studies that examined differences in pretend play between European American preschool children and Korean American preschool children, European American children engaged in a higher frequency of pretend play (Farver et al., 1995; Farver & Lee-Shim, 1997). However, themes within pretend play also varied. Specifically, European American children displayed a higher rate of conflict within play, including aggressive responding and disagreements, than Korean American children.

Although pretend play is observed in most cultures, differences in child-rearing beliefs, environmental demands, and socialization practices across cultural groups may affect the content, structure, and frequency of pretend play (Farver, Kim, & Lee-Shim, 2000). That is, child-rearing goals within different cultures may impact how parents interact with their children, including during play. For example, European American cultures tend to emphasize the development of autonomous behaviors in children, whereas some Latino cultures emphasize the development of respectful behavior without the assertion of one's own needs (Harwood, Leyendecker, Carlson, Asencio, & Miller, 2002). In play, European American mothers tend to engage in more object-focused play with their children to allow them to gain control over their physical environment, and Latino families engage in more person-focused play including pretend and role play (Bornstein, Haynes, Pascual, Painter, & Galperin, 1999; Harwood et al., 2002).

The examination of cross-cultural differences in play has provided clinicians and researchers with unique insights about how early socialization processes affect the development of children's play. When considering cultural differences in play, it is important to be cognizant that findings about cultural differences in play may not generalize beyond the sample studied. Within each culture, there is variation in the level of acculturation, child-rearing beliefs, SES, and environmental factors that may impact the content, structure, and frequency of children's pretend play. Given that research about cross-cultural differences in pretend play will never fully explain individual differences, it is vital that clinicians consider individual variability within the context of culture and acculturation when examining children's pretend play. For example, therapists should be particularly careful when trying to interpret meaning in the play of children who are acculturating to the United States. Some play themes from the country of origin may not translate well into the culture-of-destination. Recently immigrated children may not share common histories with other children. Clinicians who attempt to interpret the play of immigrants within a culture of destination framework may misinterpret the themes and interpersonal processes being displayed within the play (Cote & Bornstein, 2009). Misinterpretation may lead to misdiagnosis or difficulties in developing a therapeutic relationship.

In summary, the integration of objects into children's pretend play appears to be universal across cultures. However, the frequency with which children engage in pretend play varies widely. How caregivers attend to pretend play differs between cultural groups, and these differences appear to be partially explained by cultural beliefs about the socialization process. Preliminary studies have shown that European American children display higher rates of conflict in their play. This finding requires additional study to examine the mechanisms (e.g., environmental, familial) that lead to this presentation within play. Continued examination of cultural differences in pretend play is necessary to better understand how caregivers affect the quality and content of children's pretend play.

IMPLICATIONS OF PLAY RESEARCH FOR CLINICAL INTERVENTION

> For as these are different in him, so are your methods to be different, and your authority must hence take measures to apply itself different ways to him.
>
> —JOHN LOCKE (1693/1890)

In the 17th century, Locke recommended that individual differences in children's play be used to inform the development of education interventions. It has only been much more recently that basic play research has begun to inform the development of evidence-based mental health prevention and intervention programs. As this chapter and the other chapters in this section illustrate, much evidence links play to important developmental processes. Deficits in interpersonal processes, such as perspective taking and empathy, have been related to increased risk for peer rejection, poor school adjustment, and externalizing behavior problems. Understanding the links between play and children's interpersonal functioning can facilitate the development of interventions meant to ameliorate emotional and behavioral pathology.

The development of innovative intervention programs requires consideration of the specific mechanisms required to bring about change in children's functioning (Shirk & Russell, 1996). If play is to be a component of an intervention, it should be used in a deliberate way after taking into consideration (1) the goals of the intervention program (e.g., reduce depression, increase positive peer interactions), (2) the ages of the children for whom the intervention is designed (e.g., preschool, school-age), (3) the mechanisms likely to bring about change (e.g., skill building, schema transformation), and (4) the empirical links among those mechanisms and play. Developmental theory is a valuable starting point in the creation of new interventions, but theory alone is insufficient. Interventions should be based on empirically evaluated relationships. Consider the finding that pretend play with peers has more impact on children's socioemotional functioning than play with adults (Fisher, 1992). While most interventions are delivered individually and many identify the therapist as the primary facilitator of change, based on this finding, a group intervention with a peer play component might offer promise as a medium for skill building among children with interpersonal deficits.

As Part III of this volume illustrates, play is already integrated into a number of evidence-based mental health interventions that aim to increase healthy interpersonal functioning. For instance, in parent–child interaction therapy (PCIT; Niec, Gering, & Abbenante, Chapter 6, this volume), dyadic play is used as a medium to promote positive interactions between children with conduct problems and their parents. Parents practice child-centered interaction skills during play with their children, while therapists provide immediate, live feedback to parents. Cognitive-behavioral play therapy (CBPT; see Knell & Dasari,, Chapter 10, this volume) uses therapist-guided pretend play to translate behavioral skill-building exercises into fun, engaging, and developmentally appropriate exercises for children. For example, children may practice emotion regulation strategies in the context of play with other characters. In trauma-focused cognitive-behavioral therapy (TF-CBT; see Briggs, Runyon, & Deblinger, Chapter 7, this volume) children's creation of the trauma narrative is conceptualized as a key mechanism of change. Children may initially develop their trauma narrative through the use of pretend play or through other creative mechanisms (e.g., stories; Cohen & Mannarino, 2008). Once the child establishes the narrative, the therapist can guide the child through processing cognitive distortions that may be contributing to negative affect states (Cohen & Mannarino, 2008). Specifically, the creation of the narrative within play provides children the opportunity to create situational models that are revisable (Harris, 2000). Through learning how reality could be different (i.e., cognitive challenging), children may be able to evaluate the trauma differently and potentially reduce negative affect (Harris, 2000).

RECOMMENDATIONS FOR FUTURE RESEARCH

Russ (2004, p. 77) suggests that "specific play interventions with specific populations and specific situations" be evaluated to determine the best interventions for specific contexts. That is, clinicians implement play therapy for a wide range of presenting problems, yet only a limited empirical base exists for the use of play interventions for specific populations. Using play interventions in an unsystematic manner or using unsupported interventions may not lead to improvements in children's social and emotional functioning and risks wasting the limited resources for the treatment of children and families.

We would like to suggest that it is unnecessarily limiting to conceptualize interventions that use play as "play interventions" or "play therapy." Instead, we suggest play be conceptualized as a technique that may be integrated with evidence-based principles to facilitate change in interpersonal functioning and other domains. More research is needed to investigate the specific types of play that best facilitate change in specific developmental domains.

In fact, although basic play studies have benefited from significant improvements in methodology in the past century, there remains a relative lack of experimental studies and longitudinal research. Without such work, researchers and clinicians are constrained by an inability to attribute causality when examining the relationships between play and interpersonal functioning. It remains unclear how much play *fosters* healthy interpersonal development versus merely being an *expression* of healthy development fostered by other factors. The answer to this question is key if play is to continue to be conceptualized as a mechanism of change.

Upon development of evidence-based interventions that include play for specific presenting problems, these interventions should be evaluated against existing treatment models to determine the optimal treatment modality. Given cultural differences in the content and structure of play, it is particularly important to evaluate interventions across cultural groups, to consider differences in the function and meanings of play themes across groups, and to consider levels of acculturation among families.

Finally, the development of innovative interventions requires the development of efficient and effective models of dissemination. In the development of evidence-based interventions that include play, methods of dissemination to community-based providers must be created and assessed to determine the best methods for maintaining treatment fidelity and effectiveness.

REFERENCES

Anastassiou-Hadjicharalambous, X., & Warden, D. (2008). Physiologically-indexed and self-perceived affective empathy in conduct-disordered children high and low on callous–unemotional traits. *Child and Adolescent Psychiatry and Mental Health, 2,* 1–11.

Arey, A. (1941). Play life of children. In C. Skinner & P. Harriman (Eds.), *Child psychology: Child development and modern education* (pp. 373–398). New York: Macmillan.

Ariel, S. (2002). *Children's imaginative play: A visit to wonderland.* Westport, CT: Praeger.

Ashiabi, G. S. (2007). Play in the preschool classroom: Its socioemotional significance and the teacher's role in play. *Early Childhood Education Journal, 35,* 199–207.

Baldwin, J. (1992). Relational schemas and the processing of social information. *Psychological Bulletin, 112,* 461–484.

Batum, P., & Yagmurlu, B. (2007). What counts in externalizing behaviors?: The contributions of emotion and behavior regulation. *Current Psychology, 25,* 272–294.

Berk, L. E., Mann, T. D., & Ogan, A. T. (2006). Make-believe play: Wellspring for development of self-regulation. In D. G. Singer, R. M. Golinkoff, & K. Hirsh-Pasek (Eds.), *Play = learning: How play motivates and enhances children's cognitive and social-emotional growth* (pp. 74–100). New York: Oxford University Press.

Bornstein, M. H., Haynes, O. M., Pascual, L., Painter, K. M., & Galperin, C. (1999). Play in two societies: Pervasiveness of process, specificity of structure. *Child Development, 70,* 317–331.

Bowlby, J. (1973). *Attachment and loss: Vol. 2. Separation, anxiety, and anger.* New York: Basic Books.

Bridges, L. J., Denham, S. A., & Ganiban, J. M. (2004). Definitional issues in emotion regulation research. *Child Development, 75,* 340–345.

Burack, J. A., Flanagan, T., Peled, T., Sutton, H. M., Zygmuntowicz, C., & Manly, J. T. (2006). Social perspective-taking skills in maltreated children and adolescents. *Developmental Psychology, 42,* 207–217.

Burghardt, G. M. (2005). *The genesis of animal play.* Cambridge, MA: MIT Press.

Butcher, J. L., & Niec, L. N. (2005). Disruptive behaviors and creativity in childhood: The importance of affect regulation. *Creativity Research Journal, 17,* 181–193.

Cielinski, K. L., Vaughn, B. E., Seifer, R., & Contresas, J. (1995). Relations among sustained engagement during play, quality of play, and mother–child interaction in samples of children with Down syndrome and normally developing toddlers. *Infant Behavior and Development, 18,* 163–176.

Cohen, J. A., & Mannarino, A. P. (2008). Trauma-focused cognitive behavioural therapy for children and parents. *Child and Adolescent Mental Health, 13,* 158–162.

Colwell, M. J., & Lindsey, E. W. (2005). Preschool children's pretend and physical play and sex of play partner: Connections to peer competence. *Sex Roles, 52,* 497–509.

Cote, L. R., & Bornstein, M. H. (2009). Child and mother play in three U.S. cultural groups: Comparisons and associations. *Journal of Family Psychology, 23,* 355–363.

Curran, J. M. (1999). Constraints of pretend play: Implicit and explicit rules. *Journal of Research in Childhood Education, 14,* 47–55.

Cutting, A. L., & Dunn, J. (2006). Conversations with siblings and with friends: Links between relationship quality and social understanding. *British Journal of Developmental Psychology, 24,* 73–87.

Dansky, J. (1999). Play. In M. Runco & S. Pritzker (Eds.), *Encyclopedia of creativity* (pp. 393–408). San Diego: Academic Press.

Denham, S. A., Caverly, S., Schimdt, M., Blair, K., DeMulder, E., Caal, S., et al. (2002). Preschool understanding of emotions: Contributions to classroom anger and aggression. *Journal of Child Psychology and Psychiatry, 43,* 901–916.

Despert, L. (1938). *Emotional problems in children: Technical approaches used in their study and treatment.* Utica, NY: State Hospitals Press.

Downey, G., & Walker, E. (1989). Social cognition and adjustment in children at risk for psychopathology. *Developmental Psychology, 25,* 835–845.

Dunn, J., & Brown, J. (1994). Affect expression in the family, children's understanding of emotions, and their interactions with others. *Merrill–Palmer Quarterly, 40,* 120–137.

Dunn, J., & Hughes, C. (2001). "I've got some swords and you're dead!": Violent fantasy, antisocial behavior, friendship, and moral sensibility in young children. *Child Development, 72,* 491–505.

Eisenberg, N., & Fabes, R. A. (1998). Prosocial development. In N. Eisenberg (Ed.) & W. Damon (Series Ed.), *Handbook of child psychology: Vol. 3. Social, emotional, and personality development* (pp. 701–778). New York: Wiley.

Eisenberg, N., & Fabes, R. A. (2006). Emotion regulation and children's socioemotional competence. In L. Balter & C. S. Tamis-Lemonda (Eds.), *Child psychology: A handbook of contemporary issues* (2nd ed., pp. 357–381). New York: Psychology Press.

Erikson, E. (1940). Studies in the interpretation of play: Clinical observation of play disruption in young children. *Genetic Psychology Monographs, 22,* 557–671.

Erikson, E. (1977). *Childhood and society* (2nd ed.). New York: Norton. (Original work published 1963)

Fantuzzo, J., Sekino, Y., & Cohen, H. L. (2004). An examination of the contributions of interactive peer play to salient classroom competencies for urban Head Start children. *Psychology in the Schools, 41,* 323–336.

Farver, J. A. M., Kim, Y. K., & Lee, Y. (1995). Cultural differences in Korean-American and Anglo-American preschoolers' social interaction and play behaviors. *Child Development, 66,* 1088–1099.

Farver, J. A. M., Kim, Y. K., & Lee-Shim, Y. (2000). Within cultural differences: Examining individual differences in Korean-American and European-American preschoolers' social pretend play. *Journal of Cross-Cultural Psychology, 31,* 583–602.

Farver, J. A. M., & Lee-Shim, Y. (1997). Social pretend play in Korean- and European-American preschoolers. *Child Development, 68,* 544–556.

Fein, G. G. (1981). Pretend play in childhood: An integrative review. *Child Development, 52,* 1095–1118.

Fein, G. G. (1987). Pretend play: Creativity and consciousness. In P. Gorlitz & J. Wohlwill (Eds.), *Curiosity, imagination, and play* (pp. 281–304). Hillsdale, NJ: Erlbaum.

Fenson, L. (1986). The developmental progression of play. In A. W. Gottfried & C. W. Brown (Eds.), *The contribution of play materials and paren-*

tal involvement to children's development (pp. 53–66). Lexington, MA: Heath.

Findlay, L. C., Girardi, A., & Coplan, R. J. (2006). Links between empathy, social behavior, and social understanding in early childhood. *Early Childhood Research Quarterly, 21,* 347–359.

Fisher, E. P. (1992). The impact of play on development: A meta-analysis. *Play and Culture, 5,* 159–181.

Freedenfeld, R. N., Ornduff, S. R., & Kelsey, R. M. (1995). Object relations and physical abuse: A TAT analysis. *Journal of Personality Assessment, 64,* 552–568.

Fromberg, D. P. (1992). Play. In C. Seefeldt (Ed.), *Early childhood education: A review of research* (pp. 42–84). New York: Teachers College Press.

Fromberg, D. P. (2002). *Play and meaning in early childhood education.* Boston: Allyn & Bacon.

Gardner, B. P., & Bergen, D. (2006). Play development from birth to age four. In D. F. Fromberg & D. Bergen (Eds.), *Play from birth to twelve: Contexts, perspectives, and meanings* (pp. 3–12). New York: Routledge.

Gaskins, S. (2000). Children's daily activities in a Mayan village: A culturally grounded description. *Cross-Cultural Research, 34,* 375–389.

Galyer, K. T., & Evans, I. M. (2001). Pretend play and the development of emotion regulation in preschool children. *Early Childhood Development and Care, 166,* 93–108.

Giffin, H. (1984). The coordination of meaning in the creation of a shared make-believe reality. In I. Bretherton (Ed.), *Symbolic play: The development of social understanding* (pp. 73–100). New York: Academic Press.

Goncu, A., Mistry, J., & Mosier, C. (2000). Cultural variations in the play of toddlers. *International Journal of Behavioral Development, 24,* 321–329.

Gosso, Y., de Lima Salum e Morais, M., & Otta, E. (2007). Pretend play of Brazilian children: A window into different cultural worlds. *Journal of Cross-Cultural Psychology, 38,* 539–558.

Groos, K., & Baldwin, E. (1901). *The play of man.* New York: Appleton & Co.

Gross, J. J. (1998). The emerging field of emotion regulation: An integrative review. *Review of General Psychology, 2,* 271–299.

Haight, W., Black, J., Ostler, T., & Sheridan, K. (2006). Pretend play and emotion learning in traumatized mothers and children. In D. G. Singer, R. M. Golinkoff, & K. Hirsh-Pasek (Eds.), *Play = learning: How play motivates and enhances children's cognitive and social-emotional growth* (pp. 209–230). New York: Oxford University Press.

Haight, W., Wang, X., Fung, H. H., Williams, K., & Mintz, J. (1999). Universal, developmental, and variable aspects of young children's play: A cross-cultural comparison of pretending at home. *Child Development, 70,* 1477–1488.

Hall, S. (Ed.). (1995). *Aspects of child life and education.* London: Routledge/Thoemmes Press. (Original work published 1907)

Harris, P. L. (2000). *The work of the imagination.* Oxford, UK: Blackwell.

Hart, C. H., DeWolf, D. M., Wozniak, P., & Burts, D. C. (1992). Maternal and paternal disciplinary styles: Relations with preschoolers' playground behavioral orientations and peer status. *Child Development, 63,* 879–892.

Harwood, R., Leyendecker, B., Carlson, V., Asencio, M., & Miller, A. (2002). Parenting among Latino families in the U.S. In M. H. Bornstein (Ed.), *Handbook of parenting: Vol 4. Applied parenting* (2nd ed., pp. 21–46). Mahwah, NJ: Erlbaum.

Hay, D. F., Payne, A., & Chadwick, A. (2004). Peer relations in childhood. *Journal of Child Psychology and Psychiatry, 45,* 84–108.

Hill, A. L., Degnan, K. A., Calkins, S. D., & Keane, S. P. (2006). Profiles of externalizing behavior problems for boys and girls across preschool: The roles of emotion regulation and inattention. *Developmental Psychology, 42,* 913–928.

Howes, C., & Phillipsen, L. (1992). Gender and friendship: Relationships with peers. *Social Development, 7,* 340–349.

Howes, C., Unger, O., & Matheson, C. C. (1992). *The collaborative construction of pretend: Social pretend play functions.* Albany: State University of New York Press.

Howes, C., Unger, O., & Seidner, L. B. (1989). Social pretend play in toddlers: Parallels with social play and with solitary pretend. *Child Development, 60,* 77–84.

Hughes, F. P. (1999). *Children, play, and development* (3rd ed.). Needham Heights, MA: Allyn & Bacon.

Jenkins, J. M., & Astington, J. W. (2000). Theory of mind and social behavior: Casual models tested in a longitudinal model. *Merrill–Palmer Quarterly, 46,* 203–220.

Johnson, J. E. (2006). Play development from ages four to eight. In D. F. Fromberg & D. Bergen (Eds.), *Play from birth to twelve: Contexts, perspectives, and meanings* (pp. 13–20). New York: Routledge.

Kavanaugh, R., & Harris, P. (1999). Pretense and counterfactual thought in young children. In C. Tamis-LeMonda & L. Balter (Eds.), *Child psychology: A handbook of contemporary issues* (pp. 158–176). New York: Garland.

Ladd, G. W., & Price, J. M. (1987). Predicting children's social and school adjustment following the transition from preschool to kindergarten. *Child Development, 58,* 1168–1189.

Lebo, D. (1953). The present status of research on non-directive play therapy. *Journal of Consulting Psychology, 17,* 177–183.

Lehman, H. C., & Witty, P. A. (1927). Periodicity and play behavior. *Journal of Educational Psychology, 18,* 115–118.

Leslie, A. M. (1987). Pretense and representation: The origins of "theory of mind." *Psychological Review, 94,* 412–426.

Levine, L., & Tuber, S. (1993). Measures of mental representation: Clinical and theoretical considerations. *Bulletin of the Menninger Clinic, 57,* 69–87.

Levitt, E. (1957). The results of psychotherapy with children: An evaluation. *Journal of Consulting Psychology, 21,* 189–196.

Lindsey, E. W., & Colwell, M. J. (2003). Preschoolers' emotional competence: Links to pretend and physical play. *Child Study Journal, 33,* 39–52.

Locke, J. (1890). *Some thoughts concerning education* (new ed.). London: National Society's Depository. (Original work published 1693)

Maccoby, E. E. (1998). *The two sexes.* Cambridge, MA: Harvard University Press.

Manning, M. L. (2006). Play development from ages eight to twelve. In D. F. Fromberg & D. Bergen (Eds.), *Play from birth to twelve: Contexts, perspectives, and meanings* (pp. 21–30). New York: Routledge.

Marton, I., Wiener, J., Rogers, M., Moore, C., & Tannock, R. (2009). Empathy and social perspective taking in children with attention-deficit/hyperactivity disorder. *Journal of Abnormal Child Psychology, 37,* 107–118.

McEwen, F., Happe, F., Bolton, P., Rijsdik, F., Ronald, A., Dworzynski, K., et al. (2007). Origins of individual differences in imitation: Links with language, pretend play, and socially insightful behavior in two-year-old twins. *Child Development, 78,* 474–492.

Miller, P. A., & Jansen op de Haar, M. A. (1997). Emotional, cognitive, behavioral, and temperament characteristics of high-empathy children. *Motivation and Emotion, 21,* 109–125.

Moore, M., & Russ, S. W. (2006). Pretend play as a resource for children: Implications for pediatricians and health professionals. *Developmental and Behavioral Pediatrics, 27,* 237–248.

Morgenthaler, S. K. (2006). The meaning in play with objects. In D. F. Fromberg & D. Bergen (Eds.), *Play from birth to twelve: Contexts, perspectives, and meanings* (pp. 111–118). New York: Routledge.

Niec, L. N., & Russ, S. W. (2002). Children's internal representations, empathy, and fantasy play: A validity study of the SCORS-Q. *Psychological Assessment, 14,* 331–338.

Niec, L. N., Yopp, J., & Russ, S. W. (2009). *Validity of the Interpersonal Themes in Play Scale.* Unpublished manuscript, Department of Psychology, Central Michigan University, Mt. Pleasant, Michigan.

Nourot, P. M. (2006). Sociodramatic play pretending together. In D. F. Fromberg & D. Bergen (Eds.), *Play from birth to twelve: Contexts, perspectives, and meanings* (pp. 87–102). New York: Routledge.

Ornduff, S. R., Freedenfeld, R. N., Kelsey, R. M., & Critelli, J. W. (1994). Object relations of sexually abused female subjects: A TAT analysis. *Journal of Personality Assessment, 63,* 223–238.

Pellegrini, A. D. (1988). Elementary school children's rough-and-tumble play and social competence. *Developmental Psychology, 24,* 802–806.

Pellegrini, A. D. (2003). Perceptions and functioning of play and real fighting in early adolescence. *Child Development, 74,* 1522–1533.

Pellegrini, A. D. (2006). Rough-and-tumble play from childhood through adolescence: Differing perspectives. In D. F. Fromberg & D. Bergen (Eds.), *Play from birth to twelve: Contexts, perspectives, and meanings* (pp. 111–118). New York: Routledge.

Pellegrini, A. D., & Smith, P. K. (1998). Physical activity play: The nature and function of a neglected aspect of play. *Child Development, 69,* 577–598.

Piaget, J. (1962). *Play, dreams, and imitation in childhood.* London: Routledge & Kegan Paul.

Rubin, K. H., Fein, G., & Vanderberg, B. (1983). Play. In P. E. M. Mussen & E. M. Hetherington (Eds.), *Handbook of child psychology: Vol. 4. Socialization, personality, and social development* (pp. 693–774). New York: Wiley.

Rubin, K. H., & Howe, N. (1986). Social play and perspective taking. In G. Fein & M. Rivkin (Eds.), *The young child at play: Reviews of research* (pp. 113–125). Washington, DC: National Association for the Education of Young Children.

Russ, S. W. (2004). *Play in child development and psychotherapy: Toward empirically supported practice.* Mahwah, NJ: Erlbaum.

Russ, S. W., & Kaugars, A. S. (2000–2001). Emotion in children's play and creative problem solving. *Creativity Research Journal, 13*, 211–219.

Safran, J. (1990). Toward a refinement of cognitive therapy in light of interpersonal theory: Theory. *Clinical Psychology Review, 10*, 87–105.

Seja, A. L., & Russ, S. W. (1999). Children's fantasy play and emotional understanding. *Journal of Clinical Child Psychology, 28*, 269–277.

Shirk, S., & Russell, R. (1996). *Change processes in child psychotherapy: Revitalizing treatment and research.* New York: Guilford Press.

Singer, D. G., & Singer, J. L. (2005). *Imagination and play in the electronic age.* Cambridge, MA: Harvard University Press.

Singer, J. L. (1995). Imaginative play in childhood: Precursor of subjective thought, daydreaming, and adult pretending games. In A. D. Pellegrini (Ed.), *The future of play theory: A multidisciplinary inquiry into the contributions of Brian Sutton-Smith* (pp. 187–219). Albany: State University of New York Press.

Singer, J. L. (1998). Imaginative play in early childhood: A foundation for adaptive emotional and cognitive development. *International Medical Journal, 5*, 93–100.

Sroufe, L. A. (2000). Early relationships and the development of children. *Infant Mental Health Journal, 21*, 67–74.

Strayer, J., & Roberts, W. (2004). Empathy and observed anger and aggression in five-year-olds. *Social Development, 13*, 1–13.

Strayhorn, J. (2002). Self-control: Toward systematic training programs. *Journal of the American Academy of Child Psychiatry, 41*, 17–27.

Tamis-LeMonda, C. S., & Bornstein, M. H. (1991). Individual variation, correspondence, stability, and change in mother and toddler play. *Infant Behavior and Development, 14*, 143–162.

Westen, D. (1991). Social cognition and object relations. *Psychological Bulletin, 109*, 429–455.

Westen, D., Klepser, J., Ruffins, S. A., Silverman, M., Lifton, N., & Boekamp, J. (1991). Object relations in childhood and adolescence: The development of working representations. *Journal of Consulting and Clinical Psychology, 59*, 400–409.

Youngblade, L. M., & Dunn, J. (1995). Individual differences in young children's pretend play with mother and sibling: Links to relationships and understanding of other people's feelings and beliefs. *Child Development, 66,* 1472–1492.

Zhou, Q., Eisenberg, N., Losoya, S. H., Fabes, R. A., Reiser, M., Guthrie, I. K., et al. (2002). The relations of parental warmth and positive expressiveness to children's empathy-related responding and social functioning: A longitudinal study. *Child Development, 73,* 893–915.

PART II
Play in Evidence-Based Assessment

3

Assessment of Pretend Play

Astrida Seja Kaugars

Increasing attention has been devoted to evidence-based assessment in the fields of clinical child and pediatric psychology. This is illustrated by the special issues devoted to this topic by the *Journal of Clinical Child and Adolescent Psychology* (2005, Vol. 34, No. 3) and the *Journal of Pediatric Psychology* (2008, Vol. 33, No. 9). As noted in the introductions to each of these special issues, weak links exist between assessment and intervention and the role of assessment in the promotion of evidence-based treatments (Cohen et al., 2008; Mash & Hunsley, 2005). A similar dilemma is present in the fields of research and practice in play and play interventions.

Mash and Hunsley (2005) describe the challenges of the likely multiple purposes for assessment (e.g., diagnosis, treatment planning, treatment monitoring, and treatment evaluation) and how the different stages of assessment must be taken into account when considering which assessment instrument is to be used in which situation. This challenge also translates to the field of play and play interventions, where different measures of play may be appropriate across varying clinical situations. Thus, the purpose of the present chapter is to review the evidence base for existing measures of children's pretend play and their previous and potential utilization in clinical practice.

Children's ability to pretend and their engagement in pretend play begins in early childhood. Piaget (1962) claimed that symbolic play emerges at 2 years of age and increases over the next 3 or 4 years. However, by 12 months of age children may show evidence of symbolic acts and pretend, particularly when caregivers provide external support for pretending (Haight & Miller, 1993). Longitudinal data support Piaget's claim that the percentage of time young children engage in pretend play increases significantly between 1 and 4 years of age (Haight & Miller, 1993). Singer and Singer (1990) aptly characterized the preschool and early elementary school years as "the high season of imaginative play" given the potential prominence of play for children at this developmental stage.

Pretend play in young children has been defined by the following five criteria: (1) familiar activities may be performed in the absence of necessary material or a social context; (2) activities may not be carried out to their logical outcome; (3) a child may treat an inanimate object as animate; (4) one object or gesture may be substituted for another; and (5) a child may carry out an activity usually performed by someone else (Fein, 1981; Singer & Singer, 1990). When pretending, children can incorporate unique combinations of both reality and fantasy themes into their play with an understanding of their distinction. These characteristics are evident in the dimensions of pretend and fantasy play that are assessed with the measures reviewed in this chapter.

ASSESSING PLAY IN RESEARCH CONTEXTS

For research purposes, observations of children's play both individually and in groups have necessitated operationalizing the play behaviors or characteristics of interest to the investigator(s). Thus investigators have either developed their own or utilized more widely used assessments of children's pretend play. While some assessment tools have the potential to inform clinical work, as discussed below, others are primarily intended to help address specific study questions, in a particular context, with a specific participant population. Consequently, there is variability in whether or not the data that the assessment measures developed solely for research purposes provide can be useful when generalizing to other settings and other populations.

Specifically, classification of children's play by categories has been used in research contexts. A frequently used instrument for classifying preschool and elementary school-age children's classroom play behaviors is the Play Observation Scale (e.g., Rubin & Mills, 1988). The measure incorporates Smilansky's (1968) cognitive play categories (i.e., functional, constructive, dramatic, games with rules) within the social participation categories of Parten (1932; i.e., solitary, parallel, group). Other researchers (e.g., Lloyd & Howe, 2003) have added observations of additional behaviors (e.g., transitions, wandering), types of materials, and use of materials. Children are observed for a predetermined period of time (e.g., 60 seconds a day for 20 days; Lloyd & Howe, 2003). Acceptable reliability and validity for this observation have been demonstrated (see discussion in Pellegrini, 1991). The information provided by this type of assessment is undeniably rich and informative. However, there is relatively little information about the nature of children's pretend play within the dramatic play category. Yet, one can assess the relative frequency of different types of play behaviors (e.g., Lloyd & Howe, 2003), perhaps before and after interventions aimed at supporting or altering children's play behaviors. Observers can be trained to use the coding matrix reliably after 2 hours of instruction, which supports its use in applied settings (Pellegrini, 1991). Similarly, Pellegrini (1995) developed an observational scheme for assessing elementary schoolchildren's playground behavior where one category, role play, includes pretense behaviors.

ASSESSING PLAY IN CLINICAL CONTEXTS

In clinical contexts, there are multiple advantages to using play assessment (see discussion by Gitlin-Weiner, Sandgrund, & Schaefer, 2000). Play may reveal children's emotional concerns, allow them opportunities in which to demonstrate their skills that may otherwise be hindered in classic test batteries, and reduce children's reluctance to engage with examiners and testing materials. Pelligrini (1998) argues that in play children exhibit their "maximum competence" and thus that the use of play is supported in an assessment context.

However, it is important to distinguish between play-based measures that potentially assess multiple dimensions of children's development and measures that specifically assess pretense and fantasy in children's play. Play-based assessments can provide information about children's developmental functioning in numerous domains and may complement formal, standardized assessment measures. Yet children's use of pretense and fantasy may be one of many skills assessed, which emphasizes the need for assessment instruments specifically designed to assess pretense. For example, the Transdisciplinary Play-Based Assessment (TPBA; Linder, 1990) is a comprehensive assessment designed for use with infants and children through 6 years of age. A cross-disciplinary team observes a child in structured and unstructured play situations and evaluates the child's development in the domains of Cognitive Abilities, Social–Emotional Functioning, Communication and Language Skills, and Sensory–Motor Development. Aspects of play, as they represent development in the different domains, are assessed, including categories of play, symbolic and representational play, imitation, and characteristics of dramatic play. Qualitative data on the child's developmental range of functioning is used to provide functional, skill-based intervention recommendations. This method highlights the systematic use of play to conduct an in-depth evaluation with some information provided about a child's play development. While the TPBA is widely used, additional research is needed to provide information about the reliability and validity of this scale (Athanasiou, 2007).

REVIEW OF ASSESSMENT MEASURES

Recent efforts to review evidence-based assessment measures for children and adolescents have reviewed existing measures, established criteria for classifying existing measures, and examined reviewer agreement for classifications, yet not all reviews necessarily strive to classify measures according to criteria (e.g., well-established, approaching well-established, and promising assessment). Chambless and Ollendick (2001) summarized the criteria that have been used by various workgroups to define categories of empirically supported treatments, and Cohen et al. (2008) developed a hierarchy for classifying pediatric psychology assessment measures. Notably, the categorizations have taken into account the amount of publications (i.e., number of peer-reviewed articles) and the different types of research designs (e.g., between-group design experiments) utilizing the specific measures/treatments of interest, the availability of details necessary for evaluation and replication, and the level of detail offered regarding reliability and validity. These guidelines were taken into account when reviewing measures for the present chapter.

The focus of the present review is on standardized assessments of children's pretend play for children ages 4–10. Measures that are included have standardized instructions for children and standardized toys. All of the assessment measures include standardized coding systems that assess pretend or fantasy play in children, and published empirical support (i.e., reliability and validity data) exists for the measure. In addition, three measures with standardized coding systems that assess the content and process of children's play therapy are included. The focus of the review is on measures that would be useful in clinical work and those that have been empirically validated. In order to identify measures to be included in the present review, I reviewed articles, chapters, and books that discussed children's play and play assessment. In addition, PsycINFO, PubMed, and Web of Science searches were used to identify possible measures and relevant articles.

TABLE 3.1. Summary of Evidence-Based Assessments of Pretend Play

Measure	Ages (years)	Brief description	Psychometrics		
			Reliability	Validity	

Measure	Ages (years)	Brief description	Reliability	Validity
Affect in Play Scale (APS; Russ, 1993)	6–10	Children play with two puppets and three blocks for 5 minutes. A standardized scoring system quantifies the affect expression and quality of fantasy and imagination. A brief rating version has been recently developed.	Interrater reliability: $r = .67–.95$ $\alpha = .87–.99$ ICC $= .87–.99$ Internal consistency: Frequency of Affect, $r = .85$	Relationships among affective and cognitive scores on the APS and measures assessing creativity, coping and adjustment, emotional understanding, and interpersonal functioning. APS scores consistently not related to measures of verbal ability.
Affect in Play Scale—Preschool Version (APS-P; Kaugars & Russ, 2009)	4–5	Children play with plastic and stuffed animals, plastic cups, a plastic car, and a "hairy" rubber ball for 5 minutes. The APS scoring system was adapted for younger children and includes criteria for categorizing the type of children's play.	Interrater reliability: ICC $= .91–.99$ Internal consistency: Frequency of Affect, $r = .88$	Relationships among APS-P scores and measures of children's daily play behavior, creativity, affect intensity, and social competence.
Child-Initiated Pretend Play Assessment (ChIPPA; Stagnitti, 2007)	3–7	Conventional (e.g., farm set toys) and unstructured (e.g., pebbles, a tin, and a shoe box) play materials are used to assess children's elaborateness of play action, ability to substitute objects during play, and child's imitation of modeled actions of examiner. Children play for a 30-minute (4- to 7-year-olds) or an 18-minute (3-year-olds) session.	Interrater reliability: $\kappa = .96–1.00$ Test–retest reliability: ICC $= .56–.84$. Percentage agreement: 63–84%	ChIPPA scores discriminated between children who were typically developing and those with preacademic problems. No correlations between ChIPPA scores and parent report of children's socioemotional skills or pretend play. Level of pretend play ability related to interpersonal relationship capacity. Significant negative relationship found between parent-reported cooperation and sharing and ChIPPA elaborate play scores. *(continued)*

TABLE 3.1. (*continued*)

Measure	Ages (years)	Brief description	Psychometrics	
			Reliability	Validity
Structured Play Assessment (Ungerer & Sigman, 1981)	1–6	Child presented with toys (e.g., dolls and furniture, dump truck, blocks, a brush, a mirror) and observed in play for 15–20 minutes. Variables assessed include functional play types, symbolic play types, and play levels, and score for mastery. Can be used in observations of child individually or in parent–child interaction.	Interrater reliability: $r = .69 – > .80$ ICC $= .94–1.00$	Significant differences in the number of different functional and symbolic play acts among children with autism, Down syndrome, and developmental delays and typically developing children. Significant positive correlations among play variables and language skills. Relationships among functional and symbolic play acts in early childhood with peer interaction initiation in later childhood among children with autism. Used to assess outcomes in intervention study with observed changes in play variability and sophistication.
Test of Pretend Play (ToPP; Lewis & Boucher, 1997)	1–8	Children complete a series of tasks that reflect the developmental sequence of symbolic play behavior. Test items assess substituting one object for another, referring to an absent object as if it were present, and attributing a property to an object that it does not have.	Interrater reliability: $\kappa = 0.68$ ICC $= .96$ Percentage agreement: 94%	Relationships among ToPP scores, age, language abilities, and self-regulatory strategies. Support for convergent and discriminant validity with conceptual knowledge and symbolizing ability. ToPP scores discriminated among children with and without developmental delays. Used to assess outcomes in intervention studies with documented changes in ToPP scores.

Note. ICC, intraclass correlation coefficient.

TABLE 3.2. Summary of Evidence-Based Assessments of Play Therapy

Measure	Ages (years)	Brief description	Psychometrics		
			Reliability	Validity	
Children's Play Therapy Instrument (CPTI; Kernberg et al., 1998)	Not specified	Therapist/observer reviews videotaped segment of play therapy session. Scores assess descriptive, structural, and adaptive perspectives of child's play.	Interrater reliability: Segmentation of Child's Activity κ = .72 Dimensional Analysis scores: ICC = .52–.89 κ = .12–1.00 Percentage agreement: 44–100% Seven main subscales within Dimensional Analysis Individual rater agreement with consensus: ICC = .61–.96	Used in two single-case studies of children in play therapy with observed changes in CPTI score over the course of treatment.	
Play Therapy Observation Instrument (PTOI; Howe & Silvern, 1981)	Not specified	Therapist/observer scores 10- to 12-minute segments of play therapy interactions from videotape. Scores assess three areas of functioning with 13 items: emotional discomfort, quality of interaction with therapist, and use of fantasy.	Interrater reliability: 13 items ICC = .48–.95 Percentage agreement within one point: 82–100% Percentage agreement exactly: 89–100% Internal consistency: α = .74–.83 HR = .44–.54 Test–retest reliability: r = .68–.83	No significant differences in children's play with either psychodynamic or client-centered play therapy approaches. Differences in fantasy play and quality of interaction subscale scores between first and last play therapy sessions.	

(continued)

57

TABLE 3.2. (continued)

Measure	Ages (years)	Brief description	Psychometrics	
			Reliability	Validity
Trauma Play Scale (Findling et al., 2006)	5–7	Review videotaped play therapy sessions at the end of each 5-minute interval. Scores assessed in the following domains: Intense Play, Repetitive Play, Play Disruptions, Avoidant Play Behavior, and Negative Affect.	Interrater reliability: Mean r = .80–.86 Percentage agreement: 97–98% Intrarater reliability: r = .85–.98.	Children with a history of trauma had higher total scores, with the exception of repetitive play, than children with no known history of trauma.

Note. ICC, intraclass correlation; HR, Scott's homogeneity ratio.

Five measures assessing pretend play and three measures of play in the context of play therapy are reviewed in the next section and summarized in Tables 3.1 and 3.2: the Affect in Play Scale (APS), the Affect in Play Scale—Preschool Version (APS-P), the Child-Initiated Pretend Play Assessment (ChIPPA), a Structured Play Assessment, the Test of Pretend Play (ToPP), the Children's Play Therapy Instrument (CPTI), the Play Therapy Observation Instrument (PTOI), and the Trauma Play Scale.

Measures Assessing Pretend Play

Affect in Play Scale

DESCRIPTION

The APS consists of a standardized puppet task and coding system and assesses both cognitive and affective processes in play (Russ, 1993; Russ, 2004). Children ages 6–10 are given two human puppets, one boy and one girl, and three blocks. The child is instructed to play with the puppets any way that he or she wants to for 5 minutes. The play materials and instructions are standardized but also unstructured enough so that individual differences in play can emerge. Standardized prompts are used if the child stops playing and when there is 1 minute left to play. The play session is videotaped and scored according to a detailed scoring manual. After completing training in the scoring system, it takes about 15–20 minutes to score each child's play session.

The APS includes scores for quality of fantasy and imagination. Specifically, global ratings on 5-point Likert scales are made for organization of the play (Organization of Fantasy), elaboration and embellishment in the play (Elaboration of Fantasy), and imagination in play (Imagination). An Overall Quality of Fantasy score is computed using the mean of the other three fantasy scores.

The APS also measures the amount and types of affective expression in children's play using three affect scores. The Total Frequency of Affect score summarizes the number of units of affect expressed throughout the play session. An affect unit can include an expression of an affect state (e.g., "I feel happy"), an affect theme (e.g., "There's a monster over there"), or the two combined. The Variety of Affect Categories is the number of different affect categories, of 11 possible categories, expressed in the 5-minute play period. Affect categories include Happiness/Pleasure, Anxiety/Fear, Sadness/Hurt, Frustration/Disappointment, Nurturance/Affection, Aggression, Oral, Oral Aggression, Anal, Sexual, and Competition. The Mean Intensity of Affect score takes into account intensity ratings for each affect unit on a 5-point Likert scale. In addition to the cognitive and affect scores, the APS also includes a rating of Comfort on a 5-point Likert scale. An Affect Integration score results from multiplying the Quality of Fantasy score by the Frequency of Affect score.

A recent study by Cordiano, Russ, and Short (2008) detailed the development and validation of a brief rating version of the APS (APS-BR) that does not require videotaping. The APS-BR includes five scores. The Organization, Imagination, and Comfort scores are rated on 4-point scales and are similar in content to the APS scores. The Frequency of Affect Expression score is different in that in the APS-BR, the rater keeps an estimated tally of the number of units of affect expression and then assigns a score on a 4-point scale ranging from low (0–2 affect units) to high (> 15 affect units). A Positive/Negative Tone of Affect Expression score measures the overall affective tone of the affect in play. The rater tallies the number of positive and negative affect units and then assigns a score on a 4-point scale where (1) represents predominately negative affect dominating the play and (4) represents predominately positive affect dominating the play. Pearson correlations between corresponding scores on the APS and APS-BR were all significantly correlated and represented large effect sizes.

RELIABILITY

Interrater reliabilities reported in the published literature have consistently been good. The interrater reliabilities calculated using Pearson product-moment correlations across a sample of the published studies were in the following ranges (Christiano & Russ, 1996; Niec & Russ, 1996; Niec & Russ, 2002; Russ & Kaugars, 2000–2001; Russ, Robins, & Christiano, 1999; Seja & Russ, 1999): Frequency of Affect (r = .77–.95), Variety of Affect (r = .74–.92), Quality of Fantasy (r = .80–.90), Organization of Fantasy (r = .72–.82), Elaboration of Fantasy (r = .74), Imagination (r = .67–.78), and Comfort (r = .86–.90). Interrater reliabilities calculated with coefficient alpha ranged from moderate to high: Frequency of Affect α = .99; Variety of Affect α = .87, Quality of Fantasy α = .94, and Comfort α = .89 (Butcher & Niec, 2005). Russ and Schafer (2006) reported that average coefficients for intraclass coefficients (ICC) were Frequency of Affect = .99, Variety of Affect = .99, Organization of Fantasy = .98, Imagination = .97, and Comfort = .99. Interrater reliability for the APS-BR was calculated using ICCs. For the five APS-BR scores in two different samples, nine of the 10 scores met criteria for excellent reliability (Cordiano et al., 2008).

In one published study, the internal consistency of the Frequency of Affect score was examined by comparing the Frequency of Affect scores in the 2nd and 4th minutes with the 3rd and 5th minutes of the play period. An internal consistency of $r = .85$ was found using the Spearman–Brown split-half reliability formula (Seja & Russ, 1999).

VALIDITY

Affective and cognitive scores on the APS have been found to be related to scores on a divergent thinking task (Russ & Grossman-McKee, 1990; Russ & Schafer, 2006), which is one major cognitive process important in creativity. There were no gender differences in the pattern of correlations, and the relationships remained significant when IQ was partialed out. Caregiver report of children's creativity has been found to be negatively correlated with negative affect expression on the APS, even after controlling for verbal achievement (Butcher & Niec, 2005).

Children who were identified as "good" players on the APS used a greater number and variety of cognitive coping strategies during an invasive dental procedure, and they reported less procedural distress than children who expressed less affect and fantasy in play (Christiano & Russ, 1996). Children whose parents reported higher levels of disruptive behavior expressed more negative affect in their play (Butcher & Niec, 2005). When the directions of the APS were altered to instruct the children to have the puppets disagree about something, children expressed more negative affect in their play and reported more negative mood than children who were instructed to have the puppets have fun or when no instruction alterations were made (Russ & Kaugars, 2000–2001). Although the standard instructions were altered in some conditions in the study by Russ and Kaugars (2000–2001), the APS scores were sensitive to identifying changes in play due to the mood inductions.

Seja and Russ (1999) demonstrated that cognitive dimensions of play assessed with the APS were related to facets of emotional understanding. Children who were able to access and organize their fantasy and emotions in play were more likely to recall and organize memories related to emotional events and had a more sophisticated understanding of others' emotions. While Seja and Russ (1999) did not find a significant relationship between affective dimensions of play and emotional understanding, in a sample of Italian children Mazzeschi, Salcuni, Parolin, and Lis (2004) found consistent, yet modest, associations between APS affect scores and emotional understanding scores, particularly children's understanding of others' emotions.

Children who expressed a wide variety of affect categories, frequent positive affect, comfort in their play, and high-quality fantasy were more likely to include themes of people and relationships on an apperceptive storytelling task (Niec & Russ, 1996). Niec and Russ (2002) found that children whose play was more imaginative, organized, and elaborated were more likely to describe themselves as empathic and demonstrated a logical understanding of the relationships among emotions, thoughts, and behaviors in narratives. In both of the studies, there were no significant relationships between the APS scores and teacher (Niec & Russ, 1996; Niec & Russ, 2002) and peer (Niec & Russ, 1996) ratings of participants' interpersonal functioning (e.g., empathy).

Russ et al. (1999) demonstrated that APS scores when children were in the first and second grades were predictive of children's scores on an adapted version of the APS when they were in the fifth and sixth grades. The strength of the correlations suggests that cognitive and affective processes as assessed by the APS are stable over time. In addition, children's Quality of Fantasy scores in the first and second grades were significantly related to the number of different responses they generated on a measure of coping 4 years later.

In numerous studies using the APS, scores from standardized measures of intellectual or verbal ability have consistently not been related to APS scores and correlations among APS scores and theoretically relevant measures have remained significant with IQ or verbal ability partialed out (Russ & Grossman-McKee, 1990; Seja & Russ, 1999) .

Affect in Play Scale—Preschool Version

DESCRIPTION

The APS-P is an adaptation of the APS for children 4 and 5 years of age (Kaugars & Russ, 2009; Russ, Niec, & Kaugars, 2000). Age-appropriate toys were selected for the APS-P that are easy for young children to play with and that might elicit symbolic and fantasy play: plastic and stuffed animals, plastic cups, a plastic car, and a "hairy" rubber ball. Each child is introduced to the toys, shown an example of how to play with the toys, and encouraged to continue playing for 5 minutes. As needed, standardized prompts are used to encourage the child to initiate and/or continue playing and to talk louder. The task was discontinued if the child did not play within 2 minutes of starting the task. The play session is videotaped to ensure accurate scoring. A scoring manual is available.

The APS-P includes six scores from the APS that were slightly modified to take young children's developing language abilities into consideration. The Frequency of Affect Expression score is the number of 10-second intervals in the 5 minutes in which the child expresses affect. The Variety of Affect Categories score is the number of different types of affect categories the child expresses in the 5 minutes. In addition to the affect categories in the APS, an additional category, Unclear Affect, is included for the situations in which it is difficult to determine the type of affect in the child's expression (e.g., when sound effects like "vroom" are used). The criteria for rating Imagination, Organization, and Elaboration are scored on 5-point scales, which were modified to take into account younger children's play. Similar to the APS, the Quality of Fantasy score is the mean of the Imagination, Organization, and Elaboration scores, and the Comfort score is a global rating of children's enjoyment, pleasure, and involvement in the task. The APS-P also includes ratings to quantify the type of play children exhibit in each 20-second interval and reflect Smilansky's (1968) sequential play categories (as described and used by Jones & Glenn, 1991, and Rubin, Watson, & Jambor, 1978) and symbolic or pretend play criteria (Fein, 1981): Number of No Play Intervals, Number of Functional Play Intervals, and Number of Pretend Play Intervals.

RELIABILITY

Interrater reliability calculated using ICCs for the primary APS-P scores and play categories are high: Frequency of Affect = .95, Variety of Affect Expression = .91, Imagination = .97, Organization = .96, Elaboration = .92, Comfort = .94, Number of No Play Intervals = .95, Number of Functional Play Intervals = .99, and Number of Pretend Play Intervals = .95 (Kaugars & Russ, 2009).

The Spearman–Brown split half reliability formula was used to compare the Frequency of Affect scores in the 2nd and 4th minutes with the Frequency of Affect scores in the 3rd and 5th minutes to evaluate internal consistency, r = .88 (Kaugars & Russ, 2009).

VALIDITY

Preliminary evidence demonstrates that APS-P scores are related to children's daily play behavior, creativity, affect intensity, and social competence (Kaugars & Russ, 2009). Evidence for the face validity of the APS-P comes from results demonstrating that children who expressed more emotion in their play, a greater range of emotions, a higher quality of fantasy, and more instances of pretense in their play were more likely to be rated by their teachers as displaying enjoyment and make-believe in their daily play.

Convergent validity for the APS-P derives from findings of association between APS-P scores and measures of children's creativity, affect intensity, and social competence. Children who expressed more emotion in play, were comfortable playing, and demonstrated more pretend play offered more responses and more original responses on a divergent thinking task assessing ideational fluency. Children who expressed a variety of types of affect in their play, were more comfortable playing, and included more pretense in their play were rated by their teachers as demonstrating more intense positive emotions in their daily behavior. Similarly, children who expressed affect in their play and had higher quality of fantasy were regarded by their teachers as well integrated in their peer group and capable of functioning well with little adult supervision.

Child-Initiated Pretend Play Assessment

DESCRIPTION

The ChIPPA is a standardized assessment of children's ability to initiate and sustain pretend play during a 30-minute session for children ages 4–7 and during an 18-minute session for 3-year-old children (Stagnitti, Unsworth, & Rodger, 2000; Swindells & Stagnitti, 2006). The child and the examiner sit on the floor in a play area prepared by covering two chairs with a sheet to make a house. The assessment includes two 15-minute segments: one with conventional toys and one with symbolic toys. The first play segment assesses conventional imaginative play using one tractor, one trailer, one man doll, one girl doll, 12 fences, one wrench, three goats, two horses, four sheep, three cows, one rooster, and two pigs. The second play segment assesses symbolic play; children are presented with one small box, one large box, one plastic cone, one dowel stick, one flat stick, one tea towel, one face washer, one tin, two cloth dolls, and three smooth pebbles. Each 15-minute play segment is divided into three 5-minute sections. In the first 5-minute section, the examiner encourages the child to play without providing directions for playing. In the second 5-minute section, the examiner models five play actions. In the third 5-minute section, the examiner encourages the child to play again but does not give the child play direction or instruction (Stagnitti et al., 2000). A study by Stagnitti, Rodger, and Clarke (1997) demonstrated that both the conventional imaginative and the symbolic toys are gender-neutral.

There are three items assessed with the ChIPPA; each item is calculated separately for the conventional and symbolic toys, and total scores across the entire play assessment can be obtained. The Percentage of Elaborate Pretend Play Actions (PEPA) score represents the elaborateness, complexity, and organization of a child's play. This includes the child's ability to maintain play themes, sequences, and narratives during the play. The Number of Object Substitutions (NOS) score reflects the number of times a child pretends a toy or object is something else than its functional use. The Number of Imitated Actions (NIA) score describes the number of times a child initiates the play actions that have been demonstrated by the examiner in the second 5-minute play section. A scoring manual is available (Stagnitti, 2007).

Normative data is available to evaluate a child's performance on the ChIPPA. Standard scores can be calculated for the three Percentage of Elaborate Pretend Play Actions items and the Number of Object Substitution with symbolic toys items, and a child's z scores can be compared to those of other children his or her age. For the other items (i.e., Number of Object Substitutions with conventional toys and Number of Imitated Actions items), the child's raw scores are compared to the range and the mode of the normative sample. Typically children score 0 for these items since they play with the conventional toys in conventional ways and do not imitate the examiner (Swindells & Stagnitti, 2006).

RELIABILITY

Good-to-excellent agreement was found using Cohen's kappa to evaluate interrater agreement for the nine scores: Percentage of Elaborate Play Action scores, $\kappa = .96$ (conventional imaginative toys), .98 (symbolic toys), and .96 (combined); Number of Object Substitutions scores, $\kappa = 1.00$ (conventional imaginative toys), .97 (symbolic toys), and 1.00 (combined); and Number of Imitated Actions scores, $\kappa = 1.00$ (conventional imaginative toys), .97 (symbolic toys), and .98 (combined) (Stagnitti et al., 2000). Swindells and Stagnitti (2006) reported $\kappa = .70$ when two raters assessed a child's play simultaneously, but it is unclear which score(s) this represents.

Test–retest reliability over a 2-week interval was examined with a sample of children ages 4–5 years, which included four children with developmental delay (Stagnitti & Unsworth, 2004). ICCs were calculated for five scores: Percentage of Elaborate Play Actions conventional imaginative toys = .73, Percentage of Elaborate Play Actions symbolic toys = .77, Percentage of Elaborate Play Actions combined = .84, Number of Object Substitutions symbolic toys = .56, and Number of Object Substitutions combined = .57. For the remaining scores (i.e., Number of Object Substitutions conventional imaginative toys, and three Number of Imitated Actions scores), the majority of children scored 0, and there were no significant differences on these scores between the testing and retesting sessions. Percentage of agreement for these scores ranged from 64 to 84%.

The ChIPPA scores distinguished between children who were typically developing and those with preacademic problems (Stagnitti et al., 2000). Specifically, the elaborateness of a child's play and the child's ability to substitute objects discriminated between children in the two groups. In addition, the typically developing children imitated the examiner less frequently. The authors described three play profiles based on the ChIPPA scores that consider high versus low scores on each of the items.

Contrary to hypotheses, Swindells and Stagnitti (2006) did not find statistically significant correlations between children's play scores on the ChIPPA and parent report of children's socioemotional skills or pretend play. However, children who scored above the average range in elaborate play actions were reported by their parents as more competent in interpersonal relationships as compared to children who scored in the normal range for elaborate pretend play actions. Swindells and Stagnitti also found a significant negative relationship between parents' reports of children's cooperation and sharing and children's ChIPPA elaborate play scores. The authors suggested that perhaps children who have limited pretend play skills may be passive in their daily play interactions and thus may be perceived by their parents as sharing and cooperating well with other children.

Structured Play Assessment

DESCRIPTION

In this standardized play assessment introduced by Ungerer and Sigman (1981), the child is presented with a standard set of toys and observed in play for 15–20 minutes. Ungerer and Sigman described the unstructured assessment beginning with the experimenter using toys to model four different symbolic acts, and then the child playing alone with the toys for 16 minutes. The toys used in the assessment include three different-sized dolls, doll furniture, baby bottles, a tea set, a dump truck, a garage, blocks, a piece of paper, three pieces of sponge, a telephone, a brush, and a mirror (Kasari, Freeman, & Paparella, 2006; Ungerer & Sigman, 1981). The child's play is videotaped and scoring can be completed either during the assessment or later.

Different types of children's play behaviors are assessed including simple manipulation, relational play, functional play, and symbolic play. Simple Manipulation describes instances of the child mouthing, waving, banging, or fingering a toy. Relational Play includes situations in which the child makes nonfunctional combinations of objects (e.g., touching or banging two objects together). Functional Play describes the number of different, novel child-initiated functional play acts that are observed. Symbolic Play instances include the number of instances of different novel, child-initiated symbolic play acts that might include substitution play, agent play, or imaginary play. By recording the number of different sequences of the Functional and Symbolic Play (i.e., duration of play by category) as well as the number of different types or examples of the sequence (i.e., diversity of play), it is possible to calculate Play Level, which represents the highest, most frequent, and flexible level at which the child plays with mastery (i.e., highest spontaneous play level with at least three different types/exemplars of that level and eight different frequencies; Kasari et al., 2006; Ungerer & Sigman, 1981). The play behaviors can be scored for a child's independent play or play interaction with a caregiver.

RELIABILITY

In the original study using this assessment, Ungerer and Sigman (1981) reported that the mean correlation among two raters for the duration of play by category was .90, and the mean correlation for the diversity of play for each category was .85. The reliabilities of the individual scores ranged from .69 to greater than .80. These calculations excluded the scores for relational play stacking objects.

Kasari and colleagues (2006) calculated ICCs between two coders and found ICCs ranging from .94 to 1.00 with a mean of .97 for types of play and 1.00 for mastery (Play Level).

VALIDITY

Several studies have used the structured assessment to compare the play of children with autism to play in children who are developing typically. Ungerer and Sigman (1981) described how the range of play behaviors and the time spent in different forms of play differed for children with autism in comparison to typically developing children of comparable mental age. In addition, they found differences in the play of children with autism due to differences in language comprehension. Sigman and Ungerer (1984) examined whether there were differences in the play behaviors of children who were diagnosed with autism or mental retardation and children who were typically developing. They found that children with autism used less diverse functional play and less symbolic play both in spontaneous play and after receiving verbal cues. In a longitudinal study, Sigman and Ruskin (1999) assessed children with autism, Down syndrome, and developmental delays and typically developing children in early childhood and prior to adolescence, on average 8 years later. At the initial assessment, there were significant differences across groups in the number of different functional and symbolic play acts. There were significant positive correlations among play variables and language skills, with differences in correlations across groups for associations between nonverbal communication and play skills. Also, children with autism who demonstrated more functional and symbolic play acts in early childhood were more likely to initiate peer interactions and engage with peers in later childhood.

The Structured Play Assessment rating was used by Kasari and colleagues (2006) to assess the play of children with autism before and after an intervention and to help define goals for the treatment intervention. Children with autism who received a play intervention showed greater variability in the types of play they demonstrated and more sophisticated play. There was also evidence of generalization of play skills from individual to parent–child interaction contexts.

Test of Pretend Play

DESCRIPTION

The ToPP is a standardized version of the Warwick Symbolic Play Test described by Doswell, Lewis, Sylva, and Boucher (1994). The ToPP is a structured test that assesses symbolic play in typically developing children ages 1–6 and in children with developmental disabilities up to 8 years of age (Lewis, Boucher, Lupton, & Watson, 2000). The structured test has a Nonverbal Version and a Verbal Version. The Nonverbal Version is intended to be used with children up to 3 years of age or with older children who have difficulties comprehending the Verbal Version language. In the Nonverbal Version, symbolic play is modeled for children to copy and children's symbolic play is assessed. In addition, nonverbal means and short phrases are used to elicit original symbolic play in children. The Verbal Version is intended for use with children 3 years of age and older who have adequate language comprehension skills. In this version, symbolic play is modeled for children to copy and simple language is used to verbally instruct the child to demonstrate specific play actions and to elicit original symbolic play.

The ToPP has four sections (as described in Lewis, Boucher, et al., 2000). In Section I (self with everyday objects), the child is asked to make reference to an absent object (e.g., eat "food") when provided with everyday objects (e.g., bowl and spoon). In Section II there are four items that involve using a doll and one or more nonrepresentational materials (e.g., top, counter, box, stick, tub, cloth, reel, board, box, and cotton wool).

Children are asked to make one, two, three, or four substitutions of the nonrepresentational material for pretend objects. For the items with two or more pieces, children are asked to substitute the nonrepresentational materials for pretend objects in a related way. In Section III, the child is presented with a teddy bear and asked to complete four items: make the teddy bear do something to or with an imaginary object with no other play materials present, make the teddy bear feel something, make the teddy bear be something else, and make the teddy bear carry out a series of activities without supporting materials present. In Section IV, the child is not presented with any play materials, and in the context of four test items, he or she is asked to be something else, to do something to or with an imaginary object, to feel something, and to carry out a series of activities. Adaptations of specific items are described by O'Toole and Chiat (2006). Children's overall ToPP performance is assessed with a total score that can range from 0 to 34. Raw scores can be converted to age equivalents using the test manual (Lewis & Boucher, 1997).

RELIABILITY

Clift, Stagnitti, and DeMello (1998) assessed interrater reliability using Cohen's kappa statistic among two raters and found κ = .68. A very high level of interrater agreement (ICC = .96) was found by Lewis, Norgate, Collis, and Reynolds (2000). O'Toole and Chiat (2006) reported the percentage of interrater agreement as 94.0%.

VALIDITY

ToPP scores have been found to be positively related to age (Clift et al., 1998; Lewis, Boucher, et al., 2000; Lewis, Norgate, et al., 2000) and language scores (Clift et al., 1998; Lewis, Boucher, et al., 2000; Lewis, Norgate, et al., 2000; O'Toole & Chiat, 2006). Partial correlations between ToPP scores and language scores remained statistically significant with age partialed out (Clift et al., 1998; Lewis, Boucher, et al., 2000; Lewis, Norgate, et al., 2000; O'Toole & Chiat, 2006). O'Toole and Chiat (2006) found interesting changes in the patterns of correlations between ToPP and language scores in a cross-sectional sample of children with Down syndrome ages 2–7. Although there were strong correlations among ToPP scores and both expressive and receptive language scores among the youngest children (ages 2–3), in the oldest group (ages 6–7) only expressive language scores were significantly correlated with ToPP scores, which the authors suggest could exemplify a dissociation of language from other cognitive skills. Lewis, Boucher, and colleagues (2000) found that partialing out age reduced previously statistically significant correlations between the ToPP and children's performance on the Symbolic Play Test (Lowe & Costello, 1988) and the Leiter International Performance Test (Leiter, 1980). The authors argue that the ToPP is an assessment of both conceptual knowledge and symbolizing ability, which is why they found evidence of both convergent and discriminant validity in their results. O'Toole and Chiat (2006) found that the scores on the ToPP and a symbolic comprehension task were significantly correlated with each other in a sample of children with Down syndrome.

The ToPP score was found to correctly classify 75.9% of children in a study whose teachers identified them as developing normally or exhibiting developmental problems (Clift et al., 1998). In addition, the ToPP correctly identified 80% of children with problems in development.

Using a French adaptation of the ToPP, Vieillevoye and Nader-Grosbois (2008) did not find any significant differences in ToPP scores between children who were developing normally and children with intellectual disabilities. Across all participants, higher ToPP scores were associated with greater use of various self-regulatory strategies during dyadic play interactions, although there was variability in the pattern of correlations for the two groups. The ToPP scores, together with the ratings of the participants' dyadic pretend play, were used to create subgroups representing differences in play behavior.

With a sample of 18 children with visual impairment (ages 21–86 months), Lewis, Norgate, and colleagues (2000) found that symbolic play (as assessed with the ToPP) was not impaired in children with visual impairments after excluding children who met diagnostic criteria for autism. However, the children with visual impairments had significantly poorer performance than sighted children in the ToPP standardization sample on Section II of the ToPP, which assesses children's ability to substitute one, two, three, and four nonrepresentational materials for pretend objects as children play with a doll.

Three published studies describe the use of the ToPP to assess the effectiveness of interventions with children with autism. The ToPP was used to examine whether there were changes in play over time for children with autism who participated in either home-based early intensive behavioral interventions in a community setting or in autism-specific nursery provision (Magiati, Charman, & Howlin, 2007). The ToPP was only used at the second assessment time point, and age-equivalent scores were calculated. The study found variable improvements in children's play over time by examining changes in age-equivalent scores when the change was categorized as deterioration/minimal change, minor improvement, or moderate improvement.

In two single-case studies of children with autism who were receiving a virtual reality intervention to teach understanding of pretend play, the ToPP was administered prior to and after the intervention (Herrera et al., 2008). Four observers scored the ToPP, including two research team members and two individuals independent from the research team. Both participants demonstrated improvements in their ToPP scores. The authors describe challenges due to participants' familiarity with the ToPP when the postintervention assessment was completed.

A classroom-based study with five children with autism examined the impact of an intervention to teach children to use symbolic pretend play (Sherratt, 2002). The ToPP was administered before and after the intervention, and the four children who were assessed at both time points showed changes in their ToPP scores (i.e., age-equivalent scores increased).

Play Therapy Assessment Measures

Children's Play Therapy Instrument

DESCRIPTION

The CPTI is intended to be used to both aid in diagnosis and to measure change and outcome in child treatment (Kernberg, Chazan, & Normandin, 1998). Therapists/observers review videotaped play therapy sessions. The length of videotaped session segments ranged from 4–11 minutes in the study by Kernberg and colleagues (1998). Fifteen hours of training were provided to observers in the initial reliability study (Kernberg et al., 1998).

The CPTI includes assessment at three levels. In the first level, Segmentation, the therapist/observer classifies the child's activities into four categories: Non-Play (i.e., engagement in an activity other than play), Pre-Play (i.e., preparing for play), Play Activity, and Interruption (i.e., any abrupt cessation in a play activity). Activities assessed in the first level are summarized in a "play narrative" that describes in an integrated manner the distinctive features of the child's play. The second level, Dimensional Analysis, includes three types of analysis with subdomains. Descriptive Analysis includes a description of the category of play (e.g., gross motor activity, construction fantasy, and game play), a description of the script (i.e., the child's initiative, adult contributions, child's autonomy and reciprocity, and therapeutic alliance), and a description of where the play takes place (i.e., body, small toys, actual surroundings). Structural Analysis assesses affective components (i.e., type and range of affect), cognitive components (i.e., level of symbolic and role representation), dynamic components (i.e., play topic), and developmental components (i.e., comparisons with other children in terms of age, gender, and social and emotional development). Adaptive Analysis describes a child's coping and defensive strategies as well as a child's awareness of his or her engagement in play. The third level, Pattern of Child Activity Over Time, assesses changes in treatment (e.g., differences in the length and sequence of the different segments observed in the first level).

RELIABILITY

One published article describes the evidence for the reliability of the CPTI, which included a preliminary reliability study with the scale's authors and then a second study comparing the ratings of independent raters with consensus (Kernberg et al., 1998). The results from the second study are described in this paragraph. Agreement among raters for segmentation of children's play into four categories (i.e., Pre-Play, Non-Play, Play, and Interruption) using the weighted kappa coefficient was $\kappa = .72$. For the 25 CPTI subscales in the Dimensional Analysis level, the ICCs ranged from .52 to .89 with a mean ICC = .71, kappas ranged from .12 to 1.00, and percent agreement ranged from 44 to 100%. With regard to individual rater agreement with the consensus scores for the seven main subscales of the CPTI (i.e., Script Description; Affective, Cognitive, Dynamic, and Developmental Components; Adaptive Functions; and Awareness), the ICCs ranged from .61 to .96 with the mean of ICCs ranging from .81 to .84 for the individual raters.

VALIDITY

Two single-case studies using the CPTI are published in the literature. Chazan (2000) describes using the CPTI to assess progress and outcome in the treatment of a 2-year, 5-month-old child with a diagnosis of pervasive developmental disorder with autistic features. The CPTI was used to analyze two sessions, one at the beginning of treatment and one at the end of 7-month treatment. In the second session, the child demonstrated an increased amount of time in play and decreased amount of time in nonplay and preplay activities. There were also observed changes in the major CPTI scores including affect expression, cognition, language use, developmental ratings, and adaptive functioning. An abstract of an Italian journal article by Rossi, Strik Lievers, and Gelmi (2000) describes the use of the CPTI to assess treatment progress with a 4½-year-old child over the course of 3 months of treatment. The authors report that the scores obtained by the CPTI are consistent with clinical progress.

Play Therapy Observation Instrument

DESCRIPTION

The PTOI is used to assess the process and outcome of individual child psychotherapy (Howe & Silvern, 1981; Perry & Landreth, 1991; Rosen, Faust, & Burns, 1994). Therapists/observers review videotaped segments (10–12 minutes) of play therapy sessions and complete the PTOI ratings after viewing each segment. In the original article describing the measure, Howe and Silvern (1981) report that raters completed 20 hours of training using a manual and observations of live and videotaped play therapy sessions.

The PTOI includes 13 items; for each item, the rater selects one of several (i.e., three to six) responses that best represents the child's play behavior in the selected segment (items described in Perry & Landreth, 1991). Initially Howe and Silvern (1981) reported that the items were grouped into four subscales: Emotional Discomfort, Fantasy Play, Social Inadequacy, and Maladjustment. In subsequent work with the scale, Perry and Landreth (1991) describe omitting the Maladjustment scale due to the overlap of items included in other subscales. Rosen and colleagues (1994) combined the Social Inadequacy and Maladjustment subscales and named the subscale Quality of Interaction with the Therapist.

The Emotional Discomfort scale items describe the child's comments about worries and troublesome events, inappropriate aggression toward the therapist, conflicted play, the quality and intensity of the child's affect (i.e., mood), and play disruption. The Beneficial Fantasy Play items describe the number of different fantasy stories, the number of different fantasy roles enacted, amount of time the child spends in fantasy versus reality, and time spent concentrating on characters rather than things. The Social Inadequacy scale includes items describing body stiffness in gross and fine motor movements, incoherent or bizarre play content, and the child's inclusion/rejection of the therapist and his or her interventions. The Maladjustment scale includes all of the above listed items in addition to items assessing the frequency with which behavior is expressive of conflicts, frequency and degree of play disruption, frequency and degree of aggression directed at the therapist, and quality and intensity of the child's affect. In addition, there are six items from the original scale that are not included in the three domains (Howe & Silvern, 1981).

RELIABILITY

Howe and Silvern (1981) reported that for the 13 items selected for the PTOI, each of the items needed to demonstrate adequate interrater reliability with intraclass correlations of at least .48 and percentage agreement within 1 point of 80% or better across all of the video segments that were reviewed by two undergraduate raters. Thus for the 13 items, the ICC's for the individual items ranged from .48 to .80, and the percentage agreement within 1 point ranged from 82 to 100%. Rosen and colleagues (1994) reported that for the tapes that were included in analyses, the interrater reliability ICCs ranged from .73 to .95 and the percentage agreement for exact scores ranged from 89 to 100%.

To demonstrate internal consistency of the items for the four scales identified by Howe and Silvern (1981), Cronbach alphas and Scott's homogeneity ratios (HR) were reported: Emotional Discomfort, α = .83, HR = .46; Fantasy Play, α = .83, HR = .59; Social Inadequacy Scale, α = .74, HR = .54; and Maladjustment Scale, α = .81, HR = .44.

Test–retest reliability, or the stability of scores over two sessions, was relatively stable over a 1-week period: Fantasy Play, r = .75, Social Inadequacy, r = .79, Emotional Discomfort, r = .68, and Maladjustment, r = .83 (Howe & Silvern, 1981).

VALIDITY

Rosen et al. (1994) provided preliminary information about the validity of the PTOI. The PTOI was used to assess change for six children participating in either psychodynamic or child-centered play therapy. No significant differences on PTOI subscale scores were found for the two therapeutic approaches. There were statistically significant differences in scores for fantasy play and quality of interaction subscales when comparing the first and last sessions, which provides preliminary support for the PTOI's sensitivity to change in process and content of play therapy.

Trauma Play Scale

DESCRIPTION

The Trauma Play Scale is used to assess children's play in the context of play therapy to identify characteristic play behaviors of children who have been traumatized (Findling, Bratton, & Henson, 2006). Children's play therapy sessions are videotaped and then a select number of sessions are reviewed in 5-minute intervals. At the end of each interval, the rater provides ratings in five domains.

Five subscales comprise the Trauma Play Scale, and each item is rated on a 5-point Likert scale with behavioral anchors for each scale point. The Intense Play subscale assesses how intense, compulsive, and driven children's play is. The Repetitive Play subscale assesses the repetitive nature of children's play. The Play Disruptions subscale provides an assessment of the extent of disruption in children's play. The Avoidant Play Behavior subscale is intended to measure the child's level of avoidance of the therapist as an indicator of the child's ability to cope with interpersonal relationships. Finally, the Expression of Negative Affect subscale assesses the presence of negative affect or lack of joy during play. The authors expressed concern about the Repetitive Play subscale and omitted those scores from analyses.

Multiple options exist for summarizing the scores. First, session-level scores can be obtained for each subscale (e.g., Repetitive Play) by averaging across all 5-minute rating intervals during a session. Series-level scores represent the average of session-level scores. Another option includes averaging scores from all five subscales for each rating interval to result in an Average Trauma Play Scale score for each interval. Averages of the Average Trauma Play Scale score for intervals can be used to obtain session-level and series-level scores.

RELIABILITY

The authors computed percentage agreement and correlation coefficients for ratings at two time points: 97% agreement and mean $r = .86$ at the initial training session and 98% agreement and mean $r = .80$ for the midpoint training session. Intrarater reliability was assessed by obtaining two ratings for the same videotaped play therapy session with coefficients ranging from .85 to .98 (Findling et al., 2006).

VALIDITY

Children with a history of trauma had higher total scores on the Trauma Play Scale when the Repetitive Play scores were omitted than children with no known history of trauma (Findling et al., 2006). The authors suggest that the Repetitive Play subscale may not have been different between the two groups of children due to difficulties operationalizing and identifying the construct of repetition in play or because this characteristic may not be different for children with and without histories of trauma.

CLINICAL AND RESEARCH IMPLICATIONS

The present review provides a summary of the existing evidence-based measures of children's pretend play that hold promise for helping to bridge the divide between research and clinical work with children's play. It is encouraging to see that the five measures that were reviewed represent the perspectives of multiple disciplines with regard to play assessment. Specifically, the disciplines of psychology (i.e., APS, APS-P, Structured Play Assessment), occupational therapy (i.e., ChIPPA), and speech–language pathology (i.e., ToPP) are represented in their contributions to standardized pretend play assessment measures. Notably, there are consistencies across the measures in terms of the methods and play characteristics of interest. Thus the possibility of interdisciplinary collaboration is particularly promising as members from different disciplines could appreciate the commonalities and unique contributions of the various assessment measures.

Recommendations for using the results of assessments of children's play to guide treatment planning have already been discussed in the literature for the ChIPPA and the ToPP. As reported by Stagnitti and Unsworth (2004), the use of the ChIPPA has led to the development of a treatment program, Learn to Play, which is designed to develop the imaginative play skills of children ages 1–6 years with developmental delays, autistic spectrum disorders, language disorders, and other disabilities (Stagnitti, 1998). This would be consistent with the goals of occupational therapists who can work toward facilitating children's development of pretend play skills (Stagnitti & Unsworth, 2000). However, the Learn to Play intervention appears to be geared toward a wider audience including not only occupational therapists but also speech pathologists, special education teachers, preschool fieldwork officers, and early childhood workers (Stagnitti, 1998). Molineux (2004) provides a case example of how the use of the ChIPPA in the assessment of a 4-year-old boy who was diagnosed with autism spectrum disorder helped guide occupational therapy interventions, including using the Learn to Play program. Moreover, the ChIPPA was administered 1 year, 6 months later to help document change and progress.

Lewis, Boucher, and colleagues (2000) describe how an assessment like the ToPP may help guide clinicians working with children with communication difficulties. Specifically, they outline how comparing children's performance on tests of receptive and expressive language, nonverbal abilities, and functional and symbolic play can help identify causal factors (e.g., generalized learning impairment, specific learning impairment, or mild hearing loss) and subsequently guide treatment planning and interventions.

The relationships among intellectual and language abilities and pretend play skills appear to be particularly salient for many of the reviewed measures, in particular for younger children or children with developmental delays. This would suggest that the assessment measures of pretend play must be administered together with other indicators of children's cognitive and language functioning to better understand an individual child's areas of relative strengths and weaknesses. Moreover, additional evidence of whether the specific measures of pretend play are or are not related to cognitive or language abilities is indicated.

The use of numerous assessment measures with children representing various clinical populations provide support for the clinical utility of the measures. The ChIPPA, Structured Play Assessment, and ToPP have been used with children with developmental delays, autism, and/or Down syndrome, and the scores on the measures have discriminated among children with different diagnoses. Preliminary evidence of the use of the Structured Play Assessment and the ToPP in intervention studies suggests that the measures are sensitive to change and may be useful for larger scale prevention and intervention studies.

As evidenced in the review, there is relatively little evidence-based support for the three assessment measures that have been developed specifically to assess process and change in child play therapy. As outlined by Russ (2004), potential areas for future research in play therapy include focused research on play interventions, examination of mechanisms that may underlie change processes, and comparative studies of play interventions and other interventions. For example, the work of Rosen and colleagues (1994) examining changes in play using the PTOI for children receiving two different types of play interventions represents the type of work that needs to be represented in the empirical literature with larger sample sizes and rigorous methodology.

While the evidence base for the reviewed measures is promising, significant work is necessary to continue to expand the existing empirical support. In particular, larger sample sizes, use of the measures by different investigators or investigatory teams, and additional evidence of reliability and validity will continue to build the evidence base for existing measures. Examination of the reliability and validity of the play assessment measures with children from diverse populations is also recommended. While pretend play has been identified as universal in early childhood (see review by Lillard, 2007), there is much work to be done to better understand whether the reviewed measures are reliable and valid for children from different racial/ethnic groups, socioeconomic backgrounds, and cultures. Recent cross-cultural studies (e.g., Farver, Kim, & Lee-Shin, 2000; Goss, Morais, & Otta, 2007) have examined differences and similarities in children's pretend play and whether predictors of play were similar across different cultural groups. Interestingly, Farver and colleagues (2000) found that children's socially adaptive behavioral style, frequent positive social interaction with peers, and creativity were significantly associated with social pretend play for both Korean American and European American preschoolers. Additional research is needed to investigate whether the pretend play assessment measures are reliable and valid for children from diverse backgrounds.

Numerous sources that provide recommendations and guidelines for assessing preschool and elementary school-age children espouse assessment of play and/or play-based assessments (e.g., Brassard & Boehm, 2007; Ross, 2002). However, the authors' recommendations reflect the limited number of evidence-based assessment measures that are available to assess pretend play specifically. In addition, measures with none or limited information about their psychometric characteristics are included in the reviews. This underscores the need to continue conducting and disseminating research using the evidence-based measures of children's pretend play described in the present chapter.

REFERENCES

Athanasiou, M. S. (2007). Play-based approaches to preschool assessment. In B. Bracken & R. Nagle (Eds.), *Psychoeducational assessment of preschool children* (pp. 219–238). Mahwah, NJ: Erlbaum.

Brassard, M. R., & Boehm, A. E. (2007). *Preschool assessment: Principles and practices*. New York: Guilford Press.

Butcher, J. L., & Niec, L. N. (2005). Disruptive behaviors and creativity in childhood: The importance of affect regulation. *Creativity Research Journal, 17*(2–3), 181–193.

Chambless, D. L., & Ollendick, T. H. (2001). Empirically supported psychological interventions: Controversies and evidence. *Annual Review of Psychology, 52*, 685–716.

Chazan, S. E. (2000). Using the Children's Play Therapy Instrument (CPTI) to measure the development of play in simultaneous treatment: A case study. *Infant Mental Health Journal, 21*, 211–221.

Christiano, B. A., & Russ, S. W. (1996). Play as a predictor of coping and distress in children during an invasive dental procedure. *Journal of Clinical Child Psychology, 25*(2), 130–138.

Clift, S., Stagnitti, K., & DeMello, L. (1998). A validation study of the Test of Pretend Play using correlational and classificational analyses. *Child Language Teaching and Therapy, 14*, 199–209.

Cohen, L. L., LaGreca, A. M., Blount, R. L., Kazak, A. E., Holmbeck, G. N., & Lemanek, K. L. (2008). Introduction to special issue: Evidence-based assessment in pediatric psychology. *Journal of Pediatric Psychology, 33*(9), 911–915.

Cordiano, T. J. S., Russ, S. W., & Short, E. J. (2008). Development and validation of the Affect in Play Scale—Brief Rating Version (APS-BR). *Journal of Personality Assessment, 90*(1), 52–60.

Doswell, G., Lewis, V., Sylva, K., & Boucher, J. (1994). Validation data on the Warwick Symbolic Play Test. *European Journal of Disorders of Communication, 29*, 289–298.

Farver, J. A. M., Kim, Y. K., & Lee-Shin, Y. (2000). Within cultural differences: Examining individual differences in Korean American and European American preschoolers' social pretend play. *Journal of Cross-Cultural Psychology, 31*(5), 583–602.

Fein, G. G. (1981). Pretend play in childhood: An integrative review. *Child Development, 52*, 1095–1118.

Findling, J. H., Bratton, S. C., & Henson, R. K. (2006). Development of the Trauma Play Scale: An observation-based assessment of the impact of trauma on the play therapy behaviors of young children. *International Journal of Play Therapy, 15*(1), 7–36.

Gitlin-Weiner, K., Sandgrund, A., & Schaefer, C. (2000). Introduction. In K. Gitlin-Weiner, A. Sandgrund, & C. Schaefer (Eds.), *Play diagnosis and assessment* (2nd ed., pp. 1–12). New York: Wiley.

Goss, Y., Morais, M. L. S., & Otta, E. (2007). Pretend play of Brazilian children: A window into different cultural worlds. *Journal of Cross-Cultural Psychology, 38*(5), 539–558.

Haight, W. L., & Miller, P. J. (1993). *Pretending at home.* Albany: State University of New York Press.

Herrera, G., Alcantud, F., Jordan, R., Blanquer, A., Labajo, G., & De Pablo, C. (2008). Development of symbolic play through the use of virtual reality tools in children with autistic spectrum disorders. *Autism, 12*(2), 143–157.

Howe, P. A., & Silvern, L. E. (1981). Behavioral observation of children during play therapy: Preliminary development of a research instrument. *Journal of Personality Assessment, 45*(2), 168–182.

Jones, A., & Glenn, S. M. (1991). Gender differences in pretend play in a primary school group. *Early Child Development and Care, 72*, 61–67.

Kasari, C., Freeman, S., & Paparella, T. (2006). Joint attention and symbolic play in young children with autism: A randomized controlled intervention study. *Journal of Child Psychology and Psychiatry, 47*(6), 611–620.

Kaugars, A. S., & Russ, S. W. (2009). Assessing preschool children's pretend play: Preliminary validation of the Affect in Play Scale—Preschool Version. *Early Education and Development, 20*(5), 733–755.

Kernberg, P. F., Chazan, S. E., & Normandin, L. (1998). The Children's Play Therapy Instrument: Description, development, and reliability studies. *Journal of Psychotherapy Practice and Research, 7*, 196–207.

Leiter, R. G. (1980). *Leiter International Performance Scale.* Chicago: Stoelting.

Lewis, V., & Boucher, J. (1997). *The test of pretend play.* London: Harcourt Brace.

Lewis, V., Boucher, J., Lupton, L., & Watson, S. (2000). Relationships between symbolic play, functional play, verbal and non-verbal ability in young children. *International Journal of Language and Communication Disorders, 35*(1), 117–127.

Lewis, V., Norgate, S., Collis, G., & Reynolds, R. (2000). The consequences of visual impairment for children's symbolic and functional play. *British Journal of Developmental Psychology, 18*, 449–464.

Lillard, A. (2007). Pretend play in toddlers. In C. A. Brownell & C. B. Kopp

(Eds.), *Socioemotional development in the toddler years: Transitions and transformation* (pp. 149–176). New York: Guilford Press.

Linder, T. W. (1990). *Trandisciplinary play-based assessment: A functional approach to working with young children.* Baltimore: Brookes.

Lloyd, B., & Howe, N. (2003). Solitary play and convergent and divergent thinking skills in preschool children. *Early Childhood Research Quarterly, 18,* 22–41.

Lowe, M., & Costello, A. J. (1988). *Symbolic Play Test* (2nd ed.). Windsor, Ontario, Canada: NFER-Nelson.

Magiati, I., Charman, T., & Howlin, P. (2007). A two-year prospective follow-up study of community-based early intensive behavioural intervention and specialist nursery provision for children with autism spectrum disorders. *Journal of Child Psychology and Psychiatry, 48*(8), 803–812.

Mash, E. J., & Hunsley, J. (2005). Evidence-based assessment of child and adolescent disorders: Issues and challenges. *Journal of Clinical Child and Adolescent Psychology, 34*(3), 362–379.

Mazzeschi, C., Salcuni, S., Parolin, L., & Lis, A. (2004). Two measures of affect and emotion in Italian children aged 6 to 11 years. *Psychological Reports, 95,* 115–120.

Molineux, M. (2004). *Occupation for occupational therapists.* Malden, MA: Blackwell.

Niec, L. N., & Russ, S. W. (1996). Relationships among affect in play, interpersonal themes in fantasy, and children's interpersonal behavior. *Journal of Personality Assessment, 66*(3), 645–649.

Niec, L. N., & Russ, S. W. (2002). Children's internal representations, empathy and fantasy play: A validity study of the SCORS-Q. *Psychological Assessment, 14*(3), 331–338.

O'Toole, C., & Chiat, S. (2006). Symbolic functioning and language development in children with Down syndrome. *International Journal of Language and Communication Disorders, 41*(2), 155–171.

Parten, M. B. (1932). Social participation among preschool children. *Journal of Abnormal and Social Psychology, 27,* 243–269.

Pellegrini, A. D. (1991). *Applied child study: A developmental approach* (2nd ed.). Hillsdale, NJ: Erlbaum.

Pellegrini, A. D. (1995). *School recess and playground behavior: Educational and developmental roles.* Albany: State University of New York Press.

Pellegrini, A. D. (1998). Play and the assessment of young children. In O. N. Saracho & B. Spodek (Eds.), *Multiple perspectives on play in early childhood education* (pp. 220–239). Albany: State University of New York Press.

Perry, L., & Landreth, G. (1991). Diagnostic assessment of children's play therapy behavior. In C. E. Schafer, K. Gitlin, & A. Sandgrund (Eds.), *Play diagnosis and assessment* (pp. 643–662). New York: Wiley.

Piaget, J. (1962). *Play, dreams, and imitation in childhood.* New York: Norton.

Rosen, C., Faust, J., & Burns, W. J. (1994). The evaluation of process and outcome in individual child psychotherapy. *International Journal of Play Therapy, 3*(2), 33–43.

Ross, R. P. (2002). Best practices in the use of play for assessment and intervention with young children. In A. Thomas & J. Grimes (Eds.), *Best practices in school psychology IV* (Vol. 2, pp. 1263–1280). Washington, DC: National Association of School Psychologists.

Rossi, G., Strik Lievers, L., & Gelmi, V. (2000). The Children's Play Therapy Instrument: Longitudinal analysis of a clinical case. *Minerva Psichiatrica, 41*(3), 155–163.

Rubin, K. H., & Mills, R. S. L. (1988). The many faces of social isolation in childhood. *Journal of Consulting and Clinical Psychology, 56*(6), 916–924.

Rubin, K. H., Watson, K. S., & Jambor, T. W. (1978). Free-play behaviors in preschool and kindergarten children. *Child Development, 49*, 534–536.

Russ, S. W. (1993). *Affect and creativity: The role of affect and play in the creative process.* Hillsdale, NJ: Erlbaum.

Russ, S. W. (2004). *Play in child development and psychotherapy: Toward empirically supported practice.* Mahwah, NJ: Erlbaum.

Russ, S. W., & Grossman-McKee, A. (1990). Affective expression in children's fantasy play, primary process thinking on the Rorschach, and divergent thinking. *Journal of Personality Assessment, 54*, 756–771.

Russ, S. W., & Kaugars, A. S. (2000–2001). Emotion in children's play and creative problem solving. *Creativity Research Journal, 13*, 211–219.

Russ, S. W., Niec, L., & Kaugars, A. S. (2000). Play assessment of affect: The Affect in Play Scale. In K. Gitlin-Weiner, A. Sandgrund, & C. Schaefer (Eds.), *Play diagnosis and assessment* (2nd ed., pp. 722–749). New York: Wiley.

Russ, S. W., Robins, A. L., & Christiano, B. A. (1999). Pretend play: Longitudinal prediction of creativity and affect in fantasy in children. *Creativity Research Journal, 12*, 129–139.

Russ, S. W., & Schafer, E. D. (2006). Affect in fantasy play, emotion in memories, and divergent thinking. *Creativity Research Journal, 18*(3), 347–354.

Seja, A. L., & Russ, S. W. (1999). Children's fantasy play and emotional understanding. *Journal of Clinical Child Psychology, 28*(2), 269–277.

Sherratt, D. (2002). Developing pretend play in children with autism. *Autism, 6*(2), 169–179.

Sigman, M., & Ruskin, E. (1999). Continuity and change in the social competence of children with autism, Down syndrome, and developmental delays. *Monographs of the Society for Research in Child Development, 64*(1).

Sigman, M., & Ungerer, J. A. (1984). Cognitive and language skills in autistic, mentally retarded, and normal children. *Developmental Psychology, 20*(2), 293–302.

Singer, D. G., & Singer, J. L. (1990). *The house of make-believe: Children's play and the developing imagination.* Cambridge, MA: Harvard University Press.

Smilansky, S. (1968). *The effects of sociodramatic play on disadvantaged preschool children.* New York: Wiley.

Stagnitti, K. (1998). *Learn to play: A practical program to develop a child's imaginative play.* Melbourne, Victoria: Co-ordinates Australian Publications.

Stagnitti, K. (2007). *Manual of the Child-Initiated Pretend Play Assessment (ChIPPA).* Melbourne, Victoria: Co-ordinates Australian Publications.

Stagnitti, K., Rodger, S., & Clarke, J. (1997). Determining gender-neutral toys for assessment of preschool children's imaginative play. *Australian Occupational Therapy Journal, 44,* 119–131.

Stagnitti, K., & Unsworth, C. (2000). The importance of pretend play in child development: An occupational therapy perspective. *British Journal of Occupational Therapy, 63*(3), 121–127.

Stagnitti, K., & Unsworth, C. (2004). The test–retest reliability of the Child-Initiated Pretend Play Assessment. *American Journal of Occupational Therapy, 58,* 93–99.

Stagnitti, K., Unsworth, C., & Rodger, S. (2000). Development of an assessment to identify play behaviours that discriminate between the play of typical preschoolers and preschoolers with academic problems. *Canadian Journal of Occupational Therapy, 67*(5), 291–303.

Swindells, D., & Stagnitti, K. (2006). Pretend play and parents' view of social competence: The construct validity of the Child-Initiated Pretend Play Assessment. *Australian Occupational Therapy Journal, 53,* 314–324.

Ungerer, J. A., & Sigman, M. (1981). Symbolic play and language comprehension in autistic children. *Journal of the American Academy of Child Psychiatry, 20,* 318–337.

Vieillevoye, S., & Nader-Grosbois, N. (2008). Self-regulation during pretend play in children with intellectual disability and in normally developing children. *Research in Developmental Disabilities, 29,* 256–272.

4

Measuring Parent–Child Interactions through Play

Elizabeth Brestan-Knight and Christie A. Salamone

Although often relegated to recess or time with friends, play can be a useful clinical assessment tool. Several chapters in this volume outline how play is an important aspect of child cognitive and emotional development (Niec, Jent, & Baker, Chapter 2; Russ Fiorelli, & Spannagel, Chapter 1, this volume) and how play can be incorporated into the treatment of various childhood disorders (e.g., Briggs, Runyon, & Deblinger, Chapter 7; Kasari, Huynh, & Gulsrud, Chapter 8; Niec, Gering, & Abbernante, Chapter 6; Pincus, Chase, Chow, Weiner, & Pian, Chapter 9, this volume). The purpose of this chapter is to illustrate how, through the context of play, clinicians can observe the interactional style of parents and children and begin to develop hypotheses as to why the dyad has been referred for treatment—and how to best help the family with their presenting problems.

This chapter presents an applied aspect of play, that of assessing the functioning of parent–child dyads through a structured play-based assessment. We briefly cover the history of behavior observations, the theoretical underpinnings of behavior observations, relevant research, the pragmatics of using behavior observations as part of an evidence-based assessment battery for children with disruptive behavior, and future directions for research. Although there is a rich history of play-based assessment with other child populations, such as children with anxiety problems, autism, and attention-deficit/hyperactivity disorder (ADHD), the methods related to these additional child disorders are beyond the scope of the current chapter. Specifically, this chapter presents information related to a well-documented play-based measure of parent–child interactions, the Dyadic Parent–Child Interaction Coding System (Eyberg, Nelson, Duke, & Boggs, 2005).

A BRIEF HISTORY OF PLAY-BASED ASSESSMENT

There is a long tradition in psychology of using parent–child observations to inform treatment and research. The first documented use of behavior observations was made in Tiedemann's 1787 diary (Murchison & Langer, 1927) and several reviews of parent–child observation systems from the 1940s to the 1970s exist (Bell, 1964; Hoffman & Lippitt, 1960; Hughes & Haynes, 1978; Lytton, 1971; Wright, 1960). These early observational systems focused mainly on developmental constructs of child socialization (e.g., attachment, dependency, mood, temperament). It was not until the 1960s that clinically oriented researchers began to use observational methods to address child disruptive behavior (e.g., Hawkins, Peterson, Schweid, & Bijou, 1966; Schulman, Shoemaker, & Moelis, 1962; Wahler, Winkel, Peterson, & Morrison, 1965).

The early clinically oriented research studies varied in their research methodology and these coding systems focused broadly on child conduct problems and parenting skills. For example, Hawkins et al. (1966) provided observational data for a case study of a young boy with behavior problems (e.g., biting himself, hitting others) and Wahler et al. (1965) observed three parent–child dyads in an effort to determine which behaviors and skills could be addressed during treatment using behavior modification. Both the Hawkins et al. and the Wahler et al. studies were conducted with the main purpose of gathering information that could be used during individualized behavior modification programs; however, other researchers of the era were beginning to develop more formal coding systems. For example, Schulman et al. (1962) conducted a comprehensive observation of 41 parent–child dyads in which they coded parental behaviors related to domination, rejection, criticism, and hostility as well as child aggressive behavior. As research with child clinical populations increased, observational methods became more refined and formal coding systems were developed (e.g., Brumfield & Roberts, 1998; Forehand & McMahon, 1981; Patterson, 1982; Roberts & Powers, 1988; Robinson & Eyberg, 1981). The resultant play-based data helped to inform the development of family-based behavior therapy techniques that are still in use today.

Over the last two decades there has been an increase in the number of structured and unstructured play-based assessments available for use in the area of child disruptive behavior disorders. The wide spread availability of video-recording devices and remote sound systems assisted in the development of behavior observation techniques in that instructions can now be given to parents from a separate observation room and dyadic interactions can be recorded for later analysis. Although it is beyond the scope of the current chapter to provide an exhaustive description of all the existing play-based measures, we provide here a summary of several observational measures that can be used to inform clinical practice. The interested reader can find more information by reading an excellent review of 58 published studies in the area of parent–child direct observations by Roberts (2001). In his review, Roberts outlines the body of research for three main types of play-based measures: the Child's Game, the Parent's Game, and the Clean-Up situation. As we will discuss in more detail in a later section of this chapter, these three situations can be used during analog lab-based or home-based observations to determine the level of appropriate and inappropriate parent and child behavior displayed during an observation. Although play-based measures share the common feature of asking a parent and a child to play while the assessor records the interaction, several variables can differ depending on the specific measure employed, such as the location of the interaction (lab vs. home), the level of control that the parent is asked to exert over the situation (free play vs. the parent giving a predetermined set of commands), and the length of the observation (5 minutes vs. 45 minutes).

The Family Interaction Coding System (FICS; Patterson, 1982) is an observational system that can be used to assess child conduct problems in the home setting, as well as parent–child interactions. Because the FICS is a home-based measure several considerations need to be addressed, such as having all family members present during the observation, limiting the number of rooms they are allowed to use, not having the TV on, and restricting telephone usage and interaction with the observers. The FICS uses 29 categories that include both child behaviors and parental reactions to child behaviors, which are coded continuously and provide a sequential account of the interactions between the child and his or her parents. The child behavior codes can be summarized in a rate-per-minute variable that combines both the frequency and the duration of the behavior. A Total Aversive Behavior (TAB) score can also be calculated, which reports the sum of the number of aversive behaviors that occurred during the interaction observation.

Another play-based measure available is the Clinic Task Analog (Roberts & Powers, 1988), an adaptation of Forehand and McMahon's Parent's Game (1981), in which parents are observed while giving instructions to their children during a lab-based parent–child play interaction. The playroom is set up to include five sets of toys placed on the floor next to color-coded containers. The toys are not randomly scattered throughout the room but are instead placed together in one part of the room. During the 10-minute Clinic Task Analog, parents are instructed to use their own style of child management with their children. The procedure allows for the observation of how parents relay instructions to their children, the reinforcement contingencies parents provide to children following instructions, and whether children comply with the directives. Coding of parental verbalizations consists of two types of instructions: (1) alpha instructions, which include any parent verbalization that specifies a motor response to be obeyed (e.g., "Put the crayons in the box"), and (2) beta instructions, which include any parent verbalization that is considered too vague or uninterpretable, and therefore cannot be obeyed by the child during the analog observation (e.g., "Be careful"). Child compliance is coded within 5 seconds of the parent issuing a command, with a total compliance percentage resulting from the calculation of the number of child-compliant responses to all parent instructions divided by the total number of instructions issued and then multiplied by 100. An alpha or beta compliance percentage can also be calculated, in which the total number of child-complaint responses to parental alpha or beta instructions is divided by the total number of parental alpha or beta instructions given during the analog situation.

The Compliance Test (Beans & Roberts, 1981) is another observational system that can be used to assess child compliance to standardized parent commands during a parent–child structured play situation. The Compliance Test has been utilized for both research and clinical purposes to effectively evaluate parent training programs for children with disruptive behaviors (Brumfield & Roberts, 1998; Filcheck, Berry, & McNeil, 2004; Forehand & McMahon, 1981; Roberts, 1985; Roberts & Powers, 1988). The playroom is set up to include six types of toys, each with their accompanying toy containers, scattered randomly throughout the room. During the 10-minute Compliance Test, parents are asked to issue a total of 30 commands to their child. Parents give one command to their child accompanied by a gesture and wait 5 seconds for the child to comply. Commands can be given in either a one-step or two-step process in which the child is first instructed to pick up a toy (first step) and then asked to put it in its proper container (second step). Child compliance is indicted if the child performs the command within 5 seconds of the parent issuing the command. A total compliance percentage can be calculated, in which the number of compliant responses is divided by the total number of commands issued and then multiplied by 100. The Compliance Test is reported to be a less complicated measure to evaluate child compliance, as compared with other measures such as the Parent's Game and the Clinic Task Analog (Brumfield & Roberts, 1998; Filcheck et al., 2004; Roberts & Powers, 1988); however, the simplicity in method does yield less detailed information about the parent–child dyad in that aspects related to communication and warmth are not assessed.

As this section illustrates, play-based observations have been used for decades in the area of child development and clinical psychology. Behavior observations are widely encouraged for use in clinical practice (American Academy of Child and Adolescent Psychiatry [AACAP], 1997, 2007; McMahon & Frick, 2005; Roberts, 2001), but despite their long history they are often neglected during clinical assessment due to the time and training needed to successfully implement the procedure. Given the number of available measures, it can be daunting for the practitioner or clinical researcher to determine which measure to use. The authors suggest, however, that behavior observations of parent–child play interactions should be used as part of a comprehensive assessment battery for child disruptive behavior in light of several important developmental, theoretical, and diagnostic considerations.

CLINICALLY USEFUL ASPECTS
OF PLAY-BASED ASSESSMENT

A thorough assessment of child and family functioning is a key ingredient for all of the evidence-based treatments for child behavior problems (Eyberg, Nelson, & Boggs, 2008; McMahon & Frick, 2005). There are several benefits to using a play-based assessment of parent–child interactions during a comprehensive clinical assessment. Perhaps the most important reason to use behavioral observation methods is that they can provide valuable *multimethod, multiobserver information* about the dyad. Parents often do not have insight into the exact behavioral and cognitive issues relevant to their family situation. Thus, having a third party observe the dyad can provide valuable information about the nature of the difficulties experienced by the parents and child. In any evaluation with children and families, a multimethod approach in which a variety of techniques are used (e.g., interviews, parent report measures, self-report measures, teacher report measures, and behavioral observations) is often the best method for gathering information (LaGreca, 1990; McConaughy, 2005; Sattler & Hoge, 2006). With regard to contextual factors, children tend to vary their behavior across different environments, situations, and people (Kamphaus & Frick, 2002; McConaughy, 2005). Thus, taking into account and gathering additional information on the behavior of the child not only during an initial evaluation or therapeutic session, but also in other contexts (e.g., school, home) or across interactions with others (e.g., mother, father, siblings) can provide helpful clinical information (McConaughy, 2005; Sattler & Hoge, 2006).

Establishing rapport and developing a positive therapeutic relationship with the clinic-referred child can be a valuable aspect of family-based assessment as well (Boggs & Eyberg, 1990; Hughes & Baker, 1990; Kamphaus & Frick, 2002; Merrell, 2008; Sattler & Hoge, 2006). Children are typically not self-referred. Instead, they are brought for an evaluation by their parents; thus, they may be unmotivated or anxious about participating in the assessment process (Kamphaus & Frick, 2002). An observation of the parent–child interaction is often warranted because the child is unable to explain the complex problems that may exist in the parent–child relationship. Another benefit to using play-based assessments is that these observations can serve as an effective "icebreaker" activity for the assessment process. Specifically, a child may feel more at ease when initiating the evaluation process if he or she is first asked to play with toys rather than answer direct questions from an unfamiliar clinician. Starting an evaluation with a play-based assessment will likely serve to establish rapport and maintain cooperation from clinic-referred children (Stone & Lemanek, 1990).

Establishing rapport with the clinic-referred parent is another important assessment goal. By conducting a play-based assessment of the parent and child, the clinician can obtain useful information for case conceptualization and the development of a working alliance with the parent. For example, the clinician can use specific behavioral examples from the observation to demonstrate an understanding of the parent's core concerns during the assessment process (AACAP, 1997). Additionally, information from a play-based assessment can be used to develop a treatment plan that is appealing and motivating for the parent—because it is directly relevant to the referred dyad.

Another benefit of measuring parent–child interactions through play is that these observations can yield a high level of detailed information about the dyad. As outlined in the previous section, several coding systems are available that can provide very detailed information about the frequency of parental commands as well as the child's level of compliance in response to these directives. The high level of detail offered by behavioral observations of parent–child interactions can be extremely descriptive and helpful for both researchers and clinicians. However, behavior observations can also be very flexible in their application in that the clinician or researcher can determine which specific codes to use during a play interaction. In fact, behavior observations of play can provide a continuum of information from broad-level qualitative information (or molar-level information) to detailed analyses of behavior (or microlevel information). At the molar level, clinicians can conduct an observation and simply watch as the parent and child interact to obtain clinically relevant behavioral referents (e.g., How closely do the parent and child sit next to each other? What is the tone of the interaction?). At the microlevel, clinicians can use a specific coding scheme (such as the DPICS) to collect frequency counts for specific parent and child behaviors displayed during the observation.

We recommend that clinicians who use a play-based assessment of parent–child interactions observe both the molar and microlevels of the interaction. When conducting a play-based assessment of children with behavior problems, the broad molar-level aspects to consider are (1) the warmth provided by the parent, (2) the structure provided by the parent, and (3) the reciprocal behaviors of the child in response to the parent's warmth and structure. Other molar-level dimensions to consider include the parent's ability to regulate the child's emotional reactions during the observation, the tone of the interaction, the themes that emerge during play (e.g., aggressive, imaginative), and the child's verbal ability (AACAP, 1997).

There are also quite a few developmentally relevant aspects to consider at the molar level with regard to the child's developmental strengths and needs. Currently, a great deal of developmental research supports the crucial role of parent–child interactions in child cognitive and social development. For example, a parent's ability to modify the complexity of his or her speech patterns according to the developmental needs of the child is important for language development during the infant and toddler years (Cooper & Aslin, 1994; Liu, Kuhl, & Tsao, 2003). The strength of attachment and the attachment style demonstrated by parents and children in an unfamiliar clinic setting can provide important information about the emotional bond between parent and child (Blehar, Lieberman, & Ainsworth, 1977; Bowlby, 1988; Cassidy & Shaver, 1999; Thompson, Goodvin, & Meyer, 2006) as well as the reciprocal socialization patterns that have developed between the dyad (Ainsworth & Bowlby, 1991; Bell & Ainsworth, 1972).

Other developmental aspects to consider during a play-based observation can include the type of social modeling that a parent provides to his or her child (Thompson et al., 2006), the "goodness of fit" between the parent's perceptions of child behavior and the child's temperament (Thomas, Chess, & Birch, 1968), and whether the parent encourages child cognitive and social development by using "scaffolding" or joint problem solving during the context of play or educational tasks (Chaiklin, 2003; Vygotsky, 1926/1997). Behavioral observations can also be used to gather impressions of dyadic social reasoning abilities (McConaughy, 2005; Sattler & Hoge, 2006). In all, molar-level assessment of parent and child behavior during a play observation can provide clinicians with a unique opportunity to evaluate the developmentally sensitive—or developmentally insensitive—language, warmth, and structure displayed within the dyadic relationship.

At the microlevel, there are a variety of specific skills that are important for good parent–child communication. A play-based observation can provide the best structure to evaluate these factors at pretreatment. Clearly, the microlevel skills observed and recorded during a play-based assessment will vary depending on the specific measure used. The following examples that we provide fit well with the DPICS and the rationale for the specific skills described are closely aligned with Parent–Child Interaction Therapy (PCIT; Eyberg, 1988; Eyberg & Robinson, 1982; Hembree-Kigin & McNeil, 1995), a behavioral parent-training program described in more detail by Niec, Gering, and Abbenante (Chapter 6, this volume).

A microlevel analysis of parent behavior could address the combination of empathetic listening and responding to the child's ongoing activities (Hughes & Baker, 1990; McConaughy, 2005; Merrell, 2008; Sattler & Hoge, 2006). For example, a parent can show his or her interest in the child by reflecting a child's verbal responses or describing the child's behavior. Empathy can further be accomplished by using the child's language during the play interaction (Hughes & Baker, 1990; McConaughy, 2005). Boggs and Eyberg (1990) recommend the use of descriptive statements to further express empathy and provide feedback that the parent is listening to the child. In particular, *descriptive statements* are nonevaluative comments that describe the child and his or her ongoing activities and let the child know that the parent is paying attention. Descriptive statements can also enhance the child's attention and communication for the present topic being discussed. *Reflective statements*, which involve a repetition of what the child has said, can also be helpful in demonstrating interest, acceptance, empathy, and understanding of the child (Boggs & Eyberg, 1990; McConaughy, 2005; Sattler & Hoge, 2006). Additionally, parents can use "selective reflection" to specifically direct the child to continue to talk about certain topics (Kanfer, Eyberg, & Krahn, 1983). Finally, using *praise statements* can further increase rapport by indicating positive approval and regard toward the child and his or her activities (Boggs & Eyberg, 1990; Sattler & Hoge, 2006).

In contrast, using many questions, critical statements, and commands during interactions with children can be detrimental to rapport and relationship building (Sattler & Hoge, 2006). Sometimes questioning can be perceived by the child as exerting too much control over the interaction, particularly if the child is only given the option of forced-choice responses, in which the child is limited in what he or she can report.

Thus, parents can minimize the perception of control toward children by using few direct questions (Wood & Wood, 1983). Minimal commands should be used during a play interaction in which relationship building is the goal because these commands can be perceived by children as controlling and threatening. If commands are necessary to give, such as when parental discipline techniques are being utilized, they should be developmentally appropriate, specific instead of general to prevent child confusion or misunderstanding, and include only one request at a time because children may have difficulty remembering and complying to many commands given at once (Boggs & Eyberg, 1990). Critical statements should be avoided during play interactions with children because they show disapproval of the child and can produce negative child reactions such as anger, frustration, and decreased cooperation. In place of using criticism, parents can ignore the child's inappropriate behavior while continuing to praise good behavior, give commands for the child to engage in more appropriate behavior, or set specific rules for the child to follow during the play session (Boggs & Eyberg, 1990).

PLAY-BASED ASSESSMENT AND THE TREATMENT OF CHILD DISRUPTIVE DISORDERS

Play is an important developmental task for children, so it is probably no accident that some of the most effective treatments for child disruptive behavior disorders include a play therapy component (Eyberg et al., 2008). Family-based behavior therapies first emerged in the 1960s, partly in response to the emergence of social learning theory (Bandura, 1977) and the family coercion theory (Patterson, 1982; Patterson, Reid, & Dishion, 1992). These protocols are still used in clinical practice to treat families of children with behavior problems. Children with disruptive behavior problems often meet the diagnostic criteria for oppositional defiant disorder (ODD), which the *Diagnostic and Statistical Manual of Mental Disorders* (4th edition, text revision [DSM-IV-TR]; American Psychiatric Association, 2000) describes as a collection of externalizing behavior problems in which the child displays noncompliance, temper tantrums, and deliberate behaviors to annoy others. Children who meet the diagnostic criteria for ODD typically do not spontaneously improve without some psychological intervention that includes a behavioral component. Patterson (1982) has long suggested that a coercive family process in which parents and children reinforce each other through both negative and positive reinforcement serves to maintain the negative and coercive behavior patterns that are the hallmarks of ODD. The strength in using behavior therapy to treat families with a coercive process is that direct information is given to the parent that can enable him or her to alter the contingencies in place with his or her child. The ultimate goal of behavior therapy is to increase the positive behavior and experience that parents and children have together and decrease the negative and coercive behavior patterns.

ODD lends itself well to a play-based assessment because one of the best ways to provide feedback to parents regarding the coercive cycle is to observe them during a brief parent–child interaction, gather molar-level and microlevel data about the dyad, and then provide parents with quantitative data regarding the specific behaviors they engage in with their children. Unfortunately, many parents and children who are clinic-referred for the treatment of child disruptive behavior do not have the ability to play creatively and constructively with each other. Anecdotally, many parents report during intake assessments that they do not like to spend time with their child because the interactions are aversive; both the parent and the child are caught in a coercive cycle in which the parent and child primarily elicit negative behavior from each other (as described by Patterson, 1982). Consequently, the pretreatment observations of such parent–child dyads reveal that the parent does not know how to follow the child's lead in play, the child does not want to play with the parent, the parent does not provide developmentally appropriate direction to the child, and the child is noncompliant to parent directives. If "practice makes perfect," the benefit of using play therapy to treat children with disruptive behavior is that therapists can guide parents to provide the child with numerous opportunities to practice appropriate behaviors such as compliance, sharing toys, and playing in a respectful manner during treatment sessions and during practice at home.

A final benefit to using play-based assessment in the treatment of children with behavior problems is that the data yielded from behavior observations can provide an important measure of treatment outcome. The general purpose of behavioral parent training programs is to provide parents with the skills needed to increase their child's positive behaviors, decrease the child's negative behaviors, and manage the child during different situations. It is by conducting observations with play-based measures during parent-training sessions that clinicians are able to provide information regarding parents' progress toward treatment goals.

Several behavioral parent training models have used play and behavioral observations of parent–child interactions to address oppositional behavior or conduct problems in children (e.g., Eyberg & Robinson, 1982; Frick & McCoy, 2001; Hembree-Kigin & McNeil, 1995; Silverthorn, 2001; Webster-Stratton, 1994). One such behavioral parent training model is PCIT (Eyberg, 1988; Eyberg & Robinson, 1982; Hembree-Kigin & McNeil, 1995). Sheila Eyberg, originally developed PCIT to treat preschool-age children with ODD and their parents. Eyberg was heavily influenced by the social learning paradigm presented by Gerald Patterson (1982), the play therapy paradigm presented by Virginia Axline (1947, 1955), and a pilot program of working with families presented by Contance Hanf (1969). In essence, PCIT is a hybrid program that melds behavioral theory and relational play therapy within one treatment protocol. PCIT strives to increase warmth in parent–child relationships by using skills such as praise and reflections, as well as to teach more effective behavior management skills (e.g., reducing complex commands and parent criticisms, utilizing a specific time-out procedure). The essential components of PCIT are that the treatment includes two portions of therapy, Child Directed Interaction (similar to the Child's Game), and Parent-Directed Interaction (similar to the Parent's Game) and a therapist-lead, *in vivo* coaching component. PCIT allows parents to affect change within the parent–child interaction by practicing different contingencies following child verbal and motoric behavior, within the context of a play session. One compelling aspect of PCIT is that parents are coached by therapists to spend quality time with their child that is focused on the positive aspects of child behavior. Indeed, it is the focus on improving the warmth of the parent–child relationship that convinces many parents to try PCIT.

The Dyadic Parent–Child Interaction Coding System (DPICS; Eyberg et al., 2005; Robinson & Eyberg, 1981) is used before PCIT to assess pretreatment parent–child interactions, during PCIT to help guide treatment, and after PCIT to evaluate treatment outcome. Because behavioral parent training models such as PCIT strive to produce more positive parent–child relationships and provide parents with more effective discipline skills, the components of DPICS are well suited for the evaluation of these parent training programs.

THE DPICS

Although primarily known as a component of PCIT, the DPICS (Eyberg et al., 2005) is a well-researched, stand-alone behavioral coding system that has been widely used to assess and measure the quality of parent-child play interactions for over 25 years. The DPICS codes are particularly well suited for the assessment of children with ODD because the child codes that comprise the system directly relate to the diagnostic criteria for ODD. For example, a child who criticizes his or her parent or attempts to annoy his or her parent by using a sassy tone of voice is coded as using *Negative Talk* (NTA). Children who display disobedience and noncompliance to parent commands are coded as displaying *Noncompli-*

ance (NC). The frequent temper tantrums and attempts to gain parental attention that are hallmarks of ODD are coded as a *Yell* or *Whine* (YE and WH, respectively). Children who attempt to annoy parents by ignoring their questions may receive a code of *No Answer* (NA). Finally, if the child becomes physically aggressive toward the parent during the observation, this negative physical behavior can be coded as a *Physical Negative Touch* (NTO).

Conversely, the DPICS can also quantify the positive aspects of a parent–child interaction, such as when a parent or child praises the other or when they show physical warmth toward each other. Praise given by a parent or child toward each other, or toward a product/activity created by them, can be considered either specific (e.g., "I like your picture of the blue house"), which is coded as a *Labeled Praise* (LP), or more vague (e.g., "Nice job"), which is coded as an *Unlabeled Praise* (UP). If a parent or child shows any positive physical contact, such as by hugging or kissing one another, it would be coded as a *Physical Positive Touch* (PTO). Additionally, when a child listens to and complies with a parent command, the child would be coded as displaying *Compliance* (CO).

The DPICS procedure is the same for both clinic and research intake assessments. Parents and children are introduced to the DPICS observa-

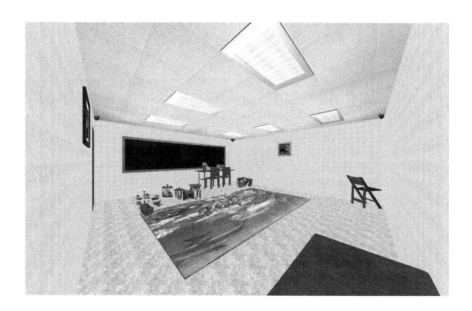

FIGURE 4.1. DPICS observation playroom set-up.

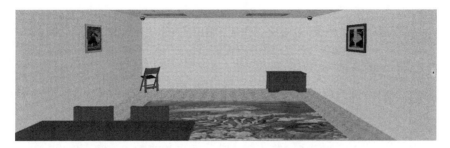

FIGURE 4.2. DPICS observation playroom view from the observation room one-way mirror from inside the observation room.

tion by explaining that they will have a chance to play together with toys for approximately 25 minutes. Parents are provided with a bug-in-the-ear device, if available, to wear during the observation by which the assessor can provide brief instructions to the parent from an observation room. If a bug-in-the-ear device is not available, the assessor can stay in the room during the observation (as far removed from the dyad as possible) and provide instructions to the parent as needed. Often children ask why the parent is wearing a bug-in-the-ear. It can be helpful to explain that the device is for the parent and not for the child.

During the DPICS observation, the parent–child dyad is observed from behind a one-way mirror while they play with a standard set of toys that encourage positive, interactive play. The observation room should have ample floor space for play, a table and two sturdy chairs within easy view of the one-way mirror, and toys with individual pieces scattered on the floor and table (see Figures 4.1 and 4.2). The same configuration of furniture and toys should be used for each assessment and the room should be cleared of any extraneous objects that children could throw or tear apart during the observation (e.g., decorative lamps, faux plants, tissue boxes, garbage containers).

Parent–child dyads are observed during three standard DPICS situations that differ in the degree of parental control required and the demands placed on the child for compliance. Directions for the first situation, *Child-Led Play*, are: "In this situation tell [child's name] that he/she may play with whatever he/she chooses. Let him/her choose any activity he/she wishes. You just follow his/her lead and play along with him/her." Directions for the second situation, *Parent-Led Play*, are: "That was fine. Please do not clean up the toys at this time. Now we'll switch to the second situation. Tell [child's name] that it is your turn to choose the game. You may choose any activity. Keep him/her playing with you according to your rules." Directions for third situation, *Clean Up*, are: "That was fine. Now please tell [child's name] that it is time to leave the playroom and the toys must be put away. Make sure you have him/her put the toys away by him/herself. Have him/her put all the toys in their containers and all the containers in the toy box."

The total time required for a comprehensive baseline or posttreatment observation of one parent–child dyad is approximately 25 minutes. For research purposes, the three situations are observed twice, usually on separate days, to increase the stability of the data. On each occasion, the *Child-Led Play* and the *Parent-Led Play* situations each take 10 minutes, with the first 5 minutes used as a warmup period to become familiar with the situation and the second 5 minutes used for actual coding of the parent–child interaction. Because cleaning up the toys may require only a few minutes with a compliant child, only 5 minutes of the *Clean-Up* situation is observed and coded. If there are multiple caregivers involved in the intake assessment, only one caretaker is observed with the child at a time. Although this may be somewhat artificial related to the typical family configuration at home, it is important to isolate the assessment of each parent–child or caretaker–child dyad to understand the interaction patterns for each dyad.

The toys used during the DPICS observation should encourage creativity and constructive play (e.g., building blocks, toy animals). Any toys that are aggressive (e.g., play guns), noisy, messy (e.g., finger paint), discourage conversation, require rules (e.g., board games), encourage pretend play (e.g., puppets), or are solitary activities (e.g., many video games) should not be included in the DPICS observation. All toys should be age-appropriate and a variety of toys (at least three different kinds) should be made available to the child in order to ensure child appeal, reduce child boredom, and provide enough options to last the duration of the observation. It is recommended that the same toys be used during the pre- and posttreatment observations and that these toys are not made available to children during treatment sessions. For a detailed list of specific appropriate and inappropriate toys used during the DPICS observations, the reader is referred to the DPICS manual (Eyberg et al., 2005).

The parent–child observations can additionally be video-recorded, pending parental consent. Video recording the DPICS observation can help clinicians or researchers to code the interaction, particularly when coding accuracy is a concern. In addition, clinicians can review video-recorded observations to help formulate treatment plans and document treatment progress. Finally, it may be helpful for parents to view the video-recorded interaction as it may help them to become more aware of their behavioral strengths and weaknesses. As part of treatment termination, parents may also benefit from viewing their pre- and posttreatment

DPICS assessment observations to demonstrate the progress they made in therapy.

In order to utilize the DPICS accurately during PCIT sessions, clinicians need to be adequately trained to understand and use the DPICS codes. Training involves a detailed process that includes reading the DPICS manual, taking quizzes on each section, coding practice transcripts or video recordings of parent–child interactions, and reaching a specific percent agreement while coding a preestablished criterion tape of a parent–child interaction. Individual or group training can be utilized in the process of becoming a reliable DPICS coder. Weekly supervision meetings with a more advanced DPICS coder to discuss coding questions are very important for the training process. For a more thorough description of the training process, the reader is again referred to the DPICS manual (Eyberg et al., 2005).

Another important distinction to make when using the DPICS is to understand the difference between the full DPICS manual (Eyberg et al., 2005) and the abridged (in-brief) version of the DPICS manual (Chase & Eyberg, 2006; both manuals are available at www.pcit.org). The full DPICS manual is primarily used for research purposes, particularly when a research project demands evaluation of sequential codes during a parent–child interaction. The research version involves the use of more parent and child codes than the abridged version and provides for a second-by-second analysis of video-recorded parent–child interactions. As such, the research version of the DPICS takes more time to learn and implement. Conversely, the abridged (in-brief) DPICS version is particularly useful for clinic purposes in that it yields frequency counts for preselected parent and child codes. The abridged version of the DPICS is typically used when coding 5-minute in-session PCIT observations that are conducted in real time. Thus, the abridged version of the DPICS is particularly well suited for evaluating whether a parent in treatment has met the specific criteria to move on to the next phase of PCIT. Deciding whether to use the research or abridged version of DPICS will likely depend on the specific goals of a parent–child observation (research or treatment).

RESEARCH SUPPORT

One criticism of behavior observation measures is the lack of psychometric data for most systems (Roberts, 2001). Unlike many coding systems used to evaluate parent–child play interactions, the DPICS has a great deal of research to support its use. The original DPICS standardization study included observations of young children (ages 2–6 years) with a diagnosis of ODD and their parents (Robinson & Eyberg, 1981). Studies using the second edition of the DPICS, or the DPICS-II, provided normative data for clinic-referred and comparison children between the ages of 3 and 6 years with both mothers (e.g., Bessmer, 1998; Bessmer & Eyberg, 1993) and fathers (Foote, 2000). More recently, the DPICS-II has been used for older children (ages 8–12 years) with a history of physical abuse (e.g., Chaffin et al., 2004; Deskins, 2005). Psychometric evidence, including correlations of categories, interobserver agreement, and test–retest reliability, has been adequate for both live and video-recorded parent–child interactions (e.g., Bessmer, 1998; Bessmer & Eyberg, 1993; Foote, 2000; Brinkmeyer, 2007; Chaffin et al., 2004; Deskins, 2005; Robinson & Eyberg, 1981). Similarly, validity evidence for the DPICS has also been adequately demonstrated with regard to discriminative validity, convergent validity, and treatment sensitivity (e.g., Bessmer, 1998; Bessmer & Eyberg, 1993; Foote, 2000; Chaffin et al., 2004; Deskins, 2005; Eyberg & Matarazzo, 1980; Eyberg & Robinson, 1982; Robinson & Eyberg, 1981; Schuhmann, Foote, Eyberg, Boggs, & Algina, 1998; Webster-Stratton, 1985; Webster-Stratton & Hammond, 1990). Specifically, the DPICS has been able to discriminate between nonreferred families and clinic-referred families (Bessmer, 1998; Foote, 2000). The DPICS has also been effectively linked to the use of other evaluation measures such as the Eyberg Child Behavior Inventory (ECBI; Eyberg & Pincus, 1999) and the Parenting Stress Index (PSI; Abidin, 1995). For a more comprehensive review of studies that have used the DPICS, as well as more detailed psychometric evidence for the coding system, see the newly revised DPICS manual (Eyberg et al., 2005).

When evaluating the wide range of research conducted on the DPICS, it is important to acknowledge the distinction between earlier versions of the DPICS (e.g., DPICS-II; Eyberg, Bessmer, Newcomb, Edwards, & Robinson, 1994) and the newly revised DPICS (Eyberg et al., 2005). PCIT researchers and clinicians are currently using the most recent version of the DPICS in lieu of the earlier versions of the coding system (i.e., DPICS-II) because the DPICS codes have been simplified and updated based on previous psychometric research studies. Current PCIT clinical procedures (e.g., mastery criteria, clinical coding sheets) have also been updated in light of the recent DPICS revision (Eyberg, 1999). As outlined by the American Psychological Association's ethical guidelines and code of conduct (2002), clinicians are strongly encouraged to utilize the most recent methods that are available when providing clinical services or designing research investigations. Thus, we encourage continued research and clinical utilization of the newly revised DPICS to better facilitate the most up-to-date empirical evidence and practice using this play-based measure.

CASE EXAMPLE

In this case example, we illustrate how a DPICS observation can be used to assist in the assessment and diagnosis of child disruptive behavior. Ms. Smith and her 6-year-old son, Sam, were recently self-referred to our PCIT clinic for the treatment of Sam's behavior problems. At intake, Ms. Smith reported that Sam had frequent temper tantrums and displayed a great deal of noncompliance at home. Ms. Smith also expressed the concern that her son may have ADHD due to his overactive behavior at school. Sam's teacher reported that he had difficulty staying seated in class and that he often interrupted others during conversations. As a recently divorced single mother, Ms. Smith expressed to us that she felt overwhelmed with her parenting duties and that she hoped therapy might help her to regain control of her son.

Ms. Smith completed several parent report measures and a DPICS observation as part of her intake assessment. On the ECBI (Eyberg & Pincus, 1999), Ms. Smith rated Sam as having an ECBI Intensity Score of 201 (*T* score = 80) and an ECBI Problem Score of 23 (*T* score = 71). On the Behavior Assessment System for Children, Second Edition Parent Rating Scales—Child (BASC-2 PRS-C; Reynolds & Kamphaus, 2004), Ms. Smith rated Sam as falling within the clinically significant range for the Aggression scale (99th percentile), Conduct Problems scale (93rd percentile), and Externalizing Problems scale (90th percentile). Sam's scores on the Depression scale (72nd percentile), Hyperactivity scale (69th percentile), and the Attention problem scales (70th percentile) were elevated and in the "at risk" range. On the PSI (Abidin, 1995), Ms. Smith reported

TABLE 4.1. Summary of Mother's Coded Behaviors during the Child-Led Play Situation

Positive codes	Total codes	Mastery
Neutral Talk (TA)	37	—
Behavior Description (BD)	0	10
Reflection (RF)	1	10
Labeled Praise (LP)	0	10
Unlabeled Praise (UP)	2	—
Avoid	Total codes	Mastery
Questions (QU)	21	0
Commands (CO)	14	0
Negative Talk (NTA)	0	0

a clinically significant level of child-related stress (99th percentile) and total stress (90th percentile). Taken together, our assessment data suggested that Ms. Smith was having significant difficulty managing Sam's behavior and that she perceived him to be a noncompliant, difficult, and aggressive child.

During the DPICS observation, Sam was observed to move quickly from one toy to another. He did not engage in cooperative play with Mrs. Smith and his vocalizations were often loud, whiny, and rude (e.g., "I want this," "You can't do this right"). At several points during the *Child-Led Play* situation, Sam was rough with the toys and he broke many crayons during the observation. Ms. Smith had difficulty engaging Sam's interest during the *Parent-Led Play* situation and he attempted to leave the room before the warmup period for the *Parent-Led Play* situation was complete. When told to clean up the toys during *Clean-Up*, Sam flatly refused to comply with his mother's commands. Instead, he continued to play with the toys until the DPICS observation concluded. Notably, Ms. Smith demonstrated more Questions (21) and Commands (14) than is recommended by the PCIT mastery criteria (0 Commands and Questions during the 5-minute *Child-Led Play* situation). She also had far fewer Labeled Praises (0), Behavior Descriptions (0), and Reflections (1) than is recommended by the PCIT mastery criteria (10 Labeled Praises, Reflections, and Behavior Descriptions during the 5-minute *Child-Led Play* situation; Eyberg, 1999). See Table 4.1 for a summary of the Abridged DPICS parent codes from this dyad's *Child-Led Play* observation.

Based on information from the intake interview, Ms. Smith's behavior report forms, a brief teacher interview, and the DPICS observation, Sam was diagnosed with ODD. We did not include a diagnosis of ADHD because his symptoms did not reach the clinically significant level and it was our hope that his overactive behavior would decrease once Ms. Smith learned to provide more consistent behavior management skills. The DPICS observation helped to clarify the treatment goals for the family in that several disruptive child behaviors and ineffective maternal behaviors were displayed during the clinic observation that helped to validate a diagnosis of ODD. Specifically, it appeared that Sam and his mother were caught in a negative interaction style consistent with Patterson's (1982) coercive family process. We predicted that Ms. Smith's frequent use of questions and ineffective commands during *Child-Led Play* and her lack of praises, reflections, and descriptions throughout the DPICS observation would be especially amenable to PCIT. After the dyad successfully completed 14 sessions of PCIT, Sam no longer met the diagnostic criteria for ODD, his school behavior problems resolved, and Ms. Smith reported decreased levels of parenting stress. Therapists first noted that Ms. Smith and Sam were making progress in therapy when Sam began to sing and include his mother in his play, which often included the theme of building toy houses with the use of construction equipment. Ms. Smith became far more positive and engaging in her play style with Sam. By the end of treatment both mother and son frequently hugged and complemented each other.

RECOMMENDATIONS FOR FUTURE RESEARCH

Research in the area of play-based assessment can be quite challenging with respect to the time, expertise, equipment, and access to populations of clinic-referred families needed to conduct this particular line of research. Despite the many challenges involved, there are numerous possibilities for interesting and clinically relevant future research projects. Just a few of the potential areas for research could include refining available coding systems, collecting more extensive psychometric data, developing new measures, developing new ways to train coders, testing the best methods for conducting play-based assessments, and expanding existing coding systems to new populations or applications. The overall theme of future research with the DPICS should be to increase the benefits of using this play-based behavioral observation method and to decrease, or minimize, the costs of using the system.

Roberts (2001) has noted that a particular weakness of the current parent–child observation literature is the lack of normative data for lab-based *Child-Led Play* observations. Roberts also points to a marked lack of psychometric evidence for the *Child-Led Play*, *Parent-Led Play*, and *Clean-Up* situations with respect to test–retest reliability, content validity, and clinical utility. With regard to the DPICS, several studies have addressed this very question (Bessmer, 1998; Foote, 2000; Deskins, 2005) and psychometric data are available to support the use of the DPICS-II. As previously mentioned, the DPICS has undergone several revisions and the current version has been available for several years. This newly revised version is widely used in clinical practice and efforts are currently underway to provide preliminary normative data for the abridged (more clinic-friendly) version of the DPICS among a sample of 8- to 12-year old children and their parents (Coursen, 2009).

Recently, researchers have studied the feasibility of using a DPICS-based observation and coding system with parents and children at home. The benefits of using direct behavioral observation coding systems to evaluate parent–child interactions, as well as the effectiveness of behavioral parent training programs, has recently led to the development of other systems that use DPICS as a foundation. For example, the Parent Instruction-Giving Game with Youngsters (PIGGY; Hupp, Reitman, Forde, Shriver, & Kelley, 2008) was developed to evaluate parent–child interactions using components of the DPICS and the Behavior Coding System (BCS; Forehand & McMahon, 1981). In capitalizing on the strengths of these previous coding systems, the PIGGY attempts to increase the structure and standardization used when coding parent–child interactions, while also making it easier to learn and administer in a variety of settings (e.g., home, clinic). Initial reliability and validity of the PIGGY are promising (Hupp et al., 2008) and suggest that this newly developed direct behavioral observation coding system can be useful when evaluating parent–child interactions, as well as the effectiveness of various behavioral parent treatment programs.

One relatively untapped area of research for play-based assessment includes an investigation into the best procedure for training observers. It is unclear whether certain prerequisites (such as a particular GPA) may help to ensure better coder accuracy among undergraduate research assistants. The level and type of graduate training (e.g., specific coursework) that is required for optimal coding by clinicians is also unknown. Although training manuals and workbooks are often involved in the training procedures for play-based assessment, the optimal length of training time and the length of time spent using different types of media (print, video, computer programs) are unclear—and likely not standard between clinics or research labs.

Other viable research alternatives could include variations in the DPICS method (e.g., analysis of optimal warmup period, the effects of using a bug-in-the-ear vs. providing instructions face to face, whether it is necessary to conduct two observations per assessment point or if one assessment is sufficient) that will help to make the assessment method even more clinically useful. Historically, there has been quite a bit of variation in whether a warmup period is used for play-based assessments as well as the number of observations conducted. Two preliminary DPICS studies (Dolbear et al., 2006; Zaremba, Carson, Salamone, & Knight, 2007) suggest that under certain parent-training conditions (such as group PCIT), the use of a warmup segment may have negatively influenced treatment outcome data in that parents used their "best" skills during the warmup period for *Child-Led Play* rather than during the typically coded second 5 minutes of *Child-Led Play*.

The DPICS also has great potential for use with alternative populations such as teachers. The Revised Edition of the School Observation Coding System (REDSOCS; Jacobs et al., 2000) is a modified version of the DPICS that has been used successfully in the classroom setting to evaluate teacher–child interactions (nonplay). The REDSOCS is an interval coding system for recording disruptive classroom behaviors of preschool- and elementary-age children in the classroom setting. Preliminary study supports both the reliability and the validity of the REDSOCS in the classroom setting (Filcheck et al., 2004; Jacobs et al., 2000).

Finally, the DPICS has even been used to evaluate adult–child play interactions beyond the traditional parent–child dyad that typically presents for clinical assessment and treatment. For example, Klinger (2007) recently used a modified version of the DPICS to evaluate parent–child interactions during popular cartoon episodes broadcast on cable television. This preliminary study resulted in the development of several new codes that were specific to cartoons (e.g., *Yell-Activity; Yell-Positive*) and research assistants were able to demonstrate adequate to good interrater reliability using kappa estimates of reliability.

CONCLUSION

Play-based measures can be a helpful adjunct to the assessment and treatment of parents and their children with disruptive behavior disorders. It is our hope that continued research in this important area will help to clarify the potential benefits of using play in the clinical setting—and that practitioners and researchers will continue to help parents and children improve their relationships, increase child compliance, and enhance child outcomes through play.

REFERENCES

Abidin, R. R. (1995). *Parenting Stress Index* (3rd ed.): *Professional manual.* Odessa, FL: Psychological Assessment Resources.

Ainsworth, M. D. S., & Bowlby, J. (1991). An ethological approach to personality development. *American Psychologist, 46,* 333–341.

American Academy of Child and Adolescent Psychiatry. (1997). Practice parameters for the psychiatric assessment of infants and toddlers (0–36 months). *Journal of the American Academy of Adolescent Psychiatry, 36*(10 Suppl.), 21S–36S.

American Academy of Child and Adolescent Psychiatry. (2007). Practice parameters for the assessment and treatment of children and adolescents with oppositional defiant disorder. *Journal of the American Academy of Adolescent Psychiatry, 46,* 126–141.

American Psychiatric Association. (2000). *Diagnostic and statistical manual of mental disorders* (4th ed., text rev.). Washington, DC: Author.

American Psychological Association (2002). *APA ethical principles of psychologists and code of conduct.* Washington, DC: Author.

Axline, V. M. (1947). *Play therapy: The inner dynamics of childhood.* Oxford, UK: Houghton Mifflin.

Axline, V. M. (1955). Play therapy procedures and results. *American Journal of Orthopsychiatry, 25,* 618–626.

Bandura, A. (1977). *Social learning theory.* Oxford, UK: Prentice-Hall.

Beans, A. W., & Roberts, M. W. (1981). The effect of time-out release contingencies on changes in child noncompliance. *Journal of Abnormal Child Psychology, 9,* 95–105.

Bell, R. Q. (1964). Structuring parent–child interaction situations for direct observation. *Child Development, 35,* 1009–1020.

Bell, S. M., & Ainsworth, M. D. (1972). Infant crying and maternal responsiveness. *Child Development, 43,* 1171–1190.

Bessmer, J. (1998). *The Dyadic Parent–Child Interaction Coding System II (DPICS II): Reliability and validity with mother–child dyads.* Unpublished doctoral dissertation, University of Florida, Gainesville, FL.

Bessmer, J. L., & Eyberg, S. M. (1993, November). *Dyadic Parent–Child Interaction Coding System-II (DPICS): Initial reliability and validity of the clinical version.* Paper presented at the Associations for the Advancement of Behavior Therapy Preconference on Social Learning and the Family, Atlanta, GA.

Blehar, M. C., Lieberman, A. F., & Ainsworth, M. D. S. (1977). Early face-to-face interaction and its relation to later infant–mother attachment. *Child Development, 48,* 182–194.

Boggs, S. R., & Eyberg, S. (1990). Interview techniques and establishing rapport. In A. M. LaGreca (Ed.), *Through the eyes of the child: Obtaining self-reports from children and adolescents* (pp. 85–108). Needham Heights, MA: Allyn & Bacon.

Bowlby, J. (1988). *A secure base: Parent–child attachment and healthy human development.* New York: Basic Books.

Brinkmeyer, M. Y. (2007). *Conduct disorder in young children: A comparison of clinical presentation and treatment outcome in preschoolers with conduct disorder versus oppositional defiant disorder.* Unpublished doctoral dissertation, University of Florida, Gainesville, FL.

Brumfield, B. D., & Roberts, M. W. (1998). A comparison of two measurements of child compliance with normal preschool children. *Journal of Clinical Child Psychology, 27*(1), 109–116.

Cassidy, J., & Shaver, P. R. (Eds.). (1999). *Handbook of attachment: Theory, research, and clinical applications.* New York: Guilford Press.

Chaffin, M., Silovsky, J. F., Funderburk, B., Valle, L. A., Brestan, E. V., Balachova, T., et al. (2004). Parent–child interaction therapy with physically abusive parents: Efficacy for reducing future abuse reports. *Journal of Consulting and Clinical Psychology, 72*(3), 500–510.

Chaiklin, S. (2003). The zone of proximal development in Vygotsky's analysis of learning and instruction. In A. Kozulin & B. Gindis (Eds.), *Vygotsky's educational theory in cultural context* (pp. 39–64). New York: Cambridge University Press.

Chase, R. M., & Eyberg, S. M. (2006). *Abridged manual for the Dyadic Parent–Child Interaction Coding System* (3rd ed.). Retrieved October 30, 2008, from *www.pcit.org.*

Cooper, R. P., & Aslin, R. N. (1994). Developmental difference in infant attention to the spectral properties of infant-directed speech. *Child Development, 65*, 1663–1677.

Coursen, L. (2009). *Frequencies of DPICS-III codes for a sample of 8 to 12 year olds.* Unpublished honor's thesis, Auburn University, Auburn, AL.

Deskins, M. M. (2005). *The Dyadic Parent–Child Interaction Coding System II: Reliability and validity with school-aged dyads.* Unpublished doctoral dissertation, Auburn University, Auburn, AL.

Dolbear, P., Flory, D., Luscomb, A., Painter, D., Stahl, K., White, E., et al. (2006, January). *An analysis of the utility of the warm-up segments of DPICS II observations.* Poster presented at the Sixth National Parent Child Interaction Therapy Conference, Gainesville, FL.

Eyberg, S. M. (1988). Behavioral assessment: Advancing methodology in pediatric psychology. *Journal of Pediatric Psychology, 10*(2), 123–139.

Eyberg, S. M. (1999). *Parent–child interaction therapy: Integrity checklists and session materials.* Unpublished treatment manual retrieved October 28, 2008, from *www.pcit.org.*

Eyberg, S. M., Bessmer, J., Newcomb, K., Edwards, D., & Robinson, E. A. (1994). *Dyadic Parent–Child Interaction Coding System–II (DPICS-II): Coder training manual* (2nd ed.). Unpublished manuscript, University of Florida, Gainesville, FL.

Eyberg, S. M., & Matarazzo, R. G. (1980). Training parents as therapists: A comparison between individual parent–child interaction training and parent group didactic training. *Journal of Clinical Psychology, 36*(2), 492–499.

Eyberg, S. M., Nelson, M. M., & Boggs, S. R. (2008). Evidence-based psychosocial treatment for children and adolescents with disruptive behavior. *Journal of Clinical Child and Adolescent Psychology, 37*(1), 215–237.

Eyberg, S. M., Nelson, M. M., Duke, M., & Boggs, S. R. (2005). *Manual for the Dyadic Parent–Child Interaction Coding System* (3rd ed.). Retrieved October 16, 2007, from *www.pcit.org.*

Eyberg, S. M., & Pincus, D. (1999). *Eyberg Child Behavior Inventory and Sutter–Eyberg Student Behavior Inventory: Professional manual.* Odessa, FL: Psychological Assessment Resources.

Eyberg, S. M., & Robinson, E. A. (1982). Parent–child interaction therapy: Effects on family functioning. *Journal of Clinical Child Psychology, 11*, 130–137.

Filcheck, H. A., Berry, T. A., & McNeil, C. B. (2004). Preliminary investigation examining the validity of the Compliance Test and a brief behavioral observation measure for identifying children with disruptive behavior. *Child Study Journal, 34*, 1–12.

Foote, R. (2000). *The Dyadic Parent–Child Interaction Coding System II (DPICS II): Reliability and validity with father–child dyads.* Unpublished doctoral dissertation, University of Florida, Gainesville, FL.

Forehand, R. L., & McMahon, R. J. (1981). *Helping the noncompliant child.* New York: Guilford Press.

Frick, P. J., & McCoy, M. G. (2001). Conduct disorder. In H. Orvaschel, J. Faust, & M. Hersen (Eds.), *Handbook of conceptualization and treatment of child psychopathology* (pp. 57–76). Oxford, UK: Pergamon.

Hanf, C. A. (1969, June). *A two-stage program for modifying maternal control-*

ling during mother–child (M–C) interaction. Paper presented at the meeting of the Western Psychological Association, Vancouver, Canada.

Hawkins, R. P., Peterson, R. F., Schweid, E., & Bijou, S. W. (1966). Behavior therapy in the home: Amelioration of problem parent–child relations with the parent in a therapeutic role. *Journal of Experimental Child Psychology, 4,* 99–107.

Hembree-Kigin, T. L., & McNeil, C. B. (1995). *Parent–child interaction therapy.* New York: Plenum Press.

Hoffman, L. W., & Lippitt, R. (1960). The measurement of family life variables. In P. H. Mussen (Ed.), *Handbook of research methods in child development* (pp. 945–1013). New York: Wiley.

Hughes, H. M., & Haynes, S. N. (1978). Structured laboratory observation in the behavioral assessment of parent–child interactions: A methodological critique. *Behavior Therapy, 9*(3), 428–447.

Hughes, J. N., & Baker, D. B. (1990). *The clinical child interview.* New York: Guilford Press.

Hupp, S. D. A., Reitman, D., Forde, D. A., Shriver, M. D., & Kelley, M. L. (2008). Advancing the assessment of parent–child interactions: Development of the parent-instruction-giving game with youngsters. *Behavior Therapy, 39,* 91–106.

Jacobs, J., Boggs, S. R., Eyberg, S. M., Edwards, D., Durning, P., Querido, J., et al. (2002). Psychometric properties and reference point data for the Revised Edition of the School Observation Coding System. *Behavior Therapy, 31,* 695–712.

Kamphaus, R. W., & Frick, P. J. (2002). *Clinical assessment of child and adolescent personality and behavior* (2nd ed.). Boston: Allyn & Bacon.

Kanfer, R., Eyberg, S. M., & Krahn, G. L. (1983). Interviewing strategies in child assessment. In C. E. Walker & M. C. Roberts (Eds.), *Handbook of clinical child psychology* (pp. 95–108). New York: Wiley.

Klinger, L. J. (2007). *What are your children watching?: A DPICS-II analysis of parent–child interactions in television cartoons.* Unpublished doctoral dissertation, Auburn University, Auburn, AL.

LaGreca, A. M. (1990). *Through the eyes of the child: Obtaining self-reports from children and adolescents.* Needham Heights, MA: Allyn & Bacon.

Liu, H., Kuhl, P. K., & Tsao, F. (2003). An association between mothers' speech clarity and infants' speech discrimination skills. *Developmental Science, 6,* F1–F10.

Lytton, H. (1971). Observational studies of parent–child interaction: A methodological review. *Child Development, 42,* 651–684.

McConaughy, S. H. (2005). *Clinical interviews for children and adolescents: Assessment to intervention.* New York: Guilford Press.

McMahon, R. J., & Frick, P. J. (2005). Evidence-based assessment of conduct problems in children and adolescents. *Journal of Clinical Child and Adolescent Psychology, 34,* 477–505.

Merrell, K. W. (2008). *Behavioral, social, and emotional assessment of children and adolescents* (3rd ed.). New York: Taylor & Francis.

Murchison, C., & Langer, S. (1927). Beobachtungen uber die entwicklung der seelenfahigkeiten bei kindern (translation of an original 1787 text by D. Tiedemann). *Pedagogical Seminary and Journal of Genetic Psychology, 34,* 205–230.

Patterson, G. R. (1982). *Coercive family process: A social learning approach.* Eugene, OR: Castalia.

Patterson, G. R., Reid, J. B., & Dishion, T. J. (1992). *Antisocial boys: A social interactional approach* (Vol. 4). Eugene, OR: Castalia.

Reynolds, C. R., & Kamphaus, R. W. (2004). *Behavior assessment system for children* (2nd ed.). Bloomington, MN: Pearson Assessments.

Roberts, M. W. (1985). Praising child compliance: Reinforcement of ritual? *Journal of Abnormal Psychology, 13*(4), 611–629.

Roberts, M. W. (2001). Clinic observations of structured parent–child interaction designed to evaluate externalizing disorders. *Psychological Assessment, 13,* 46–58.

Roberts, M. W., & Powers, S. W. (1988). The Compliance Test. *Behavioral Assessment, 10,* 375–398.

Robinson, E. A., & Eyberg, S. M. (1981). The Dyadic Parent–Child Interaction Coding System: Standardization and validation. *Journal of Consulting and Clinical Psychology, 49*(2), 245–250.

Sattler, J. M., & Hoge, R. D. (2006). *Assessment of children: Behavioral, social, and clinical foundations* (5th ed.). La Mesa, CA: Sattler.

Schuhmann, E. M., Foote, R. C., Eyberg, S. M., Boggs, S. R., & Algina, J. (1998). Efficacy of parent–child interaction therapy: Interim report of a randomized trial with short-term maintenance. *Journal of Clinical Child Psychology, 27*(1), 34–45.

Schulman, F. R., Shoemaker, D. J., & Moelis, I. (1962). Laboratory measurements of parental behavior. *Journal of Consulting Psychology, 26,* 109–114.

Silverthorn, P. (2001). Oppositional defiant disorder. In H. Orvaschel, J. Faust, & M. Hersen (Eds.), *Handbook of conceptualization and treatment of child psychopathology* (pp. 41–56). Oxford, UK: Pergamon.

Stone, W. L., & Lemanek, K. L. (1990). Developmental issues in children's self-reports. In A. M. LaGreca (Ed.), *Through the eyes of the child: Obtaining self-reports from children and adolescents* (pp. 18–56). Needham Heights, MA: Allyn & Bacon.

Thomas, A., Chess, S., & Birch, H. G. (1968). *Temperament and behavior disorders in children.* New York: New York University Press.

Thompson, R. A., Goodvin, R., & Meyer, S. (2006). Social development: Psychological understanding, self-understanding, and relationships. In J. L. Luby (Ed.), *Handbook of preschool mental health: Development, disorders, and treatment* (pp. 3–22). New York: Guilford Press.

Vygotsky, L. S. (1997). *Educational psychology.* Delray Beach, FL: St. Lucie Press. (Original text published 1926)

Wahler, R. G., Winkel, G. H., Peterson, R. F., & Morrison, D. C. (1965). Mothers as behavior therapists for their own children. *Behaviour Research and Therapy, 3,* 113–124.

Webster-Stratton, C. (1985). Mother perceptions and mother–child interactions:

Comparison of a clinic-referred and a nonclinic group. *Journal of Clinical Child Psychology, 14*(4), 334–339.

Webster-Stratton, C. (1994). Advancing videotape parent training: A comparison study. *Journal of Consulting and Clinical Psychology, 62,* 583–593.

Webster-Stratton, C., & Hammond, M. (1990). Predictors of treatment outcome in parent training for families with conduct problem children. *Behavior Therapy, 21*(3), 319–337.

Wood, H., & Wood, D. (1983). Questioning the preschool child. *Educational Review, 35,* 149–162.

Wright, H. F. (1960). Observational child study. In P. H. Mussen (Ed.), *Handbook of research methods in child development* (pp. 71–139). New York: Wiley.

Zaremba, A., Carson, A., Salamone, C., & Knight, E. B. (2007, September). *Are DPICS warm-up segments needed?: A replication.* Poster presented at the Seventh National Parent Child Interaction Therapy Conference, Oklahoma City, OK.

5

Play, Playfulness, and Creativity in Therapeutic Assessment with Children

Deborah J. Tharinger, Gina B. Christopher, and May Matson

Imagine you are planning on assessing a 9-year-old boy for whom there are serious concerns about his anger and oppositional defiant behavior (especially with his mother), evidence of self-harming behavior, and disengagement by his father pending a divorce. To lend understanding to the puzzle that the boy presents, you proceed to ask the mother and the boy to construct specific questions for the assessment, request that the mother observe and comment on all the testing sessions, invite the boy to engage in free play at the end of most of the testing sessions, and develop an idiographic sentence completion for the boy with items specific to the unfolding concerns. You also coach the boy and mother to engage in drawing, sculpting, and cartooning their family interactions together. And finally, in addition to writing a user-friendly feedback letter for the mother, you write an original fable as a major vehicle of feedback for the boy. If this description sounds unfamiliar or unusual to you, welcome to the practice of Therapeutic Assessment with children (TA-C).

Therapeutic Assessment (TA) is an innovative hybrid of psychological assessment and intervention methods that is receiving much attention. Developed by Finn and colleagues (Finn, 1996, 2007; Finn & Tonsager, 1997), TA is a collaborative endeavor between the assessor and the client, is guided by clients' questions of interest, and uses psychological assessment as the centerpiece of a potent, short-term intervention. TA is highly related to the work of Fischer (1994), Handler (2007), and Purves (2002), all of whom developed their own models of collaborative assessment independently, but who subsequently influenced and were influenced by TA. Although guided by the same underlying principles, the TA model and resultant clinical protocols have been differentially adapted to use with adults, couples, adolescents, and children. TA-C seeks to make psychological assessment a positive and beneficial experience for both parents and children through collaboratively involving them, and sometimes other relevant family members, in the assessment process. TA-C is guided by the questions constructed by the parents and the child, and the discussion of the findings with the parents is organized around their assessment questions. TA-C is somewhat distinct from the TA protocol used with adolescents. The primary difference is the greater level of parental involvement through direct observation when testing children, in contrast to greater privacy offered to adolescents. For example, unlike children, adolescents are given the opportunity to ask private assessment questions that are not shared by their parents, and are invited to participate in an intervention at which their parents are not present. This differentiation is similar to developmental differences inherent in providing psychotherapy to children versus adolescents.

TA-C has been practiced for many years and has been described by Finn (2007), Tharinger, Finn, Wilkinson, and Schaber (2007). The primary goal of TA-C is to provide a family systems intervention in the context of a collaborative child assessment. The collaboration is primarily with the parents, and therapeutic alliances are established between the assessor and the child *and* the assessor and the parents. The aims of TA-C are (1) to help parents develop a new story about their child's challenges, and as a result, become more empathic to their child; and (2) to guide parents in shifting their attitudes toward and interactions with their child in ways that will foster positive child and family development. Competences in *both* assessment and intervention are required of the assessor when applying the TA model in general, and additional specific skills are needed when working with different populations (e.g., with children, with adolescents, with adults). In TA-C, the assessor strives to provide the child with multiple opportunities and modalities to express his or her thoughts, feelings, and behaviors, and uses innovative methods to assist the parents in coming to new understandings of their child. The assessor also uses creative methods to communicate the assessment findings in a way that is meaningful and memorable to the child and the parents.

Assessment tools in TA-C include interviews with parents and children (during which assessment questions are co-constructed), selected nomothetic and idiographic testing instruments, and individualized extended inquiry methods tied to children's test responses (described in a later section). In addition, the assessor adopts a systematic and sensitive way to analyze and integrate the information gathered in relation to the assessment questions, and strives to present these findings in a collaborative manner during a discussion session with parents (Tharinger, Finn, Hersh, et al., 2008). Written feedback to parents is provided in the form of consumer-friendly letters that are organized around their assessment questions (formal reports are also made available if requested), and feedback to children is given using creative methods such as individualized fables (Tharinger, Finn, Wilkinson, et al., 2008).

Intervention tools in TA-C include working collaboratively with the parents throughout, including in the interview where questions are co-constructed and explored, using the "behind the mirror" method (described below), and during check-ins and check-outs. The assessor also works collaboratively with the child whenever possible and provides opportunities for the child to engage in play during testing sessions. The assessor also utilizes numerous *playful methods* to enhance his or her alliance with the child and the child's parents, as well as to promote the parent–child relationship. In addition, the assessor uses a variety of creative therapy/intervention techniques to guide family intervention sessions (described in a later section). Basically, the assessor in TA-C needs to be open and skilled in the use of play and play therapy techniques with children, be capable and at ease being playful with children and parents, and be creative in his or her choice of assessment methods, intervention methods, and ways of communicating findings. Thus, assessors need to be able to access playful, creative, spontaneous, and humorous approaches in response to what are often very serious concerns.

Recent publications provide an in-depth description of specific methods used in TA-C, including designing and implementing family intervention sessions (Tharinger, Finn, Austin, et al., 2008), preparing for and delivering parent feedback (Tharinger, Finn, Hersh, et al., 2008), and constructing and providing child feedback using individualized fables (Tharinger, Finn, Wilkinson, et al., 2008). In addition to these guides for practicing TA-C, research findings are accumulating that testify to its benefits and efficacy. Numerous clinical case studies have been published (Fischer, 1994; Hamilton et al., 2009; Handler, 2007; Mutchnik & Handler, 2002; Purves, 2002; Smith & Handler, in press; Tharinger et al., 2007). In these case studies, parents report gaining a better understanding of their children's problems, feeling more effective in their parenting, and becoming more motivated to pursue appropriate services following a TA-C. Parents also indicate that their children show decreased behavioral problems, improved mood, and better social functioning. A recent study reported on the efficacy of TA-C across a group of referred children (Tharinger, Finn, Gentry, et al., 2009). In that study, high treatment acceptability was found, as well as significantly decreased child symptomatology and enhanced family functioning. In addition, parents in the study demonstrated a significant increase in positive emotion and a significant decrease in negative emotion pertaining to their children's challenges and future. These findings, although limited due to the use of a noncomparison design and small sample size, support assertions from published single-case studies that TA is likely an efficacious child and family intervention.

Although research supports the likely efficacy of a comprehensive model of TA-C, it is not possible at this point to weigh the exact impact of the use of play, playfulness, and creative methods with children in the overall effectiveness of TA-C. These methods and qualities of the assessor permeate the assessment and intervention techniques used throughout TA-C, and as such their influence cannot be separated out. Nonetheless, there is no doubt that these methods and qualities allow for the assessor to enter a child's world, enhance alliance and engagement between assessors and children and children and parents, and contribute to children's understanding of themselves in a way that otherwise would not be possible. These methods also have the potential to impact parents in positive ways, such as reminding them of the power of play with their children and helping them experience how serious problems can be approached through playful means. Thus, play and playful methods are part of the fabric of TA-C, and we have every reason to believe that this fabric is necessary (but not sufficient) for the efficacy that is being found for TA-C in research efforts.

In this chapter we describe how we use play, playfulness, and other creative/expressive methods in TA-C. Following a brief overview of the importance of play in children's development, we provide a sketch of the ways play has been used in interventions with children, specifically play therapy, filial therapy, and family therapy, as these have influenced our use of play in TA-C. We then discuss how play has been used traditionally in psychological assessments with children, which sets the stage for our description of how we use it differently. Following, we detail the TA clinical protocol used with children, emphasizing how play, playfulness, and creative methods can be used in the different sessions. We acknowledge the work of Handler (2007), who perhaps more than anyone has brought play and playfulness to collaborative and therapeutic assessment with children. Throughout the discussion of the protocol, we embed a case study, illustrating the case of a 9-year-old boy and his mother. This case was drawn from the Therapeutic Assessment Project (TAP) at the University of Texas at Austin, which is codirected by Drs. Tharinger and Finn and described elsewhere (Tharinger, Finn, Gentry, et al., in press; Tharinger et al., 2007). We close by challenging assessment professionals to adopt the model and methods of TA and the modality of play in their assessments of children. In particular, we urge assessors to become comfortable assessing children through play, to model and encourage play and playfulness with the children they assess and their parents, and to be playful and creative themselves.

PLAY AND CHILDREN'S DEVELOPMENT

Play has many forms and dimensions. In its purest form, it belongs to young children who, without strictures or constraints, engage in imaginative pretend play where anything goes and they are in the moment; the form and fluidity of this type of play is ever changing and rule-free. Fantasy prevails and bounds are limitless. Ideas are tried out and problems are solved. Power is felt and mastery accomplished (Erikson, 1950).

Play is ubiquitous in early childhood. Young children are constantly at play. Play can be conceptualized as an activity that is not a means to an end but an end itself (i.e., play for the sake of play), is intrinsically motivating to the individual, and is associated with positive emotions (Lidz, 2002). Pure play reflects nonliterality, positive affect, intrinsic motivation, and flexibility (Russ, 2004). Play has long been recognized as one of the major activities of childhood, and is thought to be essential to healthy development. Preschool and early elementary schoolteachers, attuned parents, and child and educational psychologists are well informed about the purposes of play in the education, development, and socialization of children. Young children spend a great deal of time engaged in play, and begin to learn and explore their worlds through play. As they play, children develop motor, language, cognitive, social, and emotional abilities and skills (Ginsburg, Committee on Communications, & Committee on Psychosocial Aspects of Child and Family Health, 2007). Play is a favored and comfortable activity for young children and, at its most basic, is free: free of imposed meaning, time, and structure.

Play in another form, usually appearing later developmentally, is more structured and time-limited, and often meaning is made of it or imposed on it by others, such as parents and teachers. Perhaps this is more mature play, or perhaps it is compromised play, that is, play adapted to a structured, time-ruled world. Either way it seems that, even as children's language abilities become better developed and they are increasingly able to communicate through means other than play, play continues to have a major role in their lives. School-age children continue to spend large amounts of time engaged in play activities, either by themselves or with friends (Timberlake & Cutler, 2001). Older children often need to grab at the time allotted to play—after they have finished eating and chores, during 20 minutes at recess, or when school tasks are completed in the classroom. Most healthy children seem to have the ability to shift into play mode, and then shift out of it again when others, typically adults, structure them into something else. And finally, for most children, play is exhilarating, expressive, releasing, and fun.

Play as a Modality for Therapy with Children

Play can also be a modality that allows for revealing and healing when used for therapeutic purposes by trained professionals. Although impacted by time constraints and structure, child clinical, pediatric, and school psychologists (as well as psychotherapists and clinical social workers) have long utilized play as a modality to treat children who are struggling with fears, anxiety, depression, inattention, and behavioral and emotional dysregulation. These symptoms and dysfunctions are often responses to a combination of overwhelming stressors, including loss, change, illness, school failure, poor parenting, abuse/maltreatment, and a challenging temperament. As discussed, play is a natural form of expression for children; they can express their thoughts and feelings, and be accepted in a safe environment. In play therapy, the child uses play to communicate thoughts, feelings and behaviors to the therapist. The therapist works to create a safe environment, give permission for play to occur, actively facilitate the child's play, and work with the play content and affect the child provides. As the child in play therapy feels more comfortable and secure, typically more of his or her story and affect is expressed through the play. Landreth (2002), a long-time proponent of nondirective play therapy with children, notes that using the play modality in therapy allows children to be comfortable, to feel more in control and secure, to be physically active, and to express themselves more completely than they would be able to do just verbally. And although the use of play in treatment is often associated with young children, that is, children under the age of 5 or 6, who often cannot provide information in more direct ways, play can also be a useful modality for children up to age 11 or 12 and even older, depending on the emotional maturity of the child. There are also other playful, creative expressive methods that can be used with older children, such as crafts, games, psychodrama, art, music, and the sand tray.

Play is also the featured modality in filial therapy (Bratton, Ray, &

Moffit, 1998), where the therapist works with the parent and the child together, guiding the parent to play with his or her child. This model is aimed at fostering healthy parent–child relationships through training and supervising parents in the basic methodology of child-centered play therapy. Filial therapy utilizes play as a fun and developmentally appropriate means to foster interactions between parent and child. Through creating an accepting and nonjudgmental environment where children feel safe enough to express and explore their thoughts and feelings, parents learn to convey acceptance, empathy, and encouragement with their children, and to master skills of effective limit setting. The goal is to improve family interactions through increased feelings of familial affection, warmth, and trust, as well as to reduce symptoms, enhance coping strategies, increase positive feelings of self-worth and confidence, and provide a more positive perception of parents for the children.

Play has also been incorporated into family therapy. In family therapy, therapists note that play is the "language" of the child and is the most appropriate way to include him or her in the therapeutic process (Armstrong & Simpson, 2002; Bratton et al., 1998; Busby & Lufkin, 1992; Eaker, 1986; Early, 1994; Sweeney & Rocha, 2000). Family therapists have come to recognize that play is a universal language that *all* family members can speak (Busby & Lufkin, 1992). Play allows the parents to enter into the world of the child (Dermer, Olund, & Sori, 2006), and to create a lighter and playful modality from which to work on problems. Although some parents may have lost touch with the language of play due to stress and being overwhelmed, most find play accessible when it is invited and modeled by the therapist. Play is often included in family therapy as a way for families to address painful issues indirectly (Bratton et al., 1998; Busby & Lufkin, 1992; Early, 1994; Freeman, Epston, & Lobovits, 1997; Gil & Sobol, 2000), and as a way for families to build relationships and increase secure attachment (Bratton et al., 1998; Busby & Lufkin, 1992; Dermer et al., 2006; Earley, 1994). Engaging families in play can also promote the goals of therapy by giving families an opportunity to practice new skills, while allowing practitioners to observe family interactions, thereby emphasizing a systemic perspective (Busby & Lufkin, 1992; Dermer et al., 2006; Gil & Sobol, 2000; Sweeney & Rocha, 2000). We have been very influenced by this perspective in TA-C, and as will be described later, our family intervention sessions specifically reflect these goals.

Play as a Modality for Assessment of Children

Play is very commonly used in the assessment of very young children. However, despite play's continued prevalence in children's lives after preschool and the common use of play in therapy with older children, it is rarely included in individual assessments of latency-age children. Play assessment has typically been viewed as an alternative means of attaining information from children who would otherwise be "untestable" due to age, disability, or other factors (Gitlin-Weiner, Sandgrund, & Schaefer, 2000), rather than as a preferred, optimal, or enhancing methodology. Despite the limited literature on the use of play in the assessment of latency-age children, systems have been developed using play interactions between a parent and child to assess the parent–child relationship (Brooke, 2004), or using peer interactions to assess social-emotional adjustment (Welsh, Bierman, & Pope, 2000). Similarly, play is often used in family assessments conducted prior to family therapy (Deacon & Piercy, 2001), for example, by having families engage in art activities or psychodrama together. As will be seen in the forthcoming description, in TA-C play is infused throughout the assessment process, particularly in the testing sessions, and often in the family intervention session.

TA-C PROTOCOL AND CASE ILLUSTRATION OF PLAY, PLAYFULNESS, AND CREATIVE EXPRESSION AT WORK

In TA-C, we have been influenced and informed by the use of play, playfulness, and creative methods in play therapy, filial therapy, and family therapy. We also have been guided by the work of Handler (2007), who has stated, "To successfully employ therapeutic assessment approaches to assessment, the clinician must set aside some of his or her traditional training and instead focus on being more playful and imaginative.... Success in therapeutic assessment with children is facilitated if the assessor allows himself/herself to engage playfully in the assessment process with children" (p. 58). Handler describes some of his favorite playful approaches with children, including the squiggle game (Winnicott, 1953), the fantasy animal game, projective tests, and the use of photography. As will be apparent, we have integrated many of Handler's techniques into our TA-C work, as well as his call for the assessor to be playful and creative in his or her interactions with children and parents during assessment. We also have been influenced strongly by the work of Fischer (1994), who was the first clinician we know to publish an example of an individualized fable used to give assessment feedback to a child. Finn (1996) adopted Fischer's approach, as have many others working in the area of collaborative assessment (Becker, Yehia, Donatelli, & Santiago, 2002; Engelman & Allyn, 2007; Saunders & Tharinger, 2000; Schuler, 1997; Tharinger, Finn, Wilkinson, et al., 2008). We present the specific approach we have developed for writing fables in TA-C in a later section.

An overview of the comprehensive clinical protocol of TA-C, as practiced in the Therapeutic Assessment Project (TAP) (see Table 5.1), is now presented. Although it is possible to adopt only selected components of the model (Finn, 2007; Tharinger, Krumholz, Austin, & Matson, in press), we depict the complete model to illustrate the full potential for the use of play and playful and creative methods in TA-C. The TA protocol used in TAP typically involves 8–10 sessions that take place over a 2- to 3-month period, and is conducted by a team of two assessors (referred to as the Assessment Team). Although the two assessors work together with the child and parents in the initial and final sessions of the assessment, during the testing sessions one administers the testing and creative procedures with the child, while the other supports the parents in their observation of their child's testing. The function of this "observation" or "behind-the-mirror" time is detailed below. Following, we describe the various steps and sessions, illustrated by a case study and highlighting the integration of play, playfulness, and creative methods. First, we introduce the case study. The mother formally consented to written presentation of the case study.

The family we worked with on this TA-C consisted of a 9-year-old boy, David, and his mother, Nancy (names have been changed). They were Caucasian and middle class. The family had gone through a marital separation approximately 1 year before the beginning of the TA, and the final divorce settlement was pending. It appeared from initial interactions with the family that many aspects of the separation were unresolved, such as how much contact there would be between David and his father. This appeared to cause both David and Nancy significant amounts of stress. In addition, the financial structure of the family had significantly changed, and Nancy was struggling to make ends meet. She sought mental health services to address the challenges she and her son were experiencing. Although invited, the father did not participate in the TA. The TA was conducted by the second and third authors, Christopher and Matson, and supervised by Tharinger. Matson worked primarily with the mother and Christopher with the child. In the following sections, we present aspects of this case that were particularly informed by playful and creative methods. Although we also used other tests and techniques in this TA-C, we limit our discussion here to play and playful and creative methods.

Initial Meeting with Parents

In the initial meeting with the parents, the Assessment Team reviews the procedures of the assessment with the parents and addresses their questions. The team explores the parents' goals for the assessment and, with

TABLE 5.1. Therapeutic Assessment Clinical Procedures with Children

Clinical procedure and approximate time	Description
Initial meeting with parents (60–75 minutes)	• Assessment Team explores parents' goals for assessment, works with parents to generate individualized assessment questions, and explores background related to each question.
Initial meeting with child and parents (60–75 minutes)	• Parents introduce child to the Assessment Team, assessment process is explained to the child, and the child is invited to pose his or her own assessment questions. • While parents and one Assessment Team member observe through a one-way mirror via video feed, the other member of the Assessment Team engages the child in testing—often beginning with an interview/conversation, using projective drawings, and ending with free play.
Standardized testing of child (6–8 hours over 4–6 sessions; typically one session per week; total testing time varies depending on parents' assessment questions)	• The child is given standardized psychological tests that are likely to yield information relevant to the parents' assessment questions. • Following standardized administration, "extended inquiries" and discussion help illuminate the child's test responses and experience. • Parents are invited to observe all testing sessions and to offer comments during and after sessions with the Assessment Team. • Sessions often end with free play.
Family intervention session (75–90 minutes)	• Family is asked to play a game, interact in a structured format, or engage in a family assessment method. • Assessment Team observes family interactions, considers their relationship to children's emotions and behavior, and prepares parents to consider family contributions to children's problems in living.
Summary and discussion session with parents (60–75 minutes)	• Assessment results, organized around parents' assessment questions, are shared with parents. • Findings that will be most difficult for parents to hear are presented late in the session. • Parents are asked to confirm, disconfirm, or modify each assessment finding as it is presented, rather than accepting it as "absolute truth."

(continued)

TABLE 5.1. (continued)

Clinical procedure and approximate time	Description
Summary session with child (45–60 minutes)	• Assessment Team and parents meet with the child to answer the child's assessment questions and share some of the assessment findings in a developmentally appropriate way.
	• Assessment findings may be presented in the form of a personalized fable or storybook written by the Assessment Team for the child.
	• The child is invited to modify or illustrate the story and is given a copy to take home.
Written feedback sent to parents	• Within several weeks, a letter to parents summarizing the results of the assessment and addressing parents' questions is mailed.

the parents, co-constructs individualized assessment questions that capture the concerns, puzzlements, and challenges the parents have about their child and family. These questions then guide the assessment. Background information is obtained to inform the context for each assessment question (often another interview is conducted with the parents later in the assessment to more fully fill in the background of the child and family). Finally, the Assessment Team coaches the parents on preparing their child for his or her first session, which typically occurs the following week.

Case Illustration of Initial Parent Meeting

Nancy's questions for the TA revolved around how to handle David's anger and how they could work better together as a family (e.g., What is David angry about? What is making him so frustrated? How can we make things better in the family?). She also asked, "Does David continue to have questions about the separation?," "How can I keep my own frustration down?," and "What things can I do differently?" Nancy seemed very self-blaming and appeared meek during this and other initial sessions. Early within the first session, Nancy's concern regarding our practice of videotaping for research purposes became apparent. We sensed that she felt exposed and vulnerable with this setup, and appeared somewhat constrained and shut down. Although uncomfortable, Nancy accepted the situation and repeatedly told us that she knew we needed to tape the sessions; however, her unease likely affected how open she was with the Assessment Team.

Initial Meeting with Child and Parents, and "Behind-the-Mirror" Observation

The second session, typically a week following the initial meeting with the parents, starts with a brief check-in between the Assessment Team and the parents, followed by inviting the child to join. The parents are asked to introduce the child to the Assessment Team, explain the process of the assessment, and verify that the child understands the reasons for the assessment and is willing to participate. The parents and Assessment Team work together to address questions and concerns raised by the child, and the parents are asked to share with their child one or two of their assessment questions. The parents are encouraged to share a question that is systemic in nature (e.g., How can we all learn to control our anger and talk together about what bothers us?), so as not to single out the child and in order to help shift both the parents and the child to a systemic perspective. The child also is invited to contribute his or her own assessment questions, at this time or any time during the assessment. In our experience, it is hard for most children to generate their own questions at this time. They may be feeling overly self-conscious, as so much attention is being focused on them. However, we have found that more outspoken or parentified children are sometimes able to construct initial questions. Examples from recent cases in TAP include "Why do I get blamed every time something goes missing at home?" from one child, and "Why won't my parents help me more?" from another.

This session continues with the parents leaving the room with one member of the Assessment Team and going to an observation room behind a one-way mirror, or to an adjacent room with a video feed, to observe their child as he or she begins testing sessions with the other assessor. The child is made aware that the parents will be observing. The opportunity for the parents to observe the child assessment sessions with the support of an Assessment Team member is a variation on the practice originally proposed and practiced by Finn (2007), where TA-C is conducted by a single assessor in a typical office setting. Finn describes inviting parents to observe assessment sessions from the corner of his office, and then talking with the parents after each session to ascertain their reactions, respond to their questions, and make small interventions in relation to the way they perceive their child.

In our experience, this unique and creative feature of parental observation, either behind the mirror or via the video feed, greatly strengthens the intervention potential of TA-C. For example, when parents are given the opportunity to watch their child's testing, it can foster their curiosity about their child, engage them as active participants, demystify psychological assessment, and educate them about psychological tests and the assessment process. Furthermore, by discussing parents' perceptions of the testing sessions, the assessor can help them discover answers to their questions about their child and can help them begin to shift their "story" about why their child has problems. The assessor emotionally supports the parents as they reach new understandings or confirm their existing beliefs about their child. This process also allows the assessor to ascertain parental readiness and resources for change, thus informing subsequent sessions involving the parents, as well as the recommendations for future intervention. We have found that most children willingly accept their parents observing the assessment, and many of them make use of this setup to communicate to their parents either directly or through some of their test responses and play activities. Also, in a recent TAP research study (Tharinger, Finn, Gentry, et al., 2009), many parents said that the chance to observe their children's testing sessions was the most useful part of the assessment.

With the parents situated in an observation mode, the child and the assessor begin to establish their working relationship. They typically talk more about the process, and the assessor follows up with additional inquiry about any assessment questions the child may have. Next, it is common practice to invite the child to do a series of human figure drawings followed by extended inquiry procedures, and possibly an imaginary animal (Handler, 2007). This initial child session often ends with free play, to provide the child with the opportunity to engage in unstructured activity that may reveal aspects of his or her personality and life themes. Free play is also used as an opportunity for the assessor and the child to interact on a more social, creative level, and to further establish and build rapport.

Case Illustration of Initial Meeting with Parent and Child

The session began with Nancy sharing her assessment question about wanting to learn more about how she and David could work together to make things better in their family. The Assessment Team then attempted to construct assessment questions with David. David presented as extremely withdrawn and sad throughout this part of the session. He was unable to participate in creating assessment questions, which, as indicated earlier, is not unusual for a child of his age and emotional status. Christopher then introduced David to human figure drawings after his mother and Matson left to observe the session via video feed. The previous week Nancy had noted that David enjoyed drawing, and he had brought his sketchbook to the session. As predicted, starting with the drawings was a playful and creative way for David and Christopher to begin establishing rapport, as well as to get useful assessment information. David worked on drawing a person, his family, and a house. While he worked, Christopher began to see how he could become rigid, wanting the drawings to be perfect and lamenting his poor drawing ability. Nancy also picked up on this behavior while observing with Matson, and noted that he was being very hard on himself. His drawings were actually developmentally appropriate for his age, and the assessment team began to hypothesize that David might often hold himself to high standards and feel like things he does are not good enough.

David's family drawing also helped Christopher begin to see how David was coping with his parents' separation. The drawing showed David and his mother engaged in different activities in separate parts of the house, and did not include his father. After completing all of the drawings and related questions, David took out his sketchbook and began to show some of his drawings to Christopher. He told her that there were other, "inappropriate" drawings in his sketchbook that he should not show her. Christopher did not push, but rather let David share what he was comfortable with showing her. He did not show her the "inappropriate" drawings. In the adjoining room, Nancy confirmed with Matson that she had told him what drawings were "inappropriate," explaining that when he draws things such as knives or severed body parts, she worries about how such drawings would be received in other settings, such as at school. However, she said that she hoped David would show Christopher these drawings, which suggested to us that she would like some help on how to address David's aggressive fantasies.

Near the end of this session, Christopher introduced the option for free play. David was given the opportunity to explore the toy options in the room, which included puppets, Play-Doh, plastic food, plastic animals and dinosaurs, doctor toys, drawing materials, handcuffs, boxing gloves, and a toy gun. David seemed uninterested in most of the toy options until he got to the drawer containing the handcuffs, boxing gloves and gun. David took out the boxing gloves first, put one on, and began hitting his other hand. After commenting that he thought this would hurt more than it did, he quickly lost interest in the gloves. He then took out the plastic toy gun. David went on to create an elaborate game wherein he was looking for and shooting different "Kirby" characters. Kirby is the main cartoon character in a number of video games, and is generally perceived as the "hero" of the games. David identified himself as the "bad guy" in his game, and the Kirby characters as the "good guys." He became very involved in the game, crawling under a table and over chairs to find hidden Kirbys to shoot. As the game progressed, the Kirbys became more and more powerful.

When Nancy observed that David stopped playing with the boxing gloves because he said they did not hurt enough, she explained this to Matson as being "a boy thing." We were concerned, however, that this was not a "boy thing," but rather a red flag for self-harm behavior. Nancy also appeared visibly uncomfortable when David subsequently chose to spend most of the time playing with the toy gun. She began to fidget with her belongings and appeared to be less interested in watching the video feed than she had been during the drawing activities. She commented that she did not allow David to play with guns at home. This helped the team see that in contrast to David's play with Christopher, there were more limits to the play the family engaged in at home. Nancy's discomfort with this play led the team to hypothesize that she may not be able to accept David's angry or dysphoric emotions. Although Nancy appeared to accept and agree with the idea that including time for free play provided an outlet for David's emotions, it was clear that the violent play made her anxious. Matson empathized with Nancy's discomfort and explained that some therapists disagree on the inclusion of guns and violent toys in the playroom, but that we believed it was important for children to be able to express themselves in these ways if they so chose. Although Nancy accepted this idea and never asked that David's access to guns be restricted in the sessions, it was clear that she was not personally comfortable with this type of play. It is also possible that Nancy's anxieties about being observed (and, in her mind, judged) by researchers contributed to her discomfort with David displaying play themes that she may have considered socially unacceptable.

With David, Christopher let him lead the play and used the sportscasting technique to narrate his actions. In this technique, the assessor narrates what the child is doing during play, as if he or she were narrating the action in a sporting event. Christopher felt it was important to let David completely direct the play to see what themes would develop and to further build rapport. We hypothesized that David was unable to share his violent or disturbing fantasies with others and may benefit from an outlet. Although Nancy's explanation of her fears about David sharing "inappropriate" drawings at school seemed prudent given schools' heightened vigilance for signs of violence, we found ourselves wondering whether Nancy's discomfort with David's drawings and her instructions not to share them had made David feel as though the drawings were "wrong," "weird," or "bad," and by extension, so was he.

Upon subsequent discussion of this session in supervision, the Assessment Team hypothesized that it was important to allow David to express his aggressive feelings within the safe environment of the assessment and decided, whenever possible, to allow him access to free play, similar to play therapy, at the end of each testing session. Additionally, the team hypothesized that David's identification with the "bad guy" may reflect low self-esteem and low feelings of self-worth, which we wanted to explore more fully. Finally, David's disappointment when the boxing gloves did not hurt him did turn out to be an early sign of his self-harm behavior, later confirmed through his responses to self-reports and sentence completion items.

Testing Sessions (and More "Behind-the-Mirror" Observation)

The subsequent four to six sessions in TA-C consist of child testing activities, using a variety of instruments chosen according to their relevance to the assessment questions posed in each individual case. A process approach (i.e., testing the limits and extended inquiry) is used throughout in which, following standardized administration, follow-up questions are asked to select responses to projective measures, and also to responses to psychoeducational and self-report measures. We have found that this creative method allows for further exploration of surprising or concerning responses and provides a fuller understanding of the child. Test selection is individualized for each case, and potentially includes cognitive, psychoeducational, neuropsychological, behavioral, and personality (objective and performance) measures. When using sentence completion methods (which we almost always do), the items are individually constructed for each child. We have found that this technique of constructing idiographic sentence completion measures produces richer and more useful responses, has excellent face validity with the observing parents, and brings specific presenting issues directly into the room. Our test selection often includes narrative stories told to apperception cards and the Rorschach, both of which are accompanied by extended inquiry procedures (Handler, 2007). In addition, the child is often invited to engage in free or structured play, usually at the end of the testing sessions, as we have found that this provides a way for children to "communicate" in metaphor feelings they have about the session. The parents continue to observe from behind the mirror or via the video feed throughout these sessions, and are encouraged to share comments and ask questions of the assessor accompanying them. As appropriate, the parents also meet with the Assessment Team at the end of the session, without the child, for further clarification of their observations.

Case Illustration of Testing Session 1

In the next session the following week, David was asked to complete an additional human figure drawing, as well as several self-report measures. In the previous session, David had drawn his mother and himself when asked to draw his family. The Assessment Team was curious to see how he would respond to a request for a picture of his father. David had even more trouble drawing this picture than he had with the other requests during the previous session. In particular, he was very anxious about getting his father's eyes "right" and erased and redrew them several times. When he was done with the drawing, he put his head down on the table. Christopher tried to engage him in a conversation about his drawing but quickly discontinued the task due to David's profound change in mood and behavior.

At the end of the session, free play was again introduced. David went straight to the drawer with the toy gun and pulled it out along with a soft ball. He called the ball "Squishy" and used it as his partner to look for enemies in small spaces where David could not see, such as under a chair or behind the chalkboard. Again, David was very engaged in the game and enjoyed playing until the end of the session. The Assessment Team had expected David's continued use of aggressive play, and the play seemed to help David return to a more positive mood state than when he completed the drawing of his father. We interpreted David's inclusion of a partner (Squishy) in his game as a sign of his willingness to connect with others (at least others he could control).

When David again used the toy gun for his free-play activities in this session, Nancy continued to appear uncomfortable. Similar to the previous week, she began to fidget and became less talkative with Matson during the free-play period of the session. This continued to confirm our impressions that Nancy was uncomfortable with aggressive play. In our experience, other parents often become more comfortable with their children's aggressive play over time, as they begin to appreciate its usefulness in a safe environment, but this shift did not occur with Nancy.

Case Illustration of Testing Session 2

During the next testing session, again a week later, David completed a sentence completion task. The Assessment Team created idiographic stems for use with David based on Nancy's assessment questions and responses David had given earlier in the assessment. Items included "I feel like things are never right when ... " "When I think about my mom and dad's separation I ... " and "When my mom asks me to do something I.... " Based on some of David's earlier responses on a self-report measure, the following stem was included: "I think about death when.... " He finished the sentence by saying "7 hours a day." This response provided an opportunity for Christopher to ask David about self-harm in more detail, and during this discussion he revealed that he tries to "make himself bleed" on a regular basis. He reported biting himself and stabbing himself with a fork. After these responses, Nancy reported to Matson that she was somewhat surprised. She said she had seen him do these things, but not to the point that he would bleed. We thought this activity, and the responses to ideographic stems in particular, helped Nancy see how serious David's behavior was, and she became more concerned about his safety and less inclined to dismiss statements about self-harm as a "boy thing."

David was also asked to draw a fantasy animal during this session. In this technique, the child is asked to "draw a make-believe animal, one that no one has ever seen or heard of before" (Handler, 2007). The assessor then asks the child to tell a story about the animal, and the assessor responds by introducing healthy and hopeful elements into the child's story. In his drawing and story, David returned to the Kirby theme and described many of the attributes of Kirby from the videogame. Although this task did not provide the Assessment Team with new fantasy material, as David seemed to hide behind a known character and story line, it allowed them to watch him draw something easily. In comparison to his other drawings, David had no difficulty drawing Kirby and made few erasures. He enjoyed the drawing and easily told a story about what he had drawn afterward. This was in marked contrast to his mood and drawing style when working on his family drawings, confirming the source of his anxiety.

Again, the session ended with the opportunity for free play, and David went straight to the toy gun. He also pulled out a Magic 8 Ball and the boxing gloves. He gave the gloves to Christopher and told her that he and she were good Kirbys on the hunt for bad Kirbys. David and Christopher spent time looking for the Kirbys using the Magic 8 Ball to help them find where they were hiding. Upon finding the last Kirby, David said that even though the Kirby was bad, he should not die, but rather should go to the hospital and then to jail. The Assessment Team was able to see David's play mature to include Christopher, and to see him shift his aggressive play from death to imprisonment for the bad guys. The team felt hopeful about this shift, and was glad to see David finding more socially appropriate endings for the play. This confirmed our earlier decision to use free play whenever possible in the sessions, and allowed us to see David's shift in play over time. We were also glad to see that Nancy was a little more talkative while observing the play in this session, although she was still quite quiet and reserved.

Case Illustration of Testing Session 3

During the following testing session, again a week later, Christopher administered the Rorschach with David. The results supported the Assessment Team's hypotheses of David's isolation, coping deficits, depression, and attachment problems. During the inquiry phase of the administration, David did well for the first few cards, but became obviously distressed as the inquiry task went on. He even put his head down at one point while responding. Additionally, his time until giving a response noticeably slowed as the inquiry continued. Christopher asked him if he needed to take a break from the cards for a while but he preferred to continue. This was a common response from David, and demonstrated that even when situations were stressful and difficult for him, he nonetheless wanted to continue. However, the Assessment Team saw his persistence as indicating that he was not able to take appropriate self-care steps or accept offers of help and relief from others. At Rorschach card X, Christopher let him know that this was the last card. He perked up at this and was able to finish the task in a better mood. Unfortunately, due to the length of his Rorschach protocol, we were unable to end the session with free play. As Nancy watched David complete the Rorschach, she was very engaged in the task and spontaneously provided many of her own responses. This illuminated aspects of the mother's personality that would not have been available in a standard assessment.

Case Illustration of Testing Session 4

At the next session a week later, David was present for only the beginning of the session, as the majority of the time was reserved for interviewing his mother to obtain more specific details on his and their family's early life and recent stressors. In the part of the session with David, Christopher followed up on some concerns that arose from the Rorschach. David had not reported any popular responses or human representations on the Rorschach during its administration the previous week, which is unusual. Briefly returning to the Rorschach cards in this session, Christopher utilized "testing of the limits" to see if he could see the common images with help from her. David was unable to do this, and therefore this inquiry ended quickly. David's lack of flexibility when guided to see popular responses and humans affirmed our concerns about his lack of comfort in the everyday world and in interpersonal relationships. These findings also heightened our concern about the dominance of his fantasy-based world.

Following, David and Christopher again engaged in free play. David grabbed the gun, handcuffs, Magic 8 Ball, and football. He told Christopher that he was a criminal and she was the police. He instructed her to find him using only the Magic 8 Ball and the football while he had the gun. He killed Christopher many times during the game, after which she would rejoin the game as a different police officer. David seemed especially excited during this play and smiled throughout the game. The assessment team felt that allowing him to continue his aggressive play was important in order to show David acceptance of his expression of aggression. Christopher stayed within her role in the game when shot at, as it seemed important not to tell David that his play was "wrong" or "bad." When David involved Christopher in his play, Nancy was pleased at his desire to relate to Christopher, but appeared uncomfortable with Christopher's apparent enthusiasm for the violent play. At one point, Christopher elaborated David's pretend-play scenario by stating that she saw blood on the floor after David said someone had been shot. Following this comment, Nancy shuddered and appeared shocked that Christopher would say something like that. Although Matson supported Nancy's distress (and also attempted to explain the reason for Christopher's expansion), Nancy's comments and reactions continued to underscore our hypothesis that she was generally not accepting of many of his play themes and his dysphoric emotions, leaving David feeling quite rejected. This was supported by information gained from other parts of the assessment as well.

Case Illustration of Testing Session 5

The following week, Christopher and David worked on the early memory procedure (Bruhn, 1992). This procedure gave the Assessment Team more information on David's experiences of rejection and his use of fantasy to cope. Christopher then brought out the developed photographs David had taken. At the end of a session several weeks earlier, David had been given a disposable camera and invited to take pictures of people and things that were important to him (Handler, 2007). In our experience, children are usually excited to engage in this creative task. The child is asked to return the camera. After the film is developed, the child is asked to sort through the pictures and place them in order of importance. During this session, David and Christopher went through the pictures, with David telling her who everyone was in the photos. As he went through them, David often said "that one shouldn't be in there," most notably to a picture of his mom and a picture of one of his grandfathers. Then, when sorting the pictures, he placed those pictures rather low down on the list. This suggested that David did not feel close to his family, which we had hypothesized. Unfortunately, due to problems with the video feed, Nancy was unable to observe David's sorting of his family photographs, and therefore we were not able to ascertain her reactions.

After this procedure, Christopher and David engaged in structured play, playing a board game, in order to test out some ideas in preparation for planning the upcoming family intervention session. This decision and process is explained in the upcoming section on the family intervention session. Before moving on, we offer some reflection on the use of play and playfulness with David up to this point in the case study.

Reflection on the Use of Play in Testing Sessions with David

By allowing periods of free and structured play in the testing sessions with David, Christopher was able to see how he reacted within a modality that is more natural and free-form than typical assessment activities. Additionally, after responding to emotionally charged assessment measures, play was an excellent way for David to release pent-up energy and emotions. Christopher's comfort with play therapy was crucial. Even though this aspect of the assessment might seem like it would be the most difficult for an assessor, given its difference from usual assessment practices, Christopher found it to be the most rewarding and natural part of the sessions. It allowed her to "take off the white coat" and have fun with David at his level, in a more natural way. It was very useful in establishing rapport with David. It was also helpful in erasing the power differential between Christopher and David, as he was able to direct this aspect of the assessment. It was a nice contrast to how difficult it was to engage David in extended inquiry of his responses to traditional assessment measures, as he was so obviously distressed. Having the opportunity to engage with David in a different way, one that allowed him to open up, helped Christopher feel less discouraged about the assessment process with David. It sometimes seemed that David was not connecting with Christopher, but their play helped her feel more connected with him, and it seemed as though this was the case for David as well. Just as Christopher found that the opportunity to have playful interactions with David helped lighten her mood, it seemed to lighten David's mood too.

Both assessors found it difficult to be playful with Nancy throughout the assessment processes. She was somewhat rigid and constrained, and rarely seemed to "loosen up" or become comfortable, which made it difficult to interact playfully. This, as well as Nancy's apparent discomfort with watching her son play, made us speculate that she had closed off the playful part of herself in order to protect against embarrassment, avoid potentially overwhelming emotions, and maintain focus on the serious challenges she faced. This gave us a sense of what it might be like to be David, and why some of his coping mechanisms may have developed. Christopher and Matson often felt little hope that they would be able to engage Nancy in a way that would help her become more flexible and open to David. They hypothesized that this hopelessness might be what David felt when trying to engage his mother, and might be why he turned to fantasy to cope instead of turning to his mother or other people in his life.

Family Intervention Session

Following the completion of the testing sessions, an analysis of the findings, development of an initial case formulation, and construction of tentative answers to the assessment questions, a family intervention session usually is offered to the family (Tharinger, Finn, Austin, et al., 2008). The plan and format of this session is individually designed to meet the needs of the particular family and further inform the case formulation and answers to assessment questions. Generally, the parents and child are guided to interact in a structured or semistructured family activity. The goals include allowing the assessors to see the child's behavior in the family context, to test systemic hypotheses, and to provide parents with an opportunity to experience success in applying new techniques in which they might have been coached while observing the testing sessions. Additional goals include providing the child with a new experience of his or her parents, assisting the family in gaining insight into how the family contributes to the child's problems (and thus preparing parents to accept systemic feedback), inspiring the family, and imparting hope.

When planning the family session, the assessor can choose from a variety of creative techniques that help move the focus from the child to the family, yet still maintain a common purpose, that is, to continue to assess factors involved in the child's problems. There are a wide variety of possible methods and activities available for use in a family session. Tharinger, Finn, Austin, et al. (2008) describe and illustrate parent coaching, semistructured parent–child play, family drawing, family sculpture, family psychodrama, consensus TAT, and consensus Rorschach methods. Because some of these methods may evoke a high level of intensity if they are used during the family session, the assessor must carefully consider the family's readiness for that level of intensity. It is of utmost importance that the family session is mindfully and uniquely tailored to meet each family's needs, such that the targeted behavior or experience can be evoked "*in vivo*," and yet not be overwhelming.

Case Illustration of Planning and Conducting the Family Intervention Session

Based on Nancy's reactions to what she observed of David's free play, the Assessment Team decided that she would not be ready for a family intervention session focused on coaching her to respond empathically to his aggressive play themes. Instead, it was hypothesized that a better first step might be to coach her to respond empathically during a more structured activity such as a board game. To test this possibility, the last testing session (introduced above) was structured to include an opportunity for David and Christopher to play a board game together, rather than engaging in free play. Though the Assessment Team was disappointed not to have another episode of free play, they thought it would be useful to the assessment to see David's capacity for structured play, in preparation for possibly involving filial game play in the family intervention session.

Thus, at the end of the last testing session, Christopher asked David to choose among a few different board games. David picked the board game Sorry! He noted that he played it a lot at home with his mom. Although she was familiar with the game, Christopher told David she did not remember the rules in order to give him some control over the game and to see how faithful he would be to the actual rules. David played with more forgiving rules than the game typically uses. He also told Christopher that she "didn't have to" follow some of the rules in situations when it would benefit him if she did not. As they played, Christopher sometimes used sportscasting to narrate the action of the game, in order to model for Nancy a different way of interacting with David during play. David seemed to enjoy playing the structured game. This structured game playing between David and Christopher provided an opportunity for Matson to talk with Nancy about what play opportunities, if any, she and David had at home. Nancy shared that she and David frequently play the game Sorry! together. As she watched David and Christopher play the game, Nancy seemed attuned to times when David bent the rules of the game to his own advantage. She expressed frustration about him doing that at home, and explained that when he does this, she tells him that if he wants to introduce any new rules, he has to do so at the beginning of the game so that it is "fair for everyone." In our experience, children who are emotionally overwhelmed often need a more flexible structure to playing games, and Nancy's rigid approach did not seem to be amenable to that consideration. Watching Christopher's interactions with David during this activity provided an opportunity for Nancy to observe a different and more flexible way of playing a game with a child, as well as to observe David's responsiveness and engagement with Christopher as she used these techniques.

After experiencing how well David could play a structured game, and learning that he and his mother often played these games together already, the Assessment Team decided not to have them play a structured game together in the upcoming family intervention session. Thus, the team was able to test out hypotheses in the final testing session before arriving at the final plan for the family intervention session. Since David liked to draw and had mentioned enjoying drawing at home with his mom sometimes, we decided to use family drawings and family sculpture to guide the session. Family drawing is a procedure in which each member of the family is asked to draw a response to the same prompt. The family members are then asked to show and explain their drawings to the rest of the family. After that, the team planned to have Nancy and David complete a family sculpture, which is conceptually similar. In this procedure, each family member is asked to "sculpt" the other members of their family into positions that correspond to a given prompt. For example, one might ask a family to sculpt what it looks like when someone is sad in the family. Finally, the team also considered having the family complete a comic together about solving a problem in their family. Matson and Christopher prepared to be flexible in terms of David and Nancy's response to the plan, and were ready to adapt it as needed.

The family intervention session began with Christopher and Matson asking David and his mother to draw a picture of their family when they are angry. They both drew a similar situation where David was not following directions from his mom. Nancy's drawing depicted a specific event from the day before when David was walking away outside as she called to him. In David's drawing, he and his mother were inside their house, with mom telling him "No" and David saying "No fair." Nancy confirmed that these scenes portrayed a frequent problem. She appeared visibly frustrated as she described the incident that had happened the previous day, when David would not come home when they needed to get ready to go out. She explained that she does not like to raise her voice at him outside because it embarrasses her to think someone might see and hear them. She further indicated that she doesn't want to get into a power struggle by chasing him down the street, so she doesn't know what to do other than wait until he chooses to come back. David agreed that this is what usually happens. Although Nancy had talked at length about her difficulty getting David to comply with requests, it was through these drawings that the Assessment Team first saw how ineffectual she was and how significant the problem was. That is, David was disobeying her in more serious ways than the team had previously realized, like staying out for up to an hour at a time without telling Nancy where he was.

Next, Matson and Christopher asked the family to draw a picture of how they wished it would be when someone was angry. David drew himself riding his bike, with his mom telling him he could ride as long as he would like. Nancy drew a picture of David coming back and talking with her. The Assessment Team explored their very different solutions. David said he was afraid his mom would tell him no if he asked to ride his bike, and that is why he just goes out anyway. Nancy indicated that she wanted David to understand that sometimes things will not go his way and she will have to say no, but at other times she simply needs to talk to him to give him a time limit for playing outside. When the team asked what happens when David disobeys, it became clear that Nancy usually does not give him any consequences for not complying. As the team discussed their drawings, Nancy and David both appeared to be frustrated, and remained stuck in their responses, unable to agree on a realistic compromise.

Matson and Christopher then asked the family to engage in family sculptures. They asked them to sculpt what it is like when David and his mother are angry at each other. David went first, and directed Nancy to stand with her hand on her hip, pointing at him, while he stood across from her frowning. They had some difficulty staying in position, as they were both giggling about the poses. They agreed that they did not like how it felt to be in those positions. Nancy especially seemed upset at how it felt to be pointing at David. When it was her turn, she had David stand with his arms crossed and a mad face while she stood across from him, also with an upset face. Again, they both said they did not like how it felt to be in these positions. The team asked them to change positions to show how they would like it to be. David had a hard time, persisting in wanting his mother to tell him he could have whatever he wanted. He was unable to make a more realistic solution. Mom wanted to have them hugging instead, but David would not comply. She said that he does not like to hug her in front of other people.

After observing Nancy and David working on the family sculptures, the Assessment Team asked Nancy and David to give them an idea of how Nancy typically phrased her requests for him to come inside. Their examples were offered in a neutral tone of voice with no anger apparent, which seemed dissonant with their descriptions of both being angry at these times. David explained that in reality his mother would yell, which she disputed, again citing embarrassment at yelling in public. It was clear that this task was very difficult for them, as both Nancy and David appeared emotionally stirred up. The team suspected that this state was common in their everyday interactions.

In an attempt to encourage a change and a compromise solution in the session, Matson and Christopher then asked David and Nancy to draw a cartoon together of how they might be able to change the situation a little bit to be more of a compromise. David started to draw the cartoon without his mother's help. The team asked him to include Nancy more, but he continued to draw it on his own. He did not appear to be following the directions, and instead was drawing what he wanted the result to be without Nancy's input. Nancy made many quiet, ineffectual attempts to influence his drawing, which he ignored. Even when Christopher and Matson attempted to intervene to get them to work together, he paid little attention to his mother's attempts to join, and Nancy was not able to confidently insert her ideas; they were not able to collaborate. When Nancy was asked to suggest a new solution orally, she suggested that the cartoon could end by David arriving back home and asking if there was anything he could do to help her, which David rejected. The Assessment Team felt that Nancy's inclusion of David offering to help reflected an unmet need on her part rather than an age-appropriate, realistic solution. This activity again showed the team their inability to compromise, Nancy's diminished power, and her need for support.

After these activities, David and Nancy both seemed a little "down," and the Assessment Team wanted to try to end the session on a positive note. For some families it might be okay or even desirable to have them leave feeling a little down, as it might help them begin to integrate some of the affect going on in their family. However, with this family, in which both family members had indications of depression, we wanted to provide an opportunity for a different kind of interaction. The team asked them to draw a picture of their family when they are happy. David drew them at an ice cream shop. He had a giant ice cream cone (bigger than the table), and his mother had a large cone, but much smaller than his. Nancy drew them at the beach. She was reclining, Grandma (her mother) was standing on the beach near David, and David was swimming. Nancy said that she and David had just finished building a sand castle together. Although that scenario was plausible, the team was struck by her drawing the scene that followed their connection, instead of the connection itself.

The session concluded with the request for a sculpture of what the family is like when they are happy. David posed his mother standing with her hands on her head, and then started talking about his "invisible dad." Matson jumped in to stand in for his dad. David had Matson (as his dad) sit down in a chair. He then described a scene of the family making a decision about whether to go to Schlitterbahn (a local water park) or Sea World. He had shared this incident earlier in the assessment when asked to describe his memories. We thought David's response again demonstrated his longing for his family prior to the separation. When it was her turn, Nancy sculpted the two of them hugging, which David allowed. It was nice to see them in this interaction, as it gave us hope that they could connect. They appeared more relaxed and playful with each other, which showed their capacity for positive interactions, something we had not often seen in the assessment. The interaction gave the team hope that David and Nancy could connect.

Parent Feedback/Summary–Discussion Session

In the next-to-last session of TA-C, the assessors meet with parents to provide feedback in the form of answers to the parents' assessment questions, ordering the findings in a way that is most likely to foster acceptance by the parents. An in-depth description of the preparation for this session is beyond the scope of this chapter and can be found elsewhere (Tharinger, Finn, Hersh, et al., 2008). Prior to this session the assessors plan a detailed, comprehensive outline for providing feedback. During the actual session, they follow the outline yet remain flexible, accepting, and responsive to parents' comments, additions, and any disagreements. Through this process, the assessors reaffirm the collaborative nature of the assessment and the respect and value they hold for the parents. In addition to reviewing and discussing "answers" to the parents' questions for the assessment, the assessors also strive to enhance the parents' empathy for their child. Overall, the clinicians assist the parents in coming to a new explanation of, or "story" about, the child/family that leads directly to new actions.

Case Illustration of Preparing for and Providing Feedback to the Parent

Matson and Christopher, in consultation with Tharinger, spent quite a bit of time organizing the findings for Nancy. So much of the information seemed discrepant from what the team believed she could accept that they were concerned that the summary–discussion session would not go well. As described, throughout the assessment Nancy had been quiet, concerned about appearances, and generally did not seem psychologically minded. She also seemed depressed, although she assured the team that she did not consider herself depressed (Nancy indicated that she had been depressed in the past, so she knew what it was like, and that her current state was not depression). Not surprisingly, the Assessment Team had been consistently frustrated with how difficult it was to shift Nancy's thinking about David. Often, the team would leave assessment sessions feeling ineffectual. Given this history, they did not have high expectations for the feedback session with Nancy and anticipated that they would only be able to discuss the most basic findings without overwhelming her.

However, when Nancy arrived for the feedback session, there was a notable difference in her demeanor and affect. She was smiling, talkative, and eager to hear the findings. She seemed much less fearful about the future and about what the assessment would reveal. Matson and Christopher were able to discuss all of the findings with ease, and Nancy was able to hear the findings without downplaying the severity of the problems. During this session, she also spontaneously and eagerly shared a story of effectively disciplining David during the previous week. This was something the team had yet to see her do in session, and was in marked contrast to what they had observed during the previous session during the family intervention.

After completing the summary–discussion session, the Assessment Team met with Tharinger to discuss the obvious differences seen in Nancy. The team hypothesized that Nancy's participation during the family intervention session may have helped her make this shift. As was hopefully conveyed in the description of the family intervention session, Nancy had experienced repeated frustration in her attempts to effectively resolve issues with or collaborate with her son. We reasoned that this experience brought home her need to implement changes. It also seemed to us that her experience of being an effective parent during the week between the two sessions had given her increased strength, hope, and resilience. When discussing recommendations and parenting skills during the feedback session, Nancy indicated that she was well trained in most of the techniques (as she was a preschool teacher), but had lost her ability to apply her skills with her own son. She seemed proud that she was now able to do that, and was confident that she would continue to do so.

Child Feedback Session

As introduced earlier, in TA-C child feedback typically is presented in the form of an individualized story or fable written especially for the child by the assessor(s). We are grateful to Fischer (1994) and Winnicott (1953) for demonstrating how the realm of fable and fantasy can assist children in taking in the new story without overtaxing their mental and emotional capabilities or raising their defenses. In our experience, almost all children react very positively to receiving a fable. They are surprised and pleased that the assessor has written the fable just for them, and are touched that the assessor knows them so well and is hopeful about their future. Other perceived benefits of a fable format are discussed in Tharinger, Finn, Wilkinson, et al. (2008), along with several examples. We focus here on the creative feature of constructing fables.

To be creative, most assessors need to make a few adjustments; they need to free themselves from the constraints of formal professional writing in order to access their imagination and resourcefulness. We have found that once the desire is there, fables flow quite easily and are quite enjoyable to construct. Ideas for characters, settings, themes, and conflicts present themselves throughout the testing sessions, particularly through the child's play and responses to projective tasks and extended inquiries. A step-by-step guide for constructing individualized fables has been provided in Tharinger, Finn, Wilkinson, et al. (2008). The first step is to create the individualized storyboard that positions the story in a somewhat veiled context connected to the child's everyday reality. The child usually is the main character (and is often represented by an animal or fantasy figure), important family members are included, and the assessor typically is included in the fable and represented as a figure of wisdom and kindness, for example, as a wise owl, sage, respected tree in the forest, or coach. The parent characters usually have sought assistance from the wise character (as occurred during the assessment). The child's character is typically confronted with a challenge or conflict that is quite similar to one in the child's past or recent experience, and that in real life has been somewhat overwhelming. The description of the challenge and its proposed resolution is based primarily on the level of change the family appears to be ready for at the time. The goal of a fable is to model a successful step or steps toward constructive change. The steps usually are suggested by the wise character in the story and then carried out by the parental characters.

Case Illustration of Constructing and Presenting the Fable

Christopher and Matson wanted to include several themes from David's assessment in his fable, including the effect of his parents' separation on him, his reliance on fantasy-based coping, and his tendency to consider or engage in self-harm. The Assessment Team thought that weaving these themes together, along with his mother's renewed resources for helping him cope more effectively, would provide both of them with a lasting story. To create the fable, the team recalled the frequency of his perception of alien creatures on his Rorschach responses. The team decided to write a story using aliens as the main characters, as this focus would allow for a depiction of David's rich fantasy life. In the fable, the David character, named Derrick, was described as a "blob alien" from a faraway planet, "Kocab." Blob aliens were described as being able to shift shapes in order to adapt to different environments. Early in the story, Derrick's parents told him that they would be separating and he would be moving with his mother to a new planet, Earth.

> *Excerpt:* "Derrick was a blob alien. These are aliens that can shift their shape to look like all kinds of creatures. Their home planet is Kocab, but they also live on many other planets throughout the galaxy. Their ability to shift shapes helps them adapt to all the different planets. One day, Derrick's parents sat down with him at the table and told him that they had some important and hard news. Derrick would be moving to a new planet, Earth, with his mom. His dad was going to stay behind on Kocab. Derrick was shocked and was not happy about this at all. He wanted to stay on Kocab with his mom and dad together."

The fable continues to describe Derrick's difficulty with this transition and incorporates most of the main assessment concerns, such as anger toward his mom, escape to fantasy, low self-worth, and confusion around the separation.

> *Excerpt:* "On Kocab, Derrick and his mom had gotten along well, but on Earth they started to argue with each other more and more. Derrick's mom would ask him to do things, but sometimes he just ignored her, and sometimes he yelled at her. He never really got in big trouble when he did this, but he did not feel good about getting away with it."

In fables, typically the assessment is represented by a "visit to helpers." In this case, older blob aliens who had successfully moved to Earth were the identified helpers. They helped Derrick and his mother better understand Derrick's feelings and their relationship with each other.

> *Excerpt:* "So, Derrick's mom decided she would try to find help for him. She went to visit some blob aliens from Kocab who had already lived on Earth for many years. She told them about Derrick, and how angry and sad he seemed. She asked them how they had helped their children adjust to Earth."

The fable ends on a hopeful note, by referring to changes the assessment team expected David's mom to be able to incorporate in their everyday interactions.

> *Excerpt:* "That night, when they went home, Derrick's mom asked him to clean his room. He felt angry and did not want to do it. But his mom told him he had to do it or he would not be allowed to ride his bike that evening. She told him she knew he was angry, and did not want to clean his room, but he would still have to do his chores. Derrick cleaned his room quickly, and when he was done his mom gave him a big hug. She said, 'Good job, Derrick. You can go ride your bike now.' 'I would rather draw with you,' Derrick said to his mom. And Derrick and his mom really did start to work better together! She let him know what he needed to do, and they spent more time playing than arguing. Even though Derrick did not always get his way, he still got to do a lot of fun things and he knew that his mom cared about him."

After the fable was completed, Matson and Christopher asked Nancy to review it to see if she was comfortable with it and to seek her input. She said she liked it and didn't want it changed in any way. The following week, David, his mother, and the Assessment Team came together for the final time. The fable was introduced to David, and he was asked to choose who would read it. He asked his mother to read it to him. He seemed to enjoy the story, taking the opportunity to act out various scenes from the story as Nancy read it. Through his actions and comments, it was clear that he saw himself in the story. Nancy also seemed pleased that David had responded well to the fable, just as she had. The fable allowed the Assessment Team to end the assessment on a positive note, fostered by a creative method.

Written Communications to Parents

Within about 2 weeks after the final session, the Assessment Team sends written feedback to the parents, typically in the form of a personal letter rather than a traditionally organized psychological report. Finn (2007) suggests organizing written feedback to correspond to the assessment questions parents generated at the beginning of the assessment process, the same way that oral feedback is organized and presented. The assessor uses the first person and incorporates comments, examples, or disagreements that the parents offered during the feedback session into the written letter. Excerpts from a sample letter are published in Tharinger et al. (2007), and illustrate this consumer friendly and creative method.

Case Illustration of Parent Letter

Matson and Christopher used their outline for the parent summary–discussion session and their experiences from that session to tailor a letter to Nancy. They began the letter by thanking Nancy for her participation and made sure to acknowledge how appreciative they were of her openness in the face of the research videotaping, which she did not enjoy. Then the team wrote to Nancy about her specific concerns and the assessment findings.

> *Excerpt:* "When you came in you let us know that you were really concerned about David's anger, his arguing at home, and how that was affecting your family. We saw across different assessment measures that we used that he really can be disruptive at home and at school.... Because his anger and oppositional behavior can be so hard to deal with, it has given David a lot of power in your family. In our experience, children think they want that power, but they really don't. They aren't ready to handle the power and they need the adults in their life to provide structure and hold the power."

The team also addressed David's feelings of sadness and his propensity toward self-harm behavior.

> *Excerpt:* "The other main thing that stood out for us from the assessment was that David is sad, feels bad about himself, and that he thinks about, and even tries to, hurt himself. When we talked about this, you said that you had noticed his sadness at home also. What this meant to us was that these two ways he's acting are really connected. A lot of children who aren't happy can often be very irritable. Adults who are feeling sad often appear 'blue,' and those around them are able to see and identify their sadness. But children who are feeling sad often appear more irritable rather than 'blue.' People around them may see this and conclude that they are feeling angry, rather than sad. It is difficult for young children to identify and understand their feelings themselves; they may only know that they are 'not happy.' This also makes it more difficult for them to communicate and express their feelings in ways that other people can understand. And this can be very frustrating for children. But what we know about sadness in children is that these irritable behaviors are actually more related to sadness than to anger."

The team went on to address each of the assessment questions in detail, answering the specific questions Nancy had asked. The letter ended with a summary of the most important ways the team felt Nancy could help David, all of which had been discussed during the parent feedback session.

SUMMARY AND CONCLUSIONS

In this chapter we described the development of TA-C, reviewed the growing evidence for its effectiveness, and provided an in-depth description of the methods. We then specifically emphasized the importance of the assessor's capacity to use play and playfulness as an assessment and intervention tool with the child throughout the assessment. Furthermore, because parents actively participate in TA-C, we also stressed the positive impact of the assessor's ability to be playful with parents and to invite the child and parents to play together. In our experience, we have found that many parents who are frustrated with their children due to family stress and challenges have lost sight of the power of play and playfulness, that is, their power to reveal emotions that have gone unspoken, as well as to lighten and start to heal serious problems. Although it can be useful for parents to be verbally reminded of the power of play, experiencing it through observing the assessor and child at play, or through actively playing with their child in a family session, is more powerful in creating change.

We also described and illustrated how creativity can be applied to assessment methods, including collaboratively developing assessment questions and inviting parents to observe and process their child's assessment with an assessor. In addition, we illustrated many other ways the assessor can use creativity, for example, by constructing idiographic items for a sentence completion measure, using extended inquiry to address patterns in Rorschach responses, inviting the child to take and rank photographs of people and things that are important to him or her, and including unique drawing tasks such as the fantasy animal game. The case study also illustrated the power and creativity involved in planning and carrying out family intervention sessions, as well as in the construction of individualized fables.

Although we described and illustrated creating a fable for child feedback, we have also utilized other formats to communicate selected findings to children, including poems and short plays. Especially memorable are the rap songs we have written for several adolescents following their assessments. In these cases, the adolescents were very into music and the rap song modality provided a means to join them in their world. Thus, we advance that at the core of successful TA-C is the capacity of assessors to be flexible, fluid, and playful. Play and playfulness can help bring difficult issues to the forefront and can help heal them. They also let children know that we adults, as assessors or parents, can meet them in their worlds and learn from them.

At the beginning of this chapter we described the evidence for the efficacy and effectiveness of TA-C. We also noted the challenges implicit in studying comprehensive TA-C, in that it is difficult to know which of the many components or interactions of components are driving its effectiveness. We also addressed the issue that the alternative, studying components of TA-C (i.e., the parts separated from the whole), presents a different set of challenges. In general, we liken attempts to pull apart the influence of a playful attitude and creativity on the assessor's part from the actual assessment methods and techniques used to asking assessors to work with their hands tied behind their backs. We stand by our position that the capacity to be playful and creative and to work within a play modality is necessary (but not sufficient) for successful practice of TA-C.

On the one hand, our unwavering commitment to the power of play in collaborative assessment with children and parents makes us reluctant to advise studies that would separate play from the TA-C process. However, on the other hand, it complicates attempts to promote research and efforts to empirically validate our claims about the effectiveness of these methods. Thus, we propose several ideas for future research, one of which is currently underway. One of Tharinger's students, Pilgrim, currently is collecting data for her dissertation on the use of fables for child feedback. The study isolates this method so that the only difference between two groups of children receiving neuropsychological assessments is the addition of a fable as child feedback in one group, contrasted with a general description of the findings presented to the child and parents in the other group. The results of this study will contribute to our understanding of the impact of using creative methods for child feedback on consumer satisfaction and affective experience of the assessment. We can also imagine future research studies where other playful and creative components of TA-C, such as including or not including play at the end of testing sessions, are isolated and contrasted. Furthermore, within the context of research on comprehensive TA-C, we can also envision studies where parents and children are interviewed about their experiences of assessment and their sense of the effectiveness of some of the methods, including the playful and creative components. It would also be possible to compare the outcomes of assessments by assessors before and after they are more thoroughly trained to use play and playful/creative methods in their assessments. Thus, there are certainly ways to empirically examine the specific contributions of the methods we have proposed, and we plan to continue our work in this area.

Finally, we want to say that we are grateful to all the therapists who for decades have demonstrated the power of individual and filial play therapy, as well as the use of play and playfulness in family therapy. We also are indebted to Stephen Finn for his development of TA, possibly the most creative mode of psychological assessment, as well as his partnership in the study of the process of TA-C in TAP. And, as mentioned earlier, we encourage assessors interested in our work to also review the work of Handler and Fischer, also pioneers in the area of collaborative assessment with children. Without Handler's permission to be playful and Fischer's cleverness with fables, TA-C would not be so effective. Lastly, we thank the families that have participated in TAP, and in particular thank the family that allowed us to use their case in this chapter. Although the mother was particularly concerned about being exposed and found wanting, by the end of the TA she had started to regain her strengths as a parent and to be better able to support her child with his emotional needs. Although the family moved away a few weeks after the assessment, we were recently in touch and are happy to report that their lives are going well and that they are having more fun together.

REFERENCES

Armstrong, S., & Simpson, C. (2002). Expressive arts in family therapy: Including young children in the process. *TCA Journal, 30*, 2–9.

Becker, E., Yehia, G. Y., Donatelli, M. F., & Santiago, M. D. E. (2002). Interventive assessment with children and their parents in group meetings: Professional training and storybook feedback. *Humanistic Psychologist, 30*, 114–124.

Bratton, S., Ray, D., & Moffit, K. (1998). Filial/family play therapy: An intervention for custodial grandparents and their grandchildren. *Educational Gerontology, 24*, 391–406.

Brooke, S. L. (2004). Critical review of play therapy assessments. *International Journal of Play Therapy, 13*, 119–142.

Bruhn, A. R. (1992). The early memories procedure: A projective test of autobiographical memory (Part I). *Journal of Personality Assessment, 58*, 1–15.

Busby, D., & Lufkin, A. (1992). Tigers are something else: A case for family play. *Contemporary Family Therapy: An International Journal, 14*(6), 437–453.

Deacon, S. A., & Piercy, F. P. (2001). Qualitative methods in family evaluation: Creative assessment techniques. *American Journal of Family Therapy, 29*, 355–373.

Dermer, S., Olund, D., & Sori, C. (2006). Integrating play in family therapy theories. In C. F. Sori (Ed.), *Engaging children in family therapy: Creative approaches to integrating theory and research in clinical practice* (pp. 37–65). New York: Routledge/Taylor & Francis.

Eaker, B. (1986). Unlocking the family secret in family play therapy. *Child and Adolescent Social Work Journal, 3*, 235–253.

Early, J. (1994). Play therapy as a family restructuring technique: A case illustration. *Contemporary Family Therapy: An International Journal, 16*, 119–130.

Engelman, D. H., & Allen, J. B. (2007, March). Collaborative creativity: Ways in which an assessor works with a writer to craft therapeutic stories. In D. H. Engelman (Chair), *Creative approaches within therapeutic assessment.* Symposium conducted at the annual meeting of the Society for Personality Assessment, Arlington, VA.

Erikson, E. H. (1950). *Childhood and society.* New York: Norton.

Finn, S. E. (1996). *Manual for using the MMPI-2 as a therapeutic intervention.* Minneapolis: University of Minnesota Press.

Finn, S. E. (2007). *In our clients' shoes: Theory and techniques of therapeutic assessment.* Mahwah, NJ: Erlbaum.

Finn, S. E., & Tonsager, M. E. (1997). Information-gathering and therapeutic models of assessment: Complementary paradigms. *Psychological Assessment, 9*, 374–385.

Fischer, C. T. (1994). *Individualizing psychological assessment.* Mahwah, NJ: Erlbaum. (Original work published 1985)

Freeman, J., Epston, D., & Lobovits, D. (1997). *Playful approaches to serious problems: Narrative therapy with children and their families.* New York: Norton.

Gil, E., & Sobol, B. (2005). Engaging families in therapeutic play. In C. E. Bailey (Ed.), *Children in therapy: Using the family as a resource* (pp. 341–382). New York: Norton.

Ginsburg, K. R., Committee on Communications, & Committee on Psychosocial Aspects of Child and Family Health. (2001). The importance of play in promoting healthy child development and maintaining strong parent–child bonds. *Pediatrics, 119,* 182–191.

Gitlin-Weiner, K., Sandgrund, A., & Schaefer, C. (Eds.). (2000). *Play diagnosis and assessment* (2nd ed.). New York: Wiley.

Hamilton, A., Fowler, J., Hersh, B., Austin, C. A., Finn, S. E., Tharinger, D. J., et al. (2009). "Why won't my parents help me?": Therapeutic Assessment of a child and her family. *Journal of Personality Assessment, 90,* 108–120.

Handler, L. (2007). The use of Therapeutic Assessment with children and adolescents. In S. Smith & L. Handler (Eds.), *The clinical assessment of children and adolescents: A practitioner's handbook* (pp. 53–72). Mahwah, NJ: Lawrence Erlbaum Associates.

Landreth, G. L. (1991). *Play therapy: The art of the relationship.* Muncie, IN: Accelerated Development Inc.

Lidz, C. S. (2006). *Early childhood assessment.* New York: Wiley.

Mutchnick, M. G., & Handler, L. (2002). Once upon a time … : Therapeutic interactive stories. *Humanistic Psychologist, 30,* 75–84.

Purves, C. (2002). Collaborative assessment with involuntary populations: Foster children and their mothers. *Humanistic Psychologist, 30,* 164–174.

Russ, S. W. (2004). *Play in development and psychotherapy: Toward empirically supported practice.* Mahwah, NJ: Erlbaum.

Saunders, J., & Tharinger, D. J. (2000, August). *Therapeutic psychological assessment: Child and parent feedback.* Paper presented at the annual meeting of the American Psychological Association, Washington, DC.

Schuler, C. E. (1997, March). Lucy's castle: Collaborative assessment of an anxious child. In S. E. Finn (Chair), *Collaborative assessment of children and families.* Symposium conducted at the annual meeting of the Society for Personality Assessment, San Diego, CA.

Smith, J. D., & Handler, L. (2009). "Why do I get in trouble so much?": A family Therapeutic Assessment case study. *Journal of Personality Assessment, 91,* 197–210.

Sweeney, D., & Rocha, S. (2000). Using play therapy to assess family dynamics. In R. E. Watts (Ed.), *Techniques in marriage and family counseling* (Vol. 1, pp. 33–47). Alexandria, VA: American Counseling Association.

Tharinger, D. J., Finn, S. E., Austin, C., Gentry, L., Bailey, E., Parton, V., et al. (2008). Family sessions as part of child psychological assessment: Goals, techniques, clinical utility, and therapeutic value. *Journal of Personality Assessment, 90,* 547–558.

Tharinger, D., Finn, S. E., Gentry, L., Hamilton, A., Fowler, J., Matson, M., et al. (2009). Therapeutic Assessment with children: A pilot study of treatment acceptability and outcome. *Journal of Personality Assessment, 91,* 238–244.

Tharinger, D. J., Finn, S. E., Hersh, B., Wilkinson, A., Christopher, G., & Tran, A. (2008). Assessment feedback with parents and pre-adolescent children: A collaborative approach. *Professional Psychology: Research and Practice, 39,* 600–609.

Tharinger, D. J., Finn, S. E., Wilkinson, A., DeHay, T., Parton, V. T., Bailey, K. E., et al. (2008). Providing psychological assessment feedback with children through individualized fables. *Professional Psychology: Research and Practice, 39,* 610–618.

Tharinger, D. J., Finn, S. E., Wilkinson, A. D., & Schaber, P. M. (2007). Therapeutic Assessment with a child as a family intervention: Clinical protocol and a research case study. *Psychology in the Schools, 44,* 293–209.

Tharinger, D. J., Krumholz, L., Austin, C., & Matson, M. (in press). Therapeutic Assessment with children: Development, efficacy, protocol, and application to school-based assessment. In M. Bray & T. Keihl (Eds.), *Handbook of school psychology.* New York: Oxford University Press.

Tharinger, D., & Roberts, M. (in press). Human figure drawings in therapeutic assessment with children: Process, product, life context, and systemic impact. In L. Handler (Ed.), *Projective techniques: Research, innovative techniques, and case studies.*

Timberlake, E. M., & Cutler, M. M. (2001). *Developmental play therapy in clinical social work.* New York: Allyn & Bacon.

Welsh, J. A., Bierman, K. L., & Pope, A. W. (2000). Play assessment of peer interaction in children. In K. Gitlin-Weiner, A. Sandgrund, & C. Schaefer (Eds.), *Play diagnosis and assessment* (2nd ed., pp. 517–543). New York: Wiley.

Winnicott, D. W. (1953). Transitional objects and transitional phenomena. *International Journal of Psychoanalysis, 34,* 89–97.

PART III
Play in Evidence-Based Intervention

6

Parent–Child Interaction Therapy

The Role of Play in the Behavioral
Treatment of Childhood Conduct Problems

Larissa N. Niec, Cheryl Gering, and Emily Abbenante

Conduct problems in childhood include a broad range of behaviors from severe tantrums and noncompliance to physical and verbal aggression, fire setting, cruelty to animals, and intentional destruction of property. Predictors of early etiological pathways to conduct problems have been identified in children as young as 1½–2 years old (Shaw, Dishion, Supplee, Gardner, & Arnds, 2006; Shaw, Gilliom, Ingoldsby, & Nagin, 2003). These "early starters," children who manifest signs of conduct problems as toddlers and preschoolers, are at the highest risk of displaying serious, chronic, antisocial behavior later in life (Aguilar, Sroufe, Egeland, & Carlson, 2000; Moffitt, Caspi, Harrington, & Milne, 2002). Treatment, therefore, is particularly important to correct unhealthy developmental trajectories and prevent more severe impairments.

A number of efficacious treatments exist for conduct problems in young children, with the most strongly supported mode of intervention being parent management training (PMT) in which parents learn behavioral strategies to improve children's functioning (Kazdin & De Los Reyes, 2008). Parent–child interaction therapy (PCIT) is an evidence-based behavioral family intervention similar to many PMT interventions in that the primary mechanisms of change are considered to be behavioral and social learning principles. Different from many PMT models, however, play is the key medium through which parents practice new skills and parents and children engage in new, positive interaction patterns.

In this chapter we briefly review risk factors associated with childhood conduct problems, then discuss the theory underlying PCIT and provide an overview of the protocol, including the role of play in the intervention. We then review the literature on the efficacy of PCIT, discuss the case of a family who completed the intervention, and provide recommendations regarding future research. We note that to reduce redundancy throughout the chapter we use the term "parent" to identify any primary caregiver. In PCIT, it is common to work with grandparents, adoptive parents, foster parents, stepparents, and other extended family members, in addition to or instead of children's biological parents.

CHILDHOOD CONDUCT PROBLEMS

Childhood conduct problems fall within the category of disruptive behavior disorders including oppositional defiant disorder (ODD), conduct disorder (CD), and attention-deficit/hyperactivity disorder (ADHD; American Psychiatric Association, 2000). Estimates of the overall prevalence of ODD vary greatly, from 1% to more than 20%, with a median of 3%, depending on sampling methods and criteria (Lahey, Miller, Gordon, & Riley, 1999). Boys typically exhibit three to four times higher rates of conduct-disordered behavior than girls (Kazdin, 2001), with prevalence rates for boys under 18 years reported between 6 and 16% and for girls between 2 and 9% (Delligatti, Akin-Little, & Little, 2003).

Despite the difficulties inherent in diagnosing young children, preschool-age children can be reliably diagnosed with disruptive behavior disorders (Keenan & Wakschlag, 2000; Lahey et al., 1998). The continuity of conduct-disordered behavior from preschool to the early school years (Campbell & Ewing, 1990; Egeland, Kalkoske, Gottesman, & Erickson, 1990; Rose, Rose, & Feldman, 1989) and from childhood to adolescence (Campbell, 1995; Lahey et al., 1995; Offord, Boyle, & Racine, 1991) is well documented, with the early onset of conduct-disordered behavior recognized as a risk factor for later child delinquency and serious juvenile offending (Bloomquist & Schnell, 2002; Hinshaw & Lee, 2003).

A number of individual, family, and environmental factors have been associated with increased risk for the development of childhood conduct problems (see Kazdin & De Los Reyes, 2008, and McMahon, Wells, & Kotler, 2006, for reviews), but parent functioning and problematic parent–child interactions have been found to play particularly important roles. Dysfunctional caregiver–child interactions appear to mediate the link between ecological factors and child outcomes (Reid, Patterson, & Snyder, 2002). Problematic parent–child interactions identified even among infants and toddlers have been linked to later conduct problems. For example, low levels of maternal responsiveness and parent–child affection between mothers and infants as young as 6 months were associated with both parent and self-reports of aggressive behavior at 17 years (Olson, Bates, Sandy, & Lanthier, 2000). More recently, attachment security in toddlers was found to moderate the relationship between parenting and child conduct problems, with parents' use of controlling strategies and children's antisocial behavior linked in those children previously identified with insecure attachments but not in children with secure attachments (Kochanska, Barry, Stellern, & O'Bleness, 2009).

THEORY AND PRACTICE OF PCIT

PCIT directly addresses the two primary risk factors related to childhood conduct problems—dysfunctional parenting and parent–child conflict—through the implementation of behavior principles (e.g., Herschell, Calzada, Eyberg, & McNeil, 2002b). That is, problematic child behaviors are conceptualized as learned through repeated patterns of coercive parent–child interactions, and new patterns are established by altering the contingencies provided in response to both parent and child behaviors. Therapists use behavioral principles to facilitate parents' change in a way that parallels parents' use of behavioral principles to facilitate children's change.

Even before longitudinal studies of conduct problems supported the link between the parent–child relationship and later child disruptive behavior, attachment theory emphasized the importance of early parent–child bonding (Bowlby, 1970, 1980). Although many psychotherapeutic interventions interpret attachment theory by placing importance on the child–therapist bond, PCIT returns to the more direct conceptualization of attachment as the critical bond between a child and a parent. PCIT, therefore, places emphasis on the repair or enhancement of the parent–child relationship. One of the mechanisms through which the relationship is nurtured is the development of parents' child-centered play therapy skills, which will be described in more detail below.

PCIT is a goal-focused intervention in which therapists work primarily with a parent–child dyad to increase parents' positive parenting skills and reduce children's disruptive behaviors. The intervention is implemented in two primary phases: child-directed interaction (CDI), during which parents learn child-centered play skills and nonconfrontational behavior management strategies, and parent-directed interaction (PDI), during which parents learn developmentally appropriate, effective discipline techniques. Two types of sessions are used in PCIT: teaching sessions and coaching sessions. During teaching sessions, the primary education tools are didactic, discussion, and role play. Therapists conduct teaching sessions at the beginning of CDI (CDI Teach) and the beginning of PDI (PDI Teach) to expose parents to a new set of interaction skills. Central to PCIT are the coaching sessions that follow each teaching session. During coaching sessions, therapists instruct parents via a microphone and receiver while observing parent–child play through a one-way mirror. Treatment is terminated after parents have mastered the CDI and PDI skills.

PCIT is different from many other parent training interventions in several important ways. The first is the use of the *in vivo* coaching described above in which therapists provide immediate feedback to parents regarding their skills. Guiding parents in the moment to manage their children's behavior is a powerful teaching tool. In a sample of community families, therapist coaching alone increased parents' child-centered skills in two sessions (Shanley & Niec, 2010). A second characteristic of PCIT is its focus on increasing positive interactions within the parent–child relationship prior to addressing discipline concerns. Parents must demonstrate mastery of several child-centered skills prior to moving to the second phase of treatment. A third critical way in which PCIT differs from many other parent training interventions is its focus on assessment, with emphasis on actual observed behavior change in addition to parent ratings.

Assessment

Assessment of parent and child behaviors is a critical component of PCIT that is integrated into the intervention from the first contact with families until the end of treatment. Before treatment begins, assessment is used to define the problems a family is experiencing (e.g., child noncompliance, sibling aggression) and guage the severity of the target child's symptoms. Throughout treatment, assessment is used to measure the family's progress and to guide individual sessions. In addition, assessment is used to track treatment outcome as well as to determine when to terminate therapy.

The "gold standard" method of assessment in PCIT is direct observation of the parent–child interaction. Parents are observed while playing with their children in three standardized situations during pretreatment and posttreatment. In addition, a short version of the observation is administered during most coaching sessions. The parent–child interactions are coded using the Dyadic Parent–Child Interaction Coding System (DPICS-III; Eyberg, Nelson, Duke, & Boggs, 2008; see Knight and Salomone, Chapter 4, this volume). DPICS-III assesses the quality of parent–child interactions through the coding of verbal and physical behaviors (Eyberg et al., 2008).

In addition to behavior observation, rating scales are used to obtain parents' and teachers' perspectives of children's functioning and parent stress. The Eyberg Child Behavior Inventory (ECBI; Eyberg & Pincus, 1999) is a narrow-band parent-report measure of children's conduct problems used to assess treatment progress each week. Additional useful measures include a broad-band instrument of children's functioning such as the Behavior Assessment System for Children, Second Edition (BASC-II; Reynolds & Kamphaus, 2004) or the Child Behavior Checklist (CBCL; Achenbach 1991), a teacher-report form such as the Sutter–Eyberg Student Behavior Inventory (SESBI; Eyberg & Pincus, 1999), and the Parenting Stress Index—Short Form (PSI-SF; Abidin, 1995).

Child-Directed Interaction

The goal of the CDI phase of treatment is to enhance the relationship between parents and children using child-centered skills and nonconfrontational behavior modification techniques. CDI begins with a teaching session during which parents are taught a set of skills that will be used for the remainder of therapy. Parents practice the skills with their children in session while being coached and during daily 5-minute "special time" periods at home.

While in CDI, parents learn to selectively attend to appropriate child behaviors and to allow the child to maintain the lead in the interaction. For example, parents are coached to provide genuine, labeled praises for prosocial behaviors and to strategically ignore attention-seeking behaviors, like whining. Reflections of children's verbalizations and child-centered descriptions of the play are also skills parents learn to promote a warm, positive interaction. Therapists use similar differential reinforcement techniques as well as modeling to shape parents' use of the skills. Initially, parents use the child-centered skills primarily in the context of the play, but gradually the skills are generalized to other situations.

Although little research has been conducted to examine the relative importance of the components of PCIT, a meta-analysis of parent training programs identified components associated with larger effect sizes regarding positive child and parent outcomes. Teaching parents child-centered interaction skills and requiring parents to rehearse skills with their children during treatment sessions were among the components associated with the largest effect sizes (Kaminski, Valle, Filene, & Boyle, 2008).

The length of the CDI phase depends on how quickly parents master the child-centered skills. Rate of mastery depends, among other factors, on parents' consistent practice at home. As few as two CDI coaching sessions may be necessary; however, the number of sessions can vary depending on the strengths of the family. Once parents have achieved mastery of the CDI skills, the family can proceed to the PDI phase of treatment.

Parent-Directed Interaction

During PDI, the focus of treatment switches from improving child-directed interactions to improving parent-directed interactions. The goal of PDI is to increase parents' use of effective discipline using behavioral principles that emphasize consistency, predictability, and follow-through (Eyberg & University of Florida, Department of Psychology, Child Study Lab, 1999/2010). Like CDI, PDI begins with a teaching session in which parents learn a new set of skills. Parents are taught how to give children effective directions and implement a structured and developmentally appropriate discipline procedure.

As in CDI, parents practice the PDI skills during session and at home, with the goal of generalizing the skills to other settings. Again, the number of PDI coaching sessions conducted depends on how quickly parents master PDI skills. Criteria for graduation from treatment includes mastery of CDI and PDI skills, parents' report of their children's behaviors within half a standard deviation of normal on the ECBI, and parents' expression of confidence in their abilities to manage their children's behavior (Eyberg et al., 1999/2010).

THE ROLE OF PLAY IN PCIT

As discussed in the first section of this volume, children's play takes many forms: it may be solitary or social, involve the creation of dramatic narrative (e.g., fantasy play), or be structured by explicit rules and props (e.g., board games). Evidence-based psychotherapeutic interventions integrate different types of play into their protocols for different purposes. For example, in trauma-focused cognitive-behavioral therapy (TF-CBT), play may be used to help a child develop a narrative of a past trauma experience, thus becoming a component of exposure in the treatment (see Briggs, Runyon, & Deblinger, Chapter 7, this volume). Cognitive-behavioral play therapy (CBPT; see Knell & Dasari, Chapter 10, this volume) uses play as a means to implement cognitive-behavioral principles in ways that are appropriate for young children's cognitive and emotional developmental levels. In both TF-CBT and CBPT, play occurs primarily between the child and the therapist. In PCIT, rather than serving as a means of communication between children and therapists, play is the primary mode of interaction between children and their parents and serves as the medium through which parents practice new skills.

Play in PCIT is dyadic, child-centered, and constructive. That is, therapists coach parents and children to play in ways that provide opportunities for real (not fantasy-based), child-led interactions. Toys are deliberately selected to (1) promote direct parent–child communication, (2) avoid the need for parents to set limits, (3) promote children's prosocial behavior, and (4) reduce the likelihood that parents will be drawn to lead the play (Eyberg et al., 1999/2010). For example, messy toys such as paints or clay are discouraged, as well as toys likely to foster aggressive play (e.g., guns, toy soldiers) and toys that are rule-based (e.g., board games). Appropriate toys for PCIT are ones suitable for the child's developmental level and relatively unstructured: blocks, Mr. Potato Heads, Lincoln Logs, Tinker Toys, and farm and house sets are all good examples of PCIT toys.

The child-led play time of the CDI phase of PCIT serves as a means of reducing parent–child conflict, enhancing the parent–child relationship, and preparing the child to be more receptive to the new discipline techniques introduced during the second phase of treatment. By following their children's lead and using child-centered language, parents communicate that their children's activities are interesting and valuable. From an attachment theory perspective, children experience their parents as responsive and available. Over time, these types of positive interactions may become internalized as schemas in which attachment figures are represented as benevolent and children view themselves as worthy and loveable (Bowlby, 1980). During PDI, when parents are learning more direct ways to manage their children's behavior, play provides a natural context for practicing new discipline techniques and eliciting their children's compliance.

PCIT OUTCOME RESEARCH

A continuously expanding body of research provides significant support for the efficacy of PCIT for the treatment of disruptive behavior disorders in young children. Using the criteria established by the task force on promotion and dissemination of psychological procedures (Chambless et al., 1998; Chambless et al., 1996), an 11-year review of evidence-based psychosocial treatments for children and adolescents with disruptive behavior named PCIT a "probably efficacious" treatment for young children with problem behaviors (Eyberg, Nelson, & Boggs, 2008). The research on outcomes for families completing PCIT has found significant positive changes in parent functioning, child functioning, and the parent–child relationship.

Parent Functioning

After completion of PCIT, parents demonstrate an increase in a variety of positive parenting skills. They attend more positively to their children's behaviors (e.g., praises) and demonstrate more child-centered interaction (e.g., reflections and descriptions) than prior to treatment and compared to wait-listed controls (Eyberg & Robinson, 1982; Schuhmann, Foote, Eyberg, Boggs, & Algina, 1998). Parents use fewer parent-directed interaction skills (e.g., commands and questions) during child-led play than they used prior to treatment, and when instructed to lead the play, parents are able to maintain a more positive atmosphere, as evidenced by using fewer critical statements and giving more praise for children's appropriate behaviors (Eyberg & Robinson, 1982).

Parents also report less personal distress and psychopathology after participating in PCIT (Schuhmann et al., 1998), including increases in maternal adjustment as measured by changes in selected MMPI scales (Eyberg & Robinson, 1982). Such improvements are noteworthy due to the posited impact of factors such as parental, personal, and marital distress on children's problem behaviors and parenting practices (Patterson, Reid, & Dishion, 1992). After completing CDI, maternal depressive symptoms account for less of the remaining impairment in mother–child functioning than prior to CDI (Harwood & Eyberg, 2006). Remaining impairment in mother–child functioning after treatment is accounted for by pretreatment levels of impaired mother–child functioning and poor social support.

Child Functioning

Parents report statistically significant improvements in their children's disruptive behaviors after treatment (Schuhmann et al., 1998). Further, in one study, nearly 50% of parents participating in PCIT reported their children's behavior to change from the clinical and at-risk ranges to the developmentally normal range after only the child-directed phase of treatment (Harwood & Eyberg, 2006). Treatment gains for families who complete PCIT have been observed to maintain over time. Parents report similar levels of improvements in specific behavior problems up to 72 months after treatment (Hood & Eyberg, 2003) and general external-izing problems up to 2 years after treatment (Eyberg et al., 2001), as they do immediately after treatment is complete. Maintenance of children's behavioral gains over time may be associated with parents' maintained levels of parenting skills as observed during behavioral observations of parent–child play interactions 1 and 2 years after treatment (Eyberg et al., 2001).

Improvements in disruptive behaviors associated with other clinical disorders have also been found after participation in PCIT. Nixon (2001) applied PCIT to families of children who met DSM-IV criteria for ADHD before treatment and found that, after treatment, these children were less likely to meet criteria than control groups. Parents also reported reductions in their children's hyperactivity and increases in flexibility of temperament. In a case study in which PCIT was applied to a child with developmental disabilities, pretreatment and posttreatment assessments revealed behavioral ratings in the normal range, reduced parent stress, and the absence of sufficient criteria for ODD (McDiarmid & Bagner, 2005).

In addition to reporting *fewer* child disruptive behaviors after treatment, parents perceive existing behaviors as significantly *less problematic* (e.g., Eyberg et al., 2001; Eyberg & Robinson, 1982; Hood & Eyberg, 2003; McNeil, Eyberg, Eisenstadt, Newcomb, & Funderburk, 1991). These results have been demonstrated up to 30 months after treatment (e.g., Boggs et al., 2004; Eyberg et al., 2001). Parents' improved views of their children's behaviors are accompanied by reports of improved ability to manage these behaviors after treatment compared to before treatment (Hood & Eyberg, 2003) and compared to wait-listed families (Schuhmann et al., 1998). Boggs et al. (2004) reported large effect sizes between parents' pretreatment and 10- to 30-month follow-up ratings of parents' locus of control. Furthermore, parents report being highly satisfied with PCIT (e.g., Boggs et al., 2004; Brestan, Jacobs, Rayfield, & Eyberg, 1999; Schuhmann et al., 1998).

Targeting maladaptive parent–child interactions appears to improve children's functioning in areas other than conduct problems. Reduction of internalizing problems and comorbid separation anxiety disorder symptoms in particular has been reported by parents after treatment when compared to pretreatment parent reports (Chase & Eyberg, 2008). PCIT therapists teach parents how to model appropriate coping skills and interact more predictably with their children, which may reduce children's anxiety levels (Chase & Eyberg, 2008). Furthermore, children report improvements in self-esteem after treatment compared to before treatment self-reports, such that post-treatment reports improve to the normal range and are maintained

6 weeks after treatment (Eisenstadt, Eyberg, McNeil, Newcomb, & Funderburk, 1993).

Improvements in children's behaviors generalize to other settings. Children's school behaviors improve after participation in PCIT without directly intervening in the school setting. Teachers' ratings and researchers' observations of children's classroom behaviors demonstrate greater reductions in oppositional behaviors after treatment when compared to control groups (McNeil et al., 1991), reductions into the normal range on conduct problems 12 months after treatment when compared to control groups (Funderburk et al., 1998), and further improvements in social competence 12 months after treatment when compared to control groups (Funderburk et al., 1998).

Parent–Child Relationship

Mother–child functioning, defined by Harwood and Eyberg (2006) as levels of parenting stress, mothers' perceptions of their children's behaviors, and frequency of ineffective parenting practices, improves after CDI, even before problematic behaviors are addressed directly in PDI. In particular, decreases in parenting stress levels at posttreatment (e.g., Boggs et al., 2004; Eisenstadt et al., 1993; Eyberg et al., 2001; Harwood & Eyberg, 2006; Schuhmann et al., 1998) and maintenance of these levels at follow-up (e.g., Boggs et al., 2004; Eisenstadt et al., 1993; Nixon, Sweeney, Erickson, & Touyz, 2003; Querido & Eyberg, 2003; Schuhmann et al., 1998) are consistent findings across many PCIT outcome studies.

Increasing parents' awareness of their children's positive behaviors also enhances the parent–child relationship. During coaching, PCIT therapists make inductive statements regarding positive aspects of the parent–child relationships, particularly when children's behaviors are contingent on their parents' use of effective parenting skills (e.g., "Did you see Joey's smile after you imitated his play? He really likes it when you play with him"). Outcome studies have illustrated that PCIT treatment completers report more positive interactions with their children than they report prior to participation in PCIT (Schuhmann et al., 1998). Posttreatment assessments also demonstrate increases in parents' physical proximity to their children during play interactions, which suggests increased or restored warmth and genuineness (Eisenstadt et al., 1993).

Perhaps the most striking support for improvement in the parent–child relationship is demonstrated among families who have experienced relationship disruption due to child physical abuse prior to PCIT (see Borrego, Gutow, Reicher, & Barker, 2008, for a review). Physically abusive families and families at risk for physical abuse demonstrate increased positive parent–child interactions from pre- to posttreatment (Borrego, Urquiza, Rasmussen, & Zebell, 1999), have fewer rereports of physical abuse compared to families receiving standard community treatment (Chaffin et al., 2004), and are at less risk for abuse in the future (Timmer, Urquiza, Zebell, & McGrath, 2005). In particular, reduction in rereports of physical abuse from pre- to posttreatment is mediated by reduced negative parent–child interactions (Chaffin et al., 2004).

THE CASE OF LIANA H

Liana was a petite 5-year-old girl of Russian descent with large blue eyes, long curly gold hair, and a splash of freckles across her nose. She was brought to a university PCIT clinic by her adoptive parents because of high levels of oppositional behavior at home (e.g., defying adults' requests, frequent arguing, losing her temper), occasional episodes of aggression (e.g., hitting) directed toward her 4-year-old sister, and adjustment problems at school. Mr. and Mrs. H adopted Liana and her sister from a Russian orphanage when Liana was 18 months old, and much of Liana's early history was unknown. Although Liana's sister was adapting well to the adoption and displayed no behavior problems, Mr. and Mrs. H expressed concern that Liana was not developing a positive bond with them; they felt she was unresponsive to affection and worried she was unable to form a healthy relationship. The family had previously participated in "attachment therapy" with Liana, with no positive effect reported.

At the time of intake, Mr. and Mrs. H's responses on a broad-band measure of children's behavioral functioning, the BASC-II (Reynolds & Kamphaus, 2004), indicated that Liana's acting-out behaviors were significantly above average relative to other children her age. In addition, internalizing symptoms related to anxiety were also elevated. Both parents rated Liana in the clinical range on the ECBI (Eyberg & Pincus, 1999), a weekly measure of externalizing behaviors, and responses on a standardized measure of parent stress, the PSI-SF (Abidin, 1995), supported verbal reports that both Mr. and Mrs. H were experiencing high levels of stress related to parenting Liana.

Observation of parent–child interactions on the DPICS-III suggested that Liana's parents' concerns that she would reject their affection led to their inconsistent use of discipline strategies. For example, to avoid punishing Liana for misbehavior, which they feared would cause her to "hate" them, Mr. and Mrs. H frequently relented when Liana refused to comply with their requests. This pattern reinforced Liana's tantrums and escalated the level of negative interactions between her and her parents.

At the same time, Liana's quick temper and rejecting responses caused Mr. and Mrs. H to begin to avoid all types of interactions with her, which led to fewer opportunities for positive communication. As a result, the family was caught in an escalating cycle in which negative interactions were increasing in frequency and severity and there were few opportunities for warmth and enjoyment.

One of the primary goals of the CDI phase of PCIT is to enhance the parent–child relationship by teaching parents how to interact in healthy, positive ways with their children. For Liana's parents, as for most parents in PCIT, engaging in child-centered play required them to learn a set of skills that was markedly different from their typical style. For children also, child-centered time with their parents can be a significant change from the kind of interactions to which they are accustomed. Parents' regular practice of the CDI skills at home is critical, not only to improve parents' skills, but also to help children learn that the new type of interaction is enjoyable. Early in CDI, Mr. and Mrs. H each reported implementing special time at home at least five times a week; however, they reported that Liana would not remain engaged with them. Instead, she would act uninterested, tell them she did not want to play, and wander off. In day-to-day activities, Liana continued to be rejecting of her parents' offers of assistance or affection and continued to display severe tantrums. Although weekly behavioral assessment showed that both parents were progressing well in their skill development, Mr. and Mrs. H expressed frustration and concern that Liana was not responding to the changes outside of sessions. Disheartened, the family was at risk of discontinuing their practice at home or prematurely ending treatment. In reviewing the family's progress, therapists hypothesized that in this case it was not parent inconsistency that resulted in Liana's lack of engagement, rather it was Liana's early history of disrupted relationships that made it likely she needed a higher dosage of CDI. Therapists directed Mr. and Mrs. H to double the dosage by implementing special time at home twice a day with each parent.

Within 2 weeks, Liana demonstrated a significant, positive response to the increased dosage. Mr. and Mrs. H reported that their daughter not only began to participate in special time at home, she began to ask for it. A particularly poignant and important moment for Mr. H occurred when Liana asked him to help her tie her shoes and gave him a hug afterward.

By the sixth CDI coaching session, Mr. and Mrs. H mastered the child-centered skills and were ready to move to the PDI phase of treatment. During the PDI Teach session, Liana's parents expressed doubt about the likely effectiveness of the discipline strategy; however, recalling early doubts about the CDI phase of treatment and their positive outcome during that phase, they agreed to try the new discipline approach.

Key to reducing children's disruptive behaviors during PDI is parents' consistent use of discipline with successful follow-through (e.g., children cannot use tantrums to avoid parent requests). Because Mr. and Mrs. H had a history of surrendering to Liana's demands and allowing Liana to escape from tasks she did not want to complete, therapists predicted that implementing consistent discipline would be a challenge for both parents and child. As expected, Liana thoroughly tested the new discipline procedure. Initially, she refused to comply with requests, ignored warnings of consequences, and repeatedly attempted to escape from time-out. Therapists coached parents step-by-step through difficult PDI sessions with the goal of helping (1) parents to administer discipline in an effective, developmentally sensitive manner and (2) Liana to learn the new approach and to increase appropriate behaviors.

Because part of Mr. and Mrs. H's inconsistency stemmed from their fears that giving their daughter negative consequences for her inappropriate behaviors would damage their relationship with her, therapists provided the parents with psychoeducation regarding children's need for nurturing within the context of appropriate limit setting (e.g., Baumrind, 1996). During coaching, therapists reframed "punishment" as "healthy limits" and helped parents to observe Liana's ability to quickly reengage in positive interactions after receiving a consequence for negative behavior. As Mr. and Mrs. H saw how effective the new discipline strategies could be and realized that their consistency reduced Liana's disruptive behaviors without harming their relationship with her, they grew more confident in their ability to manage their daughter's behaviors. The family completed treatment after attending 16 sessions.

At treatment completion, both Mr. and Mrs. H rated Liana's behaviors within normal limits on the ECBI scales. On the BASC-II, Liana's internalizing behaviors no longer reached clinical significance. Both parents demonstrated the ability to engage with Liana using child-centered skills and to implement consistent, developmentally appropriate discipline techniques. In addition, Mr. and Mrs. H described their relationships with Liana as increasingly warm and affectionate. They reported feeling confident they could manage behavior problems that might arise in the future. Follow-up with the family at 1 month and 6 months after treatment found that Liana's behaviors remained within the range expected for her age.

FUTURE DIRECTIONS

PCIT is an evidence-based behavioral intervention that uses play as a mechanism for communication and interaction between parents and children in the treatment of childhood conduct problems. Although PCIT has demonstrated large effect sizes in the reduction of children's disruptive behaviors and the increase of positive parenting skills, numerous barriers prevent many families from benefiting from treatment. A shortage of mental health professionals trained to work with children and families means that community agencies are overburdened (Satcher, 2000). Even when families do enter treatment, many drop out prematurely or do not participate fully. Future research with evidence-based interventions such as PCIT must address problems with access, attrition, adherence, and costs in order to improve outcomes for children and families (Herschell, Calzada, Eyberg, & McNeil, 2002b; Kazdin, 2008).

PCIT can be distinguished from most other parenting interventions in its use of therapist *in vivo* coaching, its emphasis on parents' active practice with their children through play in session, its implementation of direct behavior observation to measure change, and its equal focus on repair of the parent–child relationship and parents' behavior management of children's conduct problems. These components are viewed as core to the PCIT model; however, little research has attempted to investigate the relative value of individual components, such as play, or compare the intervention to PMT models without the components. For example, although therapist coaching of parent–child interactions is considered to be an exceptionally powerful therapeutic tool and a defining component in PCIT, only one study has attempted to tease out the effect of coaching on parents' skill acquisition (Shanley & Niec, 2010).

Given the limited resources for research and the urgent need for innovative service delivery models, it may be tempting to wonder how valuable the analysis of an intervention's components may be once the intervention has been well supported as a whole. We propose this is a critical time to understand the specific mechanisms of change in PCIT, for as researchers and clinicians call for treatment models to reach greater portions of the population, there is increasing pressure to take pieces of established interventions—pieces that may be faster and less expensive to implement than the full intervention—and aim them at the problem in hopes that a little bit of an effective treatment is better than no treatment at all. Decisions about innovative models must be made deliberately, however, with data regarding the key components responsible for change. Because parenting interventions share many common behavioral principles that are well studied, a focus of future research should be to investigate the components of PCIT that distinguish it from other interventions. Such research may either serve to preserve components that are associated with greater initial costs but have significant impact (e.g., sound equipment for coaching) or suggest a need for less costly ways of implementing the model.

If our overarching goal is to reach more families more effectively, a number of other important empirical questions remain to be investigated: Do techniques such as motivational enhancement improve treatment adherence and family retention in PCIT? How can therapists better engage fathers? What is an efficient and effective model of dissemination? How do we best meet the needs of families from diverse cultures?

Although research in treatment outcome and intervention development has progressed significantly over the past 30 years, creating efficacious interventions like PCIT is in many ways just the beginning of what we must accomplish.

REFERENCES

Abidin, R. R. (1995). *Parenting stress index: Professional manual* (3rd ed.). Odessa, FL: Psychological Assessment Resources.

Achenbach, T. M. (1991). *Manual for the Child Behavior Checklist/4–18 and 1991 profile.* Burlington: University of Vermont, Department of Psychiatry.

Aguilar, D., Sroufe, L., Egeland, B., & Carlson, E. (2000). Distinguishing the life-course-persistent and adolescent-limited antisocial behavior types: From birth to 16 years. *Development and Psychopathology, 12,* 109–132.

American Psychiatric Association. (2000). *Diagnostic and statistical manual of mental disorders* (4th ed., text rev.). Washington, DC: Author.

Baumrind, D. (1996). The discipline controversy revisited. *Family Relations, 45,* 405–414.

Bloomquist, M., & Schnell, S. (2002). *Helping children with aggression and conduct problems: Best practices for intervention.* New York: Guilford Press.

Boggs, S. R., Eyberg, S. M., Edwards, D. L., Rayfield, A., Jacobs, J., Bagner, D., et al. (2004). Outcomes of parent–child interaction therapy: A comparison of treatment completers and study dropouts one to three years later. *Child and Family Behavior Therapy, 26,* 1–22.

Borrego, J. Jr., Gutow, M. R., Reicher, S., & Barker, C. H. (2008). Parent–child interaction therapy with domestic violence populations. *Journal of Family Violence, 23,* 495–505.

Borrego J. Jr., Urquiza, A. J., Rasmussen, R. A., & Zebell, N. (1999). Parent–child interaction therapy with a family at high risk for physical abuse. *Child Maltreatment, 4,* 331–342.

Bowlby, J. (1970). Disruption of affectional bonds and its effects on behavior. *Journal of Contemporary Psychotherapy, 2,* 75–86.

Bowlby, J. (1980). *Attachment and loss.* New York: Basic Books.

Brestan, E. V., Jacobs, J. R., Rayfield, A. D., & Eyberg, S. M. (1999). A consumer satisfaction measure for parent–child treatments and its relation to measures of child behavior change. *Behavior Therapy, 30,* 17–30.

Campbell, S. B. (1995). Behavior problems in preschool children: A review of recent research. *Journal of Child Psychology and Psychiatry, 36,* 113–149.

Campbell, S. B., & Ewing, L. J. (1990). Follow-up of hard-to-manage preschoolers: Adjustment at age 9 and predictors of continuing symptoms. *Journal of Child Psychology and Psychiatry, 31*, 871–889.

Chaffin, M., Silovsky, J. F., Funderburk, B., Valle, L. A., Brestan, E. V., Balachova, T., et al. (2004). Parent–child interaction therapy with physically abusive parents: Efficacy for reducing future abuse reports. *Journal of Consulting and Clinical Psychology, 72,* 500–510.

Chambless, D. L., Baker, M. J., Baucom, D. H., Beutler, L. E., Calhoun, K. S., Crits-Christoph, P., et al. (1998). Update on empirically validated therapies, II. *Clinical Psychologist, 51*, 3–16.

Chambless, D. L., Sanderson, W. C., Shoham, V., Bennett Johnson, S., Pope, K. S., Crits-Christoph, P., et al. (1996). An update on empirically validated therapies. *Clinical Psychologist, 49*, 5–18.

Chase, R. M., & Eyberg, S. M. (2008). Clinical presentation and treatment outcome for children with comorbid externalizing and internalizing symptoms. *Journal of Anxiety Disorders, 22*, 273–282.

Delligatti, N., Akin-Little, A., & Little, S. G. (2003). Conduct disorder in girls: Diagnostic and intervention issues. *Psychology in the Schools, 40,* 183–192.

Egeland, B., Kalkoske, M., Gottesman, N., & Erickson, M. F. (1990). Preschool behavior problems: Stability and factors accounting for change. *Journal of Child Psychology and Psychiatry, 31*, 891–909.

Eisenstadt, T. H., Eyberg, S. M., McNeil, S. B., Newcomb, K., & Funderburk, B. (1993). Parent–child interaction therapy with behavior problem children: Relative effectiveness of two stages and overall treatment outcome. *Journal of Clinical Child Psychology, 22,* 42–51.

Eyberg, S. M., Funderburk, B. W., Hembree-Kigin, T. L., McNeil, C. B., Querido, J. G., & Hood, K. K. (2001). Parent–child interaction therapy with behavior problem children: One and two year maintenance of treatment effects in the family. *Child and Family Behavior Therapy, 23*, 1–20.

Eyberg, S. M., Nelson, M. M., & Boggs, S. R. (2008). Evidence-based psychosocial treatments for children and adolescents with disruptive behavior. *Journal of Clinical Child and Adolescent Psychology, 37*, 215–237.

Eyberg, S. M., Nelson, M. M., Duke, M., & Boggs, S. R. (2008). *Manual for the Dyadic Parent–Child Interaction Coding System* (3rd ed.).

Eyberg, S. M., & Pincus, D. (1999). *Eyberg Child Behavior Inventory and Sutter–Eyberg Student Behavior Inventory—Revised: Professional manual.* Odessa, FL: Psychological Assessment Resources.

Eyberg, S. M., & Robinson, E. A. (1982). Parent–child interaction training: Effects on family functioning. *Journal of Clinical Child Psychology, 11*, 130–137.

Eyberg, S. M., & University of Florida, Department of Psychology, Child Study Lab (1999/2010). *Parent–child interaction therapy: Integrity checklist and session materials, V 2.10.* Unpublished manual, University of Florida, Gainesville.

Funderburk, B. W., Eyberg, S. M., Newcomb, K., McNeil, C. B., Hembree-Kigin, T., & Capage, L. (1998). Parent–child interaction therapy with behavior problem children: Maintenance of treatment effects in the school setting. *Child and Family Behavior Therapy, 20,* 17–38.

Harwood, M. D., & Eyberg, S. M. (2006). Child-directed interaction: Prediction of change in impaired mother–child functioning. *Journal of Abnormal Child Psychology, 34,* 335–347.

Herschell, A. D., Calzada, E. J., Eyberg, S., & McNeil, C. (2002a). Clinical issues in parent–child interaction therapy. *Cognitive and Behavioral Practice, 9,* 16–27.

Herschell, A. D., Calzada, E. J., Eyberg, S., & McNeil, C. (2002b). Parent–child interaction therapy: New directions in research. *Cognitive and Behavioral Practice, 9,* 9–16.

Hinshaw, S., & Lee, S. (2003). Conduct and oppositional defiant disorders. In E. Mash & R. Barkley (Eds.), *Child psychopathology* (2nd ed., pp. 144–198). New York: Guilford Press.

Hood, K. K., & Eyberg, S. M. (2003). Outcomes of parent–child interaction therapy: Mothers' reports of maintenance three to six years after treatment. *Journal of Clinical Child and Adolescent Psychology, 32,* 419–429.

Kaminski, J. W., Valle, L. A., Filene, J. H., & Boyle, C. L. (2008). A meta-analytic review of components associated with parent training program effectiveness. *Journal of Abnormal Child Psychology, 36,* 567–589.

Kazdin, A. (2001). Conduct disorders in children and adolescence. In J. Hill & B. Maughan (Eds.), *Conduct disorders in children and adolescents* (pp. 408–448). Cambridge, UK: Cambridge University Press.

Kazdin, A. (2008). Evidence-based treatments and psychological services: Shifting our emphasis to increase impact. *Psychological Services, 5,* 201–215.

Kazdin, A., & De Los Reyes, A. (2008). Conduct disorder. In R. J. Morris & T. R. Kratochwill (Eds.), *The practice of child therapy* (4th ed., pp. 207–247). Mahwah, NJ: Erlbaum.

Keenan, K., & Wakschlag, L. S. (2000). More than the terrible twos: The nature and severity of behavior problems in clinic-referred preschool children. *Journal of Abnormal Child Psychology, 28,* 33–46.

Kochanska, G., Barry, R. A., Stellern, S. A., & O'Bleness, J. J. (2009). Early attachment organization moderates the parent–child mutually coercive pathway to children's antisocial conduct. *Child Development, 80,* 1288–1300.

Lahey, B. B., Loeber, R., Hart, E. L., Frick, P. J., Applegate, B., Zhang, Q. et al. (1995). Four-year longitudinal study of conduct disorders in boys: Patterns and predictors of persistence. *Journal of Abnormal Psychology, 104,* 83–93.

Lahey, B. B., Miller, T. L., Gordon, R. A., & Riley, A. W. (1999). Developmental epidemiology of the disruptive behavior disorders. In H. C. Quay & A. E. Hogan (Eds.), *Handbook of disruptive behavior disorders* (pp. 23–48). New York: Plenum Press.

Lahey, B. B., Pelham, W. E., Stein, M. A., Loney, J., Trapani, C., Nugent, K., et al. (1998). Validity of DSM-IV attention-deficit/hyperactivity disorder for younger children. *Journal of the American Academy of Child and Adolescent Psychiatry, 37,* 695–702.

McDiarmid, M. D., & Bagner, D. M. (2005). Parent–child interaction therapy for children with disruptive behavior and developmental disabilities. *Education and Treatment of Children, 28,* 130–141.

McMahon, R. J., Wells, K. C., & Kotler, J. S. (2006). Conduct problems. In E. J. Mash & R. A. Barkley (Eds.), *Treatment of childhood disorders* (pp. 137–268). New York: Guilford Press.

McNeil, C. B., Eyberg, S., Eisenstadt, T. H., Newcomb, K., & Funderburk, B. (1991). Parent–child interaction therapy with behavior problem children: Generalization of treatment effects to the school setting. *Journal of Clinical Child Psychology, 20,* 140–151.

Moffitt, T. E., Caspi, A., Harrington, H., & Milne, B. J. (2002). Males on the life-course-persistent and adolescence-limited antisocial pathways: Follow-up at age 26 years. *Development and Psychopathology, 14,* 179–207.

Nixon, R. D. V. (2001). Changes in hyperactivity and temperament in behaviourally disturbed preschoolers after parent–child interaction therapy (PCIT). *Behaviour Change, 18,* 168–176.

Nixon, R. D. V., Sweeney, L., Erickson, D. B., & Touyz, S. W. (2003). Parent–child interaction therapy: A comparison of standard and abbreviated treatments for oppositional defiant preschoolers. *Journal of Consulting and Clinical Psychology, 71,* 251–260.

Offord, D. R., Boyle, M. H., & Racine, Y. A. (1991). The epidemiology of antisocial behavior in childhood and adolescence. In D. J. Pepler & K. H. Rubin (Eds.), *The development and treatment of childhood aggression* (pp. 31–54). Hillsdale, NJ: Erlbaum.

Olson, S., Bates, J., Sandy, J., & Lanthier, R. (2000). Early developmental precursors of externalizing behavior in middle childhood and adolescence. *Journal of Abnormal Child Psychology, 28,* 119–133.

Patterson, G. R., Reid, J. B., & Dishion, T. J. (1992). *Antisocial boys.* Eugene, OR: Castalia.

Querido, J. G., & Eyberg, S. M. (2003). *Early intervention for child conduct problems in Head Start families.* Manuscript submitted for publication.

Reid, J., Patterson, G., & Snyder, J. (2002). *Antisocial behavior in children and adolescents: A developmental analysis and model for intervention.* Washington, DC: American Psychological Association.

Reynolds, C., & Kamphaus, R. (2004). *Behavior Assessment System for Children* (2nd ed.) Circle Pines, MN: American Guidance Service.

Rose, S. L., Rose, S. A., & Feldman, J. F. (1989). Stability of behavior problems in very young children. *Development and Psychopathology, 1,* 5–19.

Satcher, D. (2000). Mental health: A report of the Surgeon General—Executive summary. *Professional Psychology: Research and Science, 31,* 5–13.

Schuhmann, E., Foote, R., Eyberg, S. M., Boggs, S., & Algina, J. (1998). Efficacy of parent–child interaction therapy: Interim report of a randomized trial with short-term maintenance. *Journal of Clinical Child Psychology, 27,* 34–45.

Shanley, J., & Niec, L. N. (2010). Coaching parents to change: The impact of in vivo feedback on parents' acquisition of skills. *Journal of Clinical Child and Adolescent Psychology, 39*, 282–287.

Shaw, D., Dishion, T., Supplee, L., Gardner, F., & Arnds, K. (2006). Randomized trial of a family-centered approach to the prevention of early conduct problems: 2-year effects of the family check-up in early childhood. *Journal of Consulting and Clinical Psychology, 74*, 1–9.

Shaw, D., Gilliom, M., Ingoldsby, E., & Nagin, D. (2003). Trajectories leading to school-age conduct problems. *Developmental Psychology, 39*, 189–200.

Timmer, S. G., Urquiza, A. J., Zebell, N. M., & McGrath, J. M. (2005). Parent–child interaction therapy: Application to maltreating parent–child dyads. *Child Abuse and Neglect, 29*, 825–842.

7

The Use of Play in Trauma-Focused Cognitive-Behavioral Therapy

Kristin M. Briggs, Melissa K. Runyon, and Esther Deblinger

Trauma-focused cognitive-behavioral therapy (TF-CBT) was originally developed over two decades ago to treat posttraumatic stress disorder (PTSD) and related difficulties in children and adolescents who experienced child sexual abuse (Deblinger, McLeer, & Henry, 1990; Cohen & Mannarino, 1996; 1998; Deblinger, Lippmann, & Steer, 1996). More recently, this treatment model has been adapted and evaluated for its efficacy in assisting youth who have suffered a wide array of traumas (e.g., traumatic loss, exposure to community and domestic violence), and it has been evaluated for its effectiveness in both individual therapy and group therapy formats (Deblinger, Stauffer, & Steer, 2001; Cohen, Deblinger, Mannarino, & Steer, 2004; Cohen, Mannarino, Perel, & Staron, 2007). In fact, now considerable evidence indicates that children need not suffer chronic PTSD or other debilitating emotional or behavioral symptoms in the aftermath of trauma. Several recent large-scale multisite studies have documented that with relatively short-term trauma-focused cognitive-behavioral treatment (i.e., 8–16 sessions), youngsters can overcome traumatic stress symptoms associated with child sexual abuse, traumatic loss, and exposure to domestic violence, as well as disasters like 9/11 and Hurricane Katrina (Lyons, Weiner, & Scheider, 2006: Hoagwood, Vogel, Levitt et al., 2007; Jaycox, Cohen, Mannarino, Langley, Walker, et al., 2010). In fact, today TF-CBT is utilized around the world to treat children and teens experiencing PTSD. In addition, it has been recognized by the U.S. Department of Health and Human Services as a model program and is listed with the National Registry of Evidence Based Practices and Programs as a scientifically supported intervention (U.S. Department of Health and Human Services, Substance Abuse and Mental Health Services Administration [USDHHS-SAMHSA], 2001, *nrepp.samhsa.gov/index.asp*).

The original formulation of TF-CBT was based on the available scientific literature examining the impact of childhood trauma on youth and their parents as well as the treatment efficacy research with respect to PTSD experienced by adult survivors of trauma (e.g., Foa, Zoellner, & Feeny, 2006). Early on, however, it became clear that children respond very differently to therapy than adults, and the element of play became a crucial ingredient in engaging children in the therapy process as did the important involvement of parents. It should be noted that cognitive-behavioral, attachment, family systems, neurobiological, and other theories have contributed significantly to the conceptualization of the TF-CBT model (Cohen, Mannarino, & Deblinger, 2006). Still, learning theories, with their emphasis on modeling, conditioning, contingencies in the environment, and cognitive factors have been most critical to the TF-CBT conceptualization of the development, maintenance, and treatment of trauma-related symptoms in youth. In fact, each of the TF-CBT treatment components has support in the empirical literature in terms of its effectiveness in targeting the cognitive-behavioral processes that appear to contribute to the maintenance and exacerbation of trauma-related symptoms over time.

DESCRIPTION OF INTERVENTION

In their TF-CBT manual *Treating Trauma and Traumatic Grief in Children and Adolescents,* Cohen, Mannarino, and Deblinger (2006) use the acronym PRACTICE to describe the educational and skill-building components that comprise TF-CBT. The PRACTICE components include Psychoeducation and parenting, Relaxation, Affective regulation, Cognitive coping, Trauma narrative, In vivo exposure, Conjoint parent–child sessions, and Enhancing safety and future development.

Typically, the PRACTICE components are delivered in 12 90-minute individual therapy sessions with the child and a supportive parent whereby the therapist meets 30–35 minutes with the parent and child separately and 5–15 minutes with the parent and child jointly to review and/or process information, skills, and/or homework assigned. Over the course of treatment and after individual preparation, increasing time may be devoted to joint parent–child time to review and process the trauma narrative. The components may also be delivered in a group format where parallel parent and children's groups are conducted for 90–110 minutes with the joint parent–child group meeting for 10–30 minutes across 12 sessions. Many of the skills learned in individual sessions can then be practiced in joint parent–child sessions, with the goal of helping the caregiver and the child to utilize the skills learned so that they can continue to practice the skills at home. The parent can also prompt the child to utilize the learned skills and offer praise and reinforcement for the appropriate use of skills. Over the course of treatment, the parent and child are learning parallel skills and education. Given that a supportive parent has been identified in the literature as one of the best predictors of a child's recovery from child trauma (Cohen & Mannarino, 1996, 1998; Mannarino & Cohen, 2000; Deblinger et al., 1996), particularly child sexual abuse, TF-CBT strongly encourages the participation of parents in the child's treatment process. The parent sessions provide interventions that parallel those of their children. Parents are taught relaxation, affect regulation, and cognitive coping skills to assist them in coping with general life stressors as well as stressors related to the abuse of their own child. These skills assist the parents in coping effectively with their own stress related to their child's traumatic experience, while also helping them to serve as a role model and ongoing coach for their children in the implementation of healthy coping skills.

During the Psychoeducation and Parenting component, the therapist provides the children and parents with education about the children's emotional (i.e., trauma symptoms, triggers, reminders, fear, depression) and behavioral (i.e., sexualized and aggressive behavior) reactions to the traumatic event(s). Children and parents are also provided with education about the event(s), such as education about child sexual abuse, domestic violence, or child physical abuse. This education may include information about common responses to the respective trauma type, how frequently the abuse or trauma happens to children, and how children might feel when they experience the trauma. Several play techniques may be useful for providing psychoeducation to children and parents. For instance, two of the authors and their colleagues have published a card game that was developed in the context of TF-CBT. The card game can infuse an element of fun to learning about child trauma (i.e., child sexual abuse, physical abuse, and/or domestic violence) as children can answer questions in a game show-fashion where bells sound to signify correct answers and points are earned for answers and praise for the other team members when conducted in a group or family format (Deblinger, Neubauer, Runyon, & Baker, 2006). The education serves as a lower-level form of exposure as it assists the child so that he or she can get comfortable learning and talking about these issues with the therapist and subsequently with his or her parents. Once the child has played the game successfully with the therapist, he or she can be encouraged to play the game with his or her parent or caregiver in a joint parent–child session. Caregivers are prepared in advance for the game to ensure that they are comfortable and knowledgeable. The therapist offers praise to the child and the parent for their participation.

The initial component also heavily emphasizes the importance of enhancing parenting skills to address children's behavioral problems. Some of these problems may be related to changes in the child's routine or an indulging parent after the abuse disclosure, while others may be related to traumatic reminders. The behavior strategies introduced include the use of praise, reinforcement/reward systems, selective attention, contingency reinforcement, and time-out procedures that are applicable to both children's general and abuse-related behavior problems. Parents are also introduced to active listening skills and coached in positive communication skills in order to facilitate communication with the child about general events as well as anxiety-provoking events.

The **R**elaxation skills component involves teaching parents and children a variety of relaxation skills to assist them in managing stress (e.g., instruction in focused breathing, progressive muscle relaxation, use of physical exercise, imagery, self-care). While relaxation skills may be utilized to cope with general stress encountered in the day-to-day environment, these skills are particularly important for decreasing the physiological hyperarousal that occurs in response to trauma reminders both at home and while a child is developing a trauma narrative during sessions. A number of creative and play strategies may be useful in introducing and producing a relaxed state in children. Some examples include relaxing "like a wet noodle" and tensing "like a tin soldier" (Deblinger & Heflin, 1996), the "Land of the Dinosaur" imagery script (Bonner, Logue, & Kees, 2003), and imagery pretending that you are a blowfish taking air in or a tree with heavy branches bending to the ground or reaching toward the sun (see Runyon, Basilio, Van Hasselt, & Hersen, 1998).

The **A**ffective expression and modulation skills interventions are useful in assisting both children and parents in recognizing, identifying, expressing, and effectively modulating emotions. Helping a child to build a feeling vocabulary will support efforts to label emotional states that can assist them in effectively expressing emotions in general, as well as those related to the traumatic or abusive experiences. This is another skill that is useful for the youth in developing a trauma narrative that incorporates diverse feelings, as this assists the clinician and the child in understanding and processing the meaning of the traumatic experience. Play strategies that assist in identifying emotions include feeling charades, fishing for feelings where the child uses a toy rod to fish feelings out of a fish bowl, and feelings bingo where feelings are called out and filled in on a bingo board and the child identifies a situation where he or she felt that particular emotional state. A variety of interventions including breathing and relaxation training, thought-stopping exercises, and mindfulness can assist children and adults with getting in touch with their feelings, while also learning to express and modulate their emotions.

Cognitive coping skills are initially introduced to help children and parents learn about the interconnections between their thoughts, feelings, and behaviors. Ultimately, children and caregivers are encouraged to identify and share thoughts, feelings, and resulting behaviors in general and in relation to traumatic experiences. This is another skill that is useful for the youth in developing a trauma narrative that is rich with thoughts as this assists the therapist and child in accessing dysfunctional thoughts that may be perpetuating PTSD and depressive symptoms. Children and parents learn to examine dysfunctional thoughts and correct them to assist them in coping with their emotions related to general life stressors and later in therapy regarding the traumas they endured. Children's books and cartoon characters with thought bubbles are useful tools to assist children in learning cognitive coping skills.

TF-CBT is grounded in cognitive-behavioral principles and emphasizes the value of *gradual exposure* throughout treatment, not just in the context of the trauma narrative and *in vivo* exposure components. Treatment begins with the psychoeducation component where the therapist models open communication and discussion about childhood trauma. As previously mentioned, other components, such as emotional expression and cognitive coping skills, help the child to begin to discuss feelings and thoughts related to his or her abusive experiences and prepare him or her for developing a trauma narrative where the child is encouraged to discuss the specific details of the trauma(s). As such, each of these components involves incremental increases in exposure to reminders of the child's traumatic experiences ("trauma reminders") as children and parents learn to tolerate increasing exposure to these reminders. The child is guided in developing a Trauma narrative that involves the child recounting the details of the traumatic/abusive experience and identifying related thoughts and feelings. This assists the child and therapist in accessing dysfunctional thoughts, such as self-blame that may be related to feelings of shame and PTSD and depressive symptoms, and provides the therapist with an opportunity to assist the child with processing and correcting these thoughts, which in turn alters his or her feelings and reduces symptoms. The written trauma narrative is reviewed with the child to repeatedly expose the child to the traumatic reminders in order to extinguish the child's generalized fears and anxiety that is often associated with thinking or talking about traumatic experience(s). A similar process is repeated with the parent in so much as the parent is asked to recount his or her experience in learning about the trauma the child has suffered. In this context, parents are also encouraged to share the thoughts and feelings they experienced at that time as well as when they are reminded of their child's traumatic experience(s). While most parents do not write a narrative per se, some parents choose to write about their experiences and others find it useful to write something at the end of treatment in preparation for expressing their thoughts and feelings of pride in their child's strength in enduring and recovering from the trauma(s) experienced to be shared at the end of treatment with their child.

Conjoint parent–child sessions are conducted with the parent and the child to assist them with practicing the skills learned over the course of therapy. These sessions also assist them with becoming increasingly comfortable in discussing the traumatic/abusive experiences in order to prepare them for sharing the child's trauma narrative and directly discussing the abusive experiences. During joint sessions, the parent is given an opportunity to praise the child for sharing about the abuse and for the use of the other skills as well. If a parent is not able to modulate his or her emotions and respond in a supportive manner to his or her child, then it would be contraindicated to share the narrative with the parent. Thus, the plan to share the narrative with the parent is not discussed with the child until the therapist has determined the therapeutic benefit of such a plan.

To Enhance the safety of the child and decrease the likelihood that clients suffer victimization experiences in the future, education and body safety skills are introduced during this component. Play is also a critical aspect of teaching these skills as youngsters enjoy reenacting experiences they have had or may have in which they can practice incorporating the personal safety skills they have learned.

TF-CBT is comprised of all of the components described above. It is important to note that while all components are introduced to all clients, depending on the client's and families' needs more or less time is devoted to each of the components. Play can be utilized to introduce many of the components and facilitate learning of the skills that are discussed below.

THE ROLE OF PLAY IN TF-CBT

"In general, children's behavior can be considered playful if it is charac-terized by flexibility, self-motivation, positive emotion, and is not strictly goal oriented" (Moore & Russ, 2006). Children's play includes a wide variety of behaviors as well as cognitive and affective processes and may be social or solitary, may involve games (with rules or unstructured), physical activity, fantasy play, art, books, cards, and more. The use of play in TF-CBT is structured and educational play versus free, nondirec-tive, or pretend play. Play is used as a way to engage children and their parents in the therapy process, to create a fun therapeutic environment, to facilitate clinician communication, and to teach specific skills. For professionals versed in the use of TF-CBT, it is understood that much of the success of the evidence-based model is founded on the creativ-ity, adaptability, and playfulness of the clinician. The use of diverse play approaches highlights the flexible and adaptable nature of TF-CBT. In addition, play provides an important vehicle for clinicians to engage and connect with children and parents in a way that increases comfort, confi-dence, and control, while also encouraging the difficult work of trauma-focused therapy. Through the use of play, new emotional and cognitive associations are made with regard to the traumas experienced, such that traumatic memories are no longer paired only with painful emotions, but often come to be associated with laughter, playful competition, pride, and feelings of courage and confidence (Deblinger & Heflin, 1996). In addition to the use of structured play to engage clients in TF-CBT, free play or nondirective play is also used at times in short intervals as a reward. To illustrate the use of structured and educational play in TF-CBT additional examples of ways to incorporate play into the PRAC-TICE components and brief case examples are provided.

Psychoeducation and Parenting

Incorporating play and already existing games into learning about sexual abuse, physical abuse, domestic violence, and healthy sexuality is a way to make the psychoeducation process fun and engaging. Not only do games add an element of fun to the psychoeducation component, but the games help to increase children's and their parents' comfort in talk-ing about highly anxiety-provoking topics (e.g., sexual abuse, physical abuse, domestic violence). Having fun and feeling anxious are competing behaviors (see Wolpe, 1985). As such, incorporating play and clinician creativity into the psychoeducation process will likely decrease the child's and the parent's anxiety and move them toward openly communicating about the child's abuse or trauma (Deblinger & Runyon, 2005).

CASE EXAMPLE

A 10-year-old male did not want to talk about sexual abuse in general or his own experience with sexual abuse. The clinician working with the child learned that he had a love for the game of football. In an effort to engage the client and to create a playful environment, the clinician created a cardboard football field and set it up in the office. The child was then asked questions about sexual abuse and when the questions were answered correctly, the player on the football field advanced across the field. When he was not willing to answer a question, the player was tackled or got sacked and did not advance. Praise, stickers, and small prizes were used as rewards for touchdowns. The clinician's ability to engage the client further built rapport and allowed the child to master and acquire accurate information about child sexual abuse.

An additional playful therapeutic tool used in psychoeducation is a card game developed by Deblinger and colleagues called "What Do You Know?" (Deblinger, Neubauer, Runyon, & Baker, 2006). It is a simple question-and-answer game designed to introduce facts and generate dialogue about sexual abuse, domestic violence, physical abuse, and personal safety. While the issues are complex and potentially anxiety-producing to discuss, the game is designed to be fun, engaging, and create a sense of empowerment. Each card has a question—for example "What can a child do if he/she has been sexually abused?," "Why don't children tell about sexual abuse?," "What is the difference between physical abuse and spanking?," and "What can children do to stay safe when grown-ups in their family are fighting?" The game allows the opportunity for clinicians to introduce educational information, as well as to assist children and their parents in identifying and correcting thoughts and/or beliefs that are dysfunctional, inaccurate, or unhelpful. Children play this game in an individual session as well as in a joint session with their parents, after parents have had an opportunity to prepare for the joint session with the clinician. The three goals for the use of the game include (1) demonstrating comfort in talking about abuse or domestic violence; (2) praising the efforts of children and parents, often through stickers, bell ringing, and points scored in a playful competition between child and parent(s); and (3) providing an opportunity for clinicians to gently correct misconceptions that may be revealed with their responses to questions. Each card has a small picture of an animal, as well as one-fourth of that animal as a larger puzzle piece in one corner, so that every four cards create a full animal of the puzzle pieces, which adds an additional play component for younger children. For older children and adolescents, the game can be made into a lighthearted competition with parent(s) to increase the fun.

Checkers is another example of a game used to facilitate the psychoeducation process that can be tailored to the clients' experiences or concerns. Clinicians may play checkers with words (i.e., *tell*, *responsible*, *vagina*, *fighting*, *curious*, *private parts*, *pornography*) taped to each checker so that when a player "jumps" another player's checker he or she must first make a comment or statement about the word written on the checker before removing the checker from the board, with the goal of increasing knowledge, dispelling myths, and increasing comfort with discussing these issues.

Similarly, the game Twister, produced by Hasbro, has been used by clinicians in implementing TF-CBT. Twister is played on a large plastic mat, like a game board, that is spread on the floor or ground. It has four rows of large colored circles on it with a different color in each row: red, yellow, blue, and green. A spinner is attached to a square board and serves as a die for the game. The spinner is divided into four labeled sections: right foot, left foot, right hand, and left hand. Each of those four sections is divided into the four colors (red, yellow, blue, and green). After spinning, the combination is called (example: right hand yellow) and players must move their matching hand or foot to a dot of the correct color. When playing for purposes of TF-CBT, only one player plays at a time to avoid any inadvertent inappropriate touches. Due to the scarcity of colored circles, an individual player often puts him- or herself in unlikely or precarious positions, eventually causing him or her to fall. A person is eliminated when he or she falls, or when his or her elbow or knee touches the mat. Suggestions for alterations made to the game to enhance knowledge about trauma and increase comfort with the topics of abuse and domestic violence include having questions taped to each of the colored circles on the Twister board so that when the child spins and is required to put a hand or a foot on a specific colored circle, he/she must first answer the question and may earn points for the question answered. Questions asked are personalized to the child playing the game and the trauma he or she experienced. Some examples of questions taped to the circles may include: "If a child tells an adult that she has been sexually abused and the adult does not believe her, what can she do?," "When parents fight by yelling and throwing things, is it ever the child's fault? Why or why not?," or "Do parents who hit their children hate them?" The child must respond to the question before being able to spin again. The clinician then enthusiastically praises the child's efforts, validates correct responses, and offers validation as well as gentle guidance and/ or corrective feedback to assist with responses that are either inaccurate, partially correct, or indicate dysfunctional thoughts. Accumulated points may be exchanged for small prizes or brief free time at the end of the session.

A third example of incorporating psychoeducation into playing a game includes the game Jenga, also produced by Hasbro. Jenga is played with wooden blocks stacked in a tower formation; each story is three blocks placed adjacent to each other along their long side, and each story is placed perpendicular to the previous one. A plastic loading tray is included to assist in stacking the blocks. Players alternate taking one and only one block from any story except the completed top story of the tower at the time of the turn, and placing it on the topmost story in order to complete it. The game ends when the tower falls. Some examples of how Jenga has been used as an educational game by clinicians implementing TF-CBT include taping questions about abuse and trauma to the Jenga blocks so that when a block is removed, the child answers the question. For example, a child may find taped to his or her Jenga block a piece of paper asking: "What are the doctor's names for girl's private parts?," "How do children feel when grown-ups call them names?," or "What is domestic violence? Give an example." The clinician personalizes the game depending on the child/family and the traumatic experience. Upon responding, the child is praised for his or her efforts, correct answers, or correct portions of responses. When a response is incorrect, partially correct, or reveals dysfunctional thoughts, the clinician is in a position to provide education and gently challenge dysfunctional thinking through probes and questioning.

With regard to the introduction of anatomically correct names for body parts, labeling body parts, and prompting discussion about privacy and the parts of the body that are private, paper dolls and blank pictures of unclothed age-appropriate children are often used. When using paper dolls, children may engage in the fun activity of designing, cutting out, and decorating bathing suits to cover private parts. Another engaging and playful way to introduce and label body parts with young children includes using a large roll of white paper and tracing the outline of the child's own body. Subsequently the child is encouraged to color a bathing suit on his or her body and, with the help of the clinician, to label all body parts including private parts.

A child and adolescent psychologist in North Dakota reported that she uses a whoopee cushion, a practical joke device designed to produce a noise resembling human flatulence when inflated and placed on a chair for an unsuspecting person to sit on. The whoopee cushion is used as a playful way to introduce to children, who have been sexually abused, education about the natural, physiological responses the body may experience when the genitals are stimulated. The psychologist indicated that she begins a session by sitting on the whoopee cushion and allowing the child to play with the cushion as she explains that the body, with it's natural physiological responses, makes a number of sounds and has a number of different natural responses that are outside of our control. Other examples include when an onion is peeled it is natural for the eyes to water or when a penis is stroked it is natural for an erection to occur (Angela Cavett, personal communication, 2008).

Relaxation

In TF-CBT, relaxation skills are taught to children to not only help them manage general feelings of stress, but also to help anxious and/or avoidant children cope with the anxiety and/or avoidance triggered by the therapy process itself. Relaxation skills help youngsters to feel a greater sense of control over the anxiety and fear they may experience when confronted with abuse reminders in the context of therapy (Deblinger & Heflin, 1996). When relaxation skills are introduced, they are geared to the child's developmental stage and are often playful in nature. Youth, particularly teenagers, may be taught progressive relaxation including guided tension-releasing exercises. The recommendation of Koeppen (1974) to include fantasy in relaxation to maintain the attention and interest of younger children is integrated into the majority of current examples of relaxation exercises with children. For example, Barbara Bonner and colleagues created a script called "The Land of Dinosaurs" which guides children back to "the time of the dinosaurs," imagining they are "huge" dinosaurs with "long necks" to stretch up to the tall trees to eat the leaves. The "dinosaurs" are guided to lie down on the ground, feeling the sun shining on them, to stretch out, to take some deep breaths and fill their "gigantic lungs" up with air, and to slowly release the air. The script continues to guide children through relaxation exercises including stretching, progressive muscle relaxation (e.g., tensing the jaw and then releasing it, lifting the shoulders as close to their ears as they can as they try to get under low hanging trees), and breathing (Bonner et al., 2003).

Simpler imagery may be used with younger children by asking them to pretend that their body is in a state of tension, like a "tin soldier" or an "uncooked piece of spaghetti" and then after a count of five to release their bodies into a state of relaxation like a "wet noodle" (Deblinger & Heflin, 1996). Another way to introduce relaxation to children includes controlled, belly breathing. For example, children are asked to imagine the expansion of their stomach on the inhale "as if it were a balloon being blown up," and then to imagine on the long exhale that the balloon is flying away as all of the air is being released from it. In another example, presented by Runyon et al. (1998), an expansion was made on a muscle relaxation sequence originated by Morris and Kratochwill (1983) to include fantasy: children are instructed to pretend they are blowfish, "take a deep breath and hold it for 10 seconds, hold it in like a big round blowfish, and let it out watching the air bubbles float up through the water. Raise both of your hands about halfway above the couch and pretend that you are reaching for a colorful rainbow, breath normally, then drop your hands and relax." Another example of a playful way to introduce controlled, belly breathing includes the use of bubbles. Children are provided a container of bubbles and are encouraged to practice slow, controlled breathing with deep inhales and long, deliberate exhales as they blow bubbles.

Affective Expression and Regulation

In TF-CBT, early in treatment, clinicians assess the child's feeling word vocabulary and work to expand the vocabulary as well as focus on emotional expression skills. During the first session of TF-CBT, children are encouraged to play a game with the clinician that includes listing as many feeling words as possible in a 1- to 2-minute period. The typical expectation is that a child will generate at most one feeling word (e.g., *angry, sad, brave, proud, happy*) per year of chronological age (Esther Deblinger, personal communication, 2008). In addition to assessing a child's capacity to link words to emotions, this activity is also a low-level gradual exposure activity because the clinician may subsequently ask the child to identify the feelings from the list that he or she was experiencing at the time of the traumatic event and that he or she still experiences when reminded of the trauma(s). The list generated is added to and referred to throughout the treatment process for discussion and ultimately may be used to assist the child during the trauma narrative when he or she is asked to describe trauma-related feelings.

When a child struggles to generate a list of feeling words, he or she is praised by the clinician for his or her effort and then other playful attempts may be made to assist the child in creating a more extensive list of feeling words, again to achieve the goal of creating a vocabulary of feeling words to be used by the child in sessions and to discuss the feelings associated with the trauma as well as for the child to use in day-to-day life to express him- or herself and regulate emotions. Examples of playful, engaging efforts for a clinician to help a child generate feeling words or expand on the list of feeling words include creating scenarios to prompt a child to think of a feeling word (e.g., "How might a child feel when he is given a new bicycle?" "How might a child feel when he sees two kids fighting on the playground at school?"), or referring to pictures in books and magazines to engage a child in identifying the emotions expressed on the faces of the people in the pictures, creating feeling face collages from magazine pictures and then labeling the feelings each person in the pictures is expressing. Children may also play feelings charades where a child and his or her parent or the clinician picks a feeling word out of a container and then acts out the feeling (e.g., by stomping his or her feet and clenching his or her fists to exemplify anger) until the other person identifies the feeling being acted out. To build additional awareness with regard to affective expression, children may also use mirrors to see their own facial expressions and make linkages to affective expression.

CASE EXAMPLE

A 6-year-old male had been severely physically abused, neglected, and exposed to domestic violence during his toddler years. He was in a foster placement when referred for TF-CBT and was accompanied to treatment by his foster mother. When he entered treatment, his emotions were dysregulated and ranged from numb dissociation to aggression to self and others. He was withdrawn and silent during most of the initial sessions, responding "I don't know" to all attempts to communicate. The clinician working with this child struggled immensely to build rapport and to establish trust and what was perceived as a safe environment to conduct TF-CBT. Gradually, with the use of feelings posters, cut-out pictures of baby faces from magazines to create a collage, the use of mirrors, and playing feelings charades, the child began to build a vocabulary for feelings. Ultimately, by the end of his treatment process, he had developed a range of feeling words to express his emotions as well as coping skills to regulate his emotions. In particular, he developed the ability to identify feelings of anger and before acting out aggressively toward himself or others to count to 10, to use deep breathing, and to give himself a "time-out" to calm down.

Variations of the commonly used sentence completion technique with feelings are used for emotional expression skills as well. A sentence stem is provided, for example, "I feel happy when … " or "I feel safe when … ," and the child completes the sentence. Some examples of ways this may be implemented in a playful way include taping the written sentence stem on a small sheet of colored paper and taping them around the clinician's office. The child is then encouraged to find as many of the colored papers as he or she can, as if in a treasure hunt, completing the thought as each sentence stem is discovered. Another variation of sentence completion for affective expression includes a game called "Fishing for Feelings," where the sentence stems are written and attached to pieces of laminated paper cut out in the shape of fish and put into a "pond" which is a plastic tub decorated on the outside to look as if it is an underwater scene. The child is then provided a "fishing pole" which is a wooden stick with yarn attached to a magnet, and the child fishes out the sentence stems by attaching the magnetic fishing pole to paper clips attached to each "fish" (Donyale Baker, personal communication, 2005).

Another game used for this component is called "Emotional Bingo," produced by Marjorie Mitlin. Children play bingo while simultaneously building feeling word vocabulary and verbalizing examples of emotions experienced. The contents of the game include a large poster with 34 different faces in boxes with different facial expressions and written feelings underneath the face (e.g., afraid, appreciated, grouchy). Each one of the 34 feelings/emotions is then represented on its' own individual card as well as on different bingo cards; 24 out of the total 34 feeling words and pictures are depicted on each bingo card in varying orders. The clinician draws one of the individual cards and reads off the emotion/feeling on the card. The child then looks for the feeling word or picture on his or her bingo card. If the word is on the child's bingo card he or she then has an opportunity to share an experience that involves that emotion. For example, a player may say, "I have *embarrassed* on my bingo card. I felt embarrassed when my teacher at school told the whole class that I got an 'F' on my quiz." This game can also be used in joint parent–child sessions to encourage active listening and empathy, such that, after a child and/or parent has shared an experience that involves the emotion they have on their bingo card, the other player(s) have an opportunity to listen, reflect back, validate the experience the person has shared, and praise him or her for sharing. For example, the parent of the child may then say, "I understand that you were embarrassed when your teacher told the whole class you got an 'F' on your quiz. Thank you for telling me about that." The game ends when any one player has a direct line (horizontal, vertical, or diagonal) of feelings that have been called off.

FACE IT!, 10 card games to learn about feelings, is another way that play is used in TF-CBT (Childswork/Childsplay, 1998). The game includes a standard deck of 52 cards, yet instead of suits, the cards are divided into four age groups identified by color: children (green), teens (blue), adults (red), and older adults (gold). The cards are numbered 1–13 and each number represents one of 13 different feelings (e.g., happy, sad, surprised) with pictures of actual people in the respective age groups expressing facially the feeling word corresponding to the number. The instructions accompanying the deck of cards describe 10 different games that can be used with the cards. One example out of the 10 games that clinicians use with TF-CBT is the game "Concentration." Two of the age groups are separated out from the entire deck of cards with matching feeling words from two different age groups written on the card (e.g., *loved, shy, tired, frustrated, happy*). Each card with a feeling word written on it has a matching card, albeit in a different age group (e.g., a child face for happy and then a teen face for happy). The cards are then turned upside down with the back of the cards showing and spaced evenly in a large square on a table or desk. The child and the clinician and/or the child and his or her parent(s) alternate turning over one card and then another card in an attempt to find two feeling cards that match. If a match is made, the two cards are removed from the table and the player tells of a time when he or she experienced that feeling. For example, if a child picks both cards with the word *afraid*, as the child removes the pair from the playing table, she may say, "I feel afraid of the dark." If no match is made, the two cards are turned back over, face down, on the table, with an effort to remember its placement for a future opportunity to make a match. The game is over when all pairs have been removed from the table.

One child adolescent psychologist who practices TF-CBT described using a play activity called "Mood Manicure" to engage adolescent or preadolescent girls in affective expression. Each child is presented with different colors of fingernail polish and is able to assign an emotion to each color. The teen then chooses which colors she will wear based on her current emotions and how strong the emotion is. The teen determines the appropriate proportion of each feeling she is experiencing and paints her fingernails accordingly (e.g., four nails are painted red if she is feeling angry that day and has identified red as the color that she identifies with anger and perhaps one is painted electric blue to express the part of herself that is feeling sassy that day) (Goodyear-Brown, personal communication, 2008).

Additional examples of affective expression activities used with younger children include four circles with semicomplete faces drawn with four prime emotions written under the faces (happy, sad, mad, scared). The child is asked to complete the drawing of the face to add expression to the circle, most often including completion of the mouth and so on, and then to describe a time he or she felt that way. A similar example used with younger children is the "Color Your Life" technique which includes provision of a blank outline of a picture of a body; the child is encouraged to assign feeling words to different colored markers (e.g., blue = sad, orange = happy, red = angry, green = brave) and asked to color in the body with the colors to indicate the proportion of the child that is feeling each of the identified feeling words and where he or she is feeling it in the body (O'Connor, 1983).

Cognitive Coping

Cognitive coping is a skill that helps children and parents dispute and correct dysfunctional, inaccurate, or unhelpful thoughts that may be associated with feelings of shame, which in turn may contribute to depression and the perpetuation of trauma symptoms (Deblinger & Runyon, 2005). It is sometimes a challenge for young children to understand what a thought is, making the connections between thoughts, feelings, and behaviors complex to explain to young children. The use of the thought bubble or think cloud is a method used by cognitive-behavioral clinicians working with children to introduce the concept of cognitions (Bernard & Joyce, 1984). Clinicians on staff at the CARES Institute sometimes use comic strips with thought bubbles coming out of a person's mind to assist in introducing the concept of thoughts to younger children. Children are then encouraged to draw their own comic strips on paper or on dry eraser boards to incorporate thought bubbles coming out of their minds and to write in what they were thinking at the time. The examples discussed initially are neutral as the general concept of cognitive coping is introduced earlier in treatment and later reviewed in the context of cognitive processing when children's thoughts about the trauma(s) experienced are reviewed and examined after the trauma narrative is written.

Once a child seems to have an understanding of what a thought is, clinicians often draw a triangle, called a "Cognitive Coping Triangle," on a piece of paper or on a dry erase board indicating that each arm of the triangle interacts with the other two arms of the triangle and labeling each of the three arms with the words *thoughts*, *feelings*, *behaviors*, indicating that the thoughts a person has impacts the way the person feels and in turn, the way the person behaves. One way of introducing cognitive coping, which includes educational play as well as physical movement and engagement, is to create a large replica of a cognitive coping triangle out of tape on the floor of an office. A large triangle is created on the floor of the office with one arm assigned thoughts, another arm assigned feelings, and the final arm assigned behaviors. The child is then asked to engage physically by jumping or leaping from one "arm of the triangle" to another while discussing thoughts, feelings, and behaviors, and the linkages.

CASE EXAMPLE

A clinician working with an 8-year-old client was introducing cognitive coping using a cognitive coping triangle made out of tape. She described an imaginary situation at school where the child is called to the principal's office. The clinician then asked the child to jump to the thought arm of the triangle and to identify what thought the child may have. The child said, "I would be thinking I must have done something wrong." The clinician praised the child, "Great job identifying a thought," then asked the child to jump to the feeling arm of the triangle and asked the child, "If you were called to the principal's office and thought to yourself, I must have done some-thing wrong, how might you be feeling?" The child responded, "Scared." The clinician validated the child, "Sure, I can understand that if you thought you had done something wrong you would feel scared," and instructed the child to jump to the behavior arm of the triangle. Once on the behavior arm of the triangle, the clinician said, "If you were called to the principal's office, thought that you must have done something wrong, and were feeling scared, what do you think you would do?" The child paused and said, "I might cry." After validating and praising the child for her efforts, the clinician then has an opportunity to re-create the same scenario probing for thoughts that are more neutral or positive (e.g., "I wonder what the principal wants?" or "Maybe the principal wants to see me to con-gratulate me for raising the most money in the class fundraiser for the school") and to solicit potential resulting feelings (e.g., curious, confident) and behaviors (e.g., hurrying to seek out the principal), teaching the skill of cognitive coping.

In TF-CBT, games are also used to help children differentiate between helpful and hurtful thoughts. For example, one clinician uses the game Jenga by writing thoughts on each block. One thought might read, "I am a beautiful, smart girl." Another thought might read, "The freckles on my face make me look ugly." The clinician coaches the child to determine which thoughts are helpful and accurate and which thoughts are unhelpful and inaccurate by asking him- or herself ques-tions like "How does that statement make me feel?" or "Would I say that to my best friend?" The clinician then encourages children to iden-tify alternative statements that are more helpful and/or accurate, for example, by asking themselves, "What can I say to myself that makes me feel better?" The statements may be neutral and/or trauma-specific such as, "I was courageous to tell about the sexual abuse," or in con-trast, "I should have told sooner, so the abuse was my fault."

In Cohen, Mannarino, and Deblinger's (2006) book, a best friend role-play is introduced where a child or parent who has a belief about him- or herself that is unhelpful or distorted is asked to role-play a dia-logue with his or her best friend.

CASE EXAMPLE

A single mother of a 7-year-old child often left her child with a man she had known for many years while she went to work at night. Upon learning that the man had fondled her daughter under her nightgown, the mother immediately notified the authorities and sought counseling services for her daughter. Despite having taken action immediately, throughout the course of treatment the mother of the young girl consistently said, "I should have known. I never should have left my daughter with him." During one session, the clinician suggested to the mother, "I want you to pretend your best friend, Sarah, who is also a single mother of a young child, is the one whose daughter was fondled by her babysitter. Imagine your friend Sarah was in the same situation you are in now and she said to you, 'I should have known. I never should have left my daughter with him,' what would you say to Sarah?" The mother paused and said, "I would say, you had no way of knowing that he would touch your child. You trusted him. He had been a part of your life and your family for many years and was never anything other than respectful toward you. Your daughter adored him. There was nothing you knew about his history that indicated he would abuse a child. And, as soon as your daughter told you what he had done, you made sure she never saw him again and got her the help she needs." Offering the opportunity for clients to respond to their own thoughts as if it were their best friend often gives a new perspective and an opportunity for a shift in dysfunctional or unhelpful thoughts because people are often more supportive of their friends than they are of themselves.

Trauma Narrative and Processing

At times when working to engage a child in the trauma narrative, a clinician is asking him- or herself, "How can I creatively engage with this child who is avoidant of the details of the traumatic experience to talk about his or her trauma?" In TF-CBT, the creation of a trauma narrative typically includes a clinician and the child determining together the significant aspects of the traumatic experience, often ranging in scope beyond the actual incident(s) of abuse to include the disclosure, being interviewed by authorities (e.g., police officers, prosecutors, child protective service representatives), medical exams, and the like, together listing "chapters" to be included in the "book" that is to be the trauma narrative. During the initial phase of writing a trauma narrative, children are instructed to recount the details of the events constituting each chapter from beginning to end including what they were thinking and feeling at the time, as if the clinician is a secretary or reporter. The timing of writing particular chapters varies depending on the degree of stress associated with the recollection of certain events. Therapists are encouraged to give children two choices as to what they would like to write about each session. Children in turn generally choose to talk or write about the least anxiety-provoking memories first, leaving the more difficult experiences to process later in treatment once they have developed more confidence, comfort, and skill. The clinician records exactly what the child is saying either in writing or at a computer. Children are encouraged to express themselves verbally while capturing the narrative, but also through art and illustrations for each chapter.

In instances where a child is not interested or resists writing a trauma narrative, other creative solutions have been utilized to allow a child to recount the details of the traumatic and/or abusive experience and identify related thoughts and feelings. At times, it is about creating an environment that is experienced by the child as safe and comfortable and identifying a vehicle (e.g., poetry, song, art project) that engages him or her in effectively exploring his or her thoughts, feelings, and developing beliefs about the trauma(s).

CASE EXAMPLE

A 9-year-old male experiencing avoidant PTSD symptoms was reluctant to complete a trauma narrative. He had completed the other components of TF-CBT and thus had experienced some gradual exposure and education about sexual abuse, but felt shame and embarrassment and refused to talk about the details of his sexual abuse. The clinician was often met with silence when attempting to engage him in creating a hierarchy and completing his narrative. The clinician knew the child had an interest in camping. In an effort to create a relaxed, comfortable environment and to incorporate creativity and play to engage her client in the trauma narrative, the clinician created an environment mimicking a campground in her office. She set up a tent and a mock campfire with flashlights creating an environment that was comfortable and associated with fun for the child, allowing the client to move past his avoidance to complete the trauma narrative.

Additional examples of playful ways to engage children in the trauma narrative include the use of microphones for interviews, talk-shows, game shows where, for example, the client recounts the details of a traumatic event as a celebrity being interviewed on a talk show (e.g., *The Oprah Winfrey Show*).

CASE EXAMPLE

A clinician at the CARES Institute discussed a client she worked with, a 9-year-old female, who took a particular interest in the tape recorder that was set up in the office to record her own sessions to be used in supervision. The clinician was adaptable and flexible and used the child's interest in the tape recorder, and an old-fashioned microphone, as a way to engage and to make TF-CBT a fun, playful experience for the child. The 9-year-old client was intelligent and creative, so she was a self-starter in the use of the tape recorder. She was creative in ways that she and the clinician could use the recorder as they proceeded through treatment with the child's self-directed play (e.g., at times she was a talk-show host, an investigator at the prosecutor's office, or a journalist reporting on sexual abuse). According to the clinician, the child often interviewed her during acquisition of education about sexual abuse as well as while developing cognitive coping skills. Further, when it came time to write her trauma narrative, the child played both the role of the interviewer and the role of the interviewee, often switching chairs and using props in the office to change her appearance (e.g., a boa, a hat) as she switched her roles. With the use of the tape recorder, the child created her entire narrative in interview format, including cognitive processing and challenging dysfunctional thoughts.

Puppets are another vehicle that engage children and at times create enough distance to reduce anxiety and avoidance, allowing children to recount the details of the traumatic event(s) experienced more readily.

CASE EXAMPLE

One clinician spoke about a 6-year-old girl who would not stay in the room and would not talk about the trauma she endured. However, she would talk to the hedge hog puppet the clinician had in her office. Another, slightly older child working with the same clinician preferred to hold the puppet himself and used a raccoon puppet who lived in a garbage can. The child raised the raccoon's head to respond to questions and report details about the abuse and when he needed to retreat, to relax and take deep breaths before continuing, he alerted the clinician by returning the raccoon to the inside of the garbage can for safety and containment.

Other examples of efforts made by clinicians to engage children in the trauma narrative process, when there is extreme reluctance to recount the trauma verbally, include the use of a doll house or sand trays to re-create a traumatic event. When using a doll house, the child uses dolls and the house to recount details of the trauma including location of the abuse in the home and the people present. For this purpose, dolls are identified, for example, as the parents who engaged in domestic violence as well as the children who were exposed to the violence. The clinician is then able to record the recounted details, allowing for further probing for thoughts and feelings as well as cognitive processing at a later time.

CASE EXAMPLE

A clinician with a psychodynamic background utilized a sand tray to encourage her client to work through the trauma narrative and processing component. She discussed working with a 7-year-old female who was shut down and too fearful to talk about the physical abuse she had endured. The child used a sand tray and figurines to set up an incident of physical abuse in the home. The child recounted the details of the abusive experience in the sand tray, with the figurines. As the child recounted the details, the clinician captured her words in writing and was able to reread the description in a later session to probe for thoughts and feelings from the child.

After the trauma narrative is complete and the clinician has probed for feelings and thoughts from the client, the clinician works with the client to process inaccurate, unhelpful, and/or dysfunctional thoughts. As was described previously, in the Cognitive Coping Section as an approach for working with parents, when processing thoughts and feelings with children after the trauma narrative is complete, best friend role plays or imagining what the client may say to another child who has been sexually abused are playful ways to target unhelpful thoughts with children.

CASE EXAMPLE

A clinician was working with a 13-year-old female who had been sexually abused by her maternal uncle at age 8. Throughout her narrative, the client repeated a theme of self-blame. Despite psychoeducation indicating that many children delay disclosure or go all the way into adulthood without disclosing incidents of sexual abuse, the client maintained a belief that she made a mistake by not disclosing the abuse sooner and therefore allowed future incidents of sexual abuse to occur in the family. After completion of the trauma narrative, and with an understanding of the origin of the client's beliefs and feelings, the clinician was able to use role play with the client to shift her belief system. The client was asked to imagine herself talking to a 10-year-old girl who had just disclosed that her uncle sexually abused her when she was 8 after she learned that a younger cousin of hers was touched in a sexually inappropriate way by the same uncle. In the role play, the 10-year-old blamed herself for the younger cousin's sexual abuse and felt that she made a big mistake by not telling sooner. Through the use of role play, the 13-year-old client was able to take on the role of the expert telling the 10-year-old child that her uncle was responsible for the sexual abuse because he is an adult and misused his power and the loving, trusting relationship he had with her. She talked about how the child's uncle used coercion and threats of harming her parents to scare her and "trick her" into not disclosing. She further informed the 10-year-old in the role play that many, many children never tell for a number of different reasons and she was brave to tell and to help her younger cousin to not feel so alone.

Conjoint Parent–Child Sessions

Conjoint parent–child sessions are incorporated into TF-CBT early in treatment to help parents practice communication and parenting skills. Later in treatment, conjoint sessions are designed to help parents and children practice skills together and openly engage in general trauma-related discussions. These educational sessions provide an opportunity to assess parent and child responses to general trauma-related discussions in order to determine the therapeutic appropriateness of engaging in later conjoint sessions in which children share their trauma narrative with parent(s). In most instances these fun, educational sessions prepare parents and children well for later reviewing and discussing the details of the trauma(s) experienced. The sessions include the exchange of praise that has been prepared in advance with the clinician and often include some sort of game, playful competition, or role play that has been previously prepared in the individual sessions. Some of the games mentioned above that are frequently used in conjoint parent–child sessions include the "What Do You Know" card game, played as a family competition with additional points given when children and/or parents praise one another, and "Emotional Bingo." Other games that have not been described in detail in this chapter, but that are great resources for conjoint parent–child sessions include Angry Animals (Mariah & Kidsrights), Survivor's Journey (Rohlfs-Burke & Kidsrights, 1994), and Peace Path (from the WPS, Creative Therapy Store), to name only a few.

In addition to already marketed games, often times encouraging role reversal is a playful way to reiterate and summarize material that has already been introduced, for example, by allowing the child to play the expert and teach the clinician and parents all the child knows about domestic violence or sexual abuse, or playing school and the child is the teacher doing a lesson on child sexual or physical abuse.

CASE EXAMPLE

One 11-year-old girl who experienced sexual abuse pretended the clinician and her parents were students at a school and she had been hired by the school district as an expert consultant on sexual abuse to come in and do a presentation about child sexual abuse to the student body. Some of the acquired information she explained to the pretend audience included children are never at fault for child sexual abuse; some adults who abuse children use tricks to get children to do what they want them to do because adults are smarter, bigger, and more powerful than children are. The child talked about how she now knows that many, many children never tell about sexual abuse well into adulthood, if at all, for a lot of reasons including fears about whether or not they will be believed, fear that they may get in trouble or may get the person that abused them in trouble, but that it is very important for children to tell. She then added, while wagging her finger, "So if anyone in this audience has ever been sexually abused, it is so important that you tell, tell, tell until someone believes you so that you can get the help you need." After she was done presenting, the "children" in the audience were able to ask her questions and offered her praise for her courage and expertise on the subject of childhood sexual abuse, which seemed to build a sense of empowerment for the young girl as she beamed with pride answering the audience's questions.

Enhancing Safety and Future Development

Role plays are used to incorporate activity and behavioral rehearsal when enhancing safety. Children are often given scenarios to consider. For example, the therapist might have the child practice how he or she would respond if an older child asked him or her to go behind the shed so they could play a "fun" touching private parts game. The child is encouraged to (1) consider whether the situation described is safe or unsafe; (2) if unsafe, to practice the skill of assertive communication using a strong voice, maintaining eye contact, and saying "NO!," and immediately getting away from the situation; and (3) seeking help from an adult. Children are, in fact, encouraged to tell and keep telling until they find an adult who understands and does something to help them feel safe. Children are also taught to differentiate between okay secrets (e.g., a surprise party where the secret will be revealed in a short amount of time and feels good) versus not okay secrets (e.g., private part touching where a child has been told to keep it a secret forever and it feels bad). Similarly, role plays are used for behavioral rehearsal for general safety skills as well as for an opportunity to practice dialogues about healthy sexuality and to practice creating physical and emotional boundaries with regard to relationships.

A clinician reported she plays a game with young children to increase awareness about predatory behavior and to help children resist unwanted or inappropriate advances, to get away, and to get help from an adult. The game she referred to is called "The Trick Hat," which begins with a dialogue about ways perpetrators trick children into sexual abuse. Included in the dialogue are examples ranging from physical threats to coercion and bribes. Examples of trickery (e.g., "I have a special game for just the two of us to play, it will be a secret just between you and me") are written down and placed into a hat. The child (or children in a therapeutic group) pull out tricks from the hat and talk about the example prior to acting out a safe response to the attempted trick.

PLAY IN TF-CBT GRADUATION

Upon graduation from TF-CBT, there is often a celebration which includes a graduation cap, a graduation certificate, and on occasion blown-up balloons. Often times, during a final graduation session, there is some time reserved for review and summary of skills learned and education acquired. One clinician described a graduation session with a family she worked with. To make the review and summary portion of the graduation session playful and engaging, she included written statements and questions covering psychoeducation about sexual abuse as well as coping skills and some praise statements on small slips of paper and enclosed them in the balloons so that the child and parents could pop the balloons to get the question and/or statement out of the balloon in summary and celebration of the accomplishment of completing TF-CBT. Graduation sessions are also often planned in advance and include time reserved for pure celebration, which may include dancing, singing, playing music, and/or sharing a prepared snack. Looking forward to this celebration can help motivate children to actively participate in therapy and may reduce the risk of premature dropout. It is important to take the time to acknowledge the hard work and accomplishments of both parent(s) and children in successfully completing therapy with a playful celebration.

In addition to the examples of the use of play in TF-CBT included in this chapter, there are many books and games that are used as support materials and ways to make TF-CBT engaging, fun, and educational for children and their families as well. Appendix 7.1 presents an extensive list of games and books that are often used to enhance and support the implementation of TF-CBT.

FUTURE RESEARCH AND CONCLUSIONS

As the scientific literature has developed, the TF-CBT model has evolved and will likely continue to do so based on the findings of ongoing and future TF-CBT trials and other relevant research in the field. While it has been well documented that many youngsters are quite resilient in the face of multiple traumas, other youth suffer emotional and behavioral difficulties that severely disrupt their healthy development and adjustment. TF-CBT, as well as other therapy models, may be greatly enhanced by research that helps us to identify those factors that support resiliency and/or decrease children's vulnerability to trauma. In fact, research that identifies the potential benefits of play in helping children cope with stress and trauma may also importantly inform efforts to provide children with natural supports as well as efficient and effective interventions. While TF-CBT has been well documented for its efficacy in supporting the recovery of traumatized youth, there is still much to be learned about the critical ingredients of this treatment model. This is particularly important in disaster relief work as there are often very limited mental health services and a great need for the most effective and efficient services in those circumstances. Thus, given the multicomponent nature of this model, it will be useful to identify the critical components of treatment given a child's posttrauma presentation. In addition, while parental support appears to critically influence a child's recovery, research further examining the necessity of parental involvement in treatment may also elucidate when school-based trauma recovery programs which do not involve parents significantly might be sufficient.

In sum, while TF-CBT is a structured treatment approach that is well documented in terms of its efficacy, its treatment components must be delivered with skill and sensitivity. The critical role of a trusting therapist–client relationship should not be underestimated, nor should the importance of engaging clients in a manner that demonstrates respect for cultural and familial values. In addition, therapists' use of play and creativity may not only enhance their success in engaging young clients, but may produce more positive outcomes and greater satisfaction overall. Finally, the use of play often naturally demonstrates a positive attitude toward life despite the hardships experienced. The therapist's "playfulness," in fact, models the importance of reengaging in the positive aspects of life, while simultaneously demonstrating confidence in clients' abilities to engage in the therapy process and overcome the traumas endured.

REFERENCES

Bernard, M. E., & Joyce, M. R. (1984). *Rational-emotive therapy with children and adolescents*. New York: Wiley.

Bonner, B. L., Logue, M. B., & Kees, M. (2003). Child maltreatment. In M. C. Roberts (Ed.), *Handbook of pediatric psychology* (3rd ed., pp. 652–663). New York: Guilford Press.

Cohen, J. A., Deblinger, E., Mannarino, A. P., & Steer, R. (2004). A multisite, randomized controlled trial for children with sexual abuse-related PTSD symptoms. *Journal of the American Academy of Child and Adolescent Psychiatry, 43*, 393–402.

Cohen, J. A., & Mannarino, A. P. (1996). A treatment outcome study for sexually abused preschool children: Initial findings. *Journal of the American Academy of Child and Adolescent Psychiatry, 35*, 42–50.

Cohen, J. A., & Mannarino, A. P. (1998). Interventions for sexually abused children: Initial treatment outcome findings. *Child Maltreatment, 3*, 17–26.

Cohen, J. A., Mannarino, A. P., & Deblinger, E. (2006). *Treating trauma and traumatic grief in children and adolescents.* New York: Guilford Press.

Cohen, J. A., Mannarino, A. P., Perel, J. M., & Staron, V. (2007). A pilot randomized controlled trial of combined trauma-focused CBT and setraline for childhood PSTD symptoms. *Journal of the American Academy of Child and Adolescent Psychiatry, 46*, 811–819.

Deblinger, E., & Heflin, A. H. (1996). *Treating sexually abused children and their nonoffending parents.* New York: Sage.

Deblinger, E., Lippmann, J., & Steer, R. (1996). Interventions for children suffering posttraumatic stress symptoms: Initial treatment outcome findings. *Child Maltreatment, 1*, 310–321.

Deblinger, E., McLeer, S. V., & Henry, D. E. (1990). Cognitive behavioral treatment for sexually abused children suffering post-traumatic stress: Preliminary findings. *Journal of the American Academy of Child and Adolescent Psychiatry, 29*, 747–752.

Deblinger, E., Neubauer, F., Runyon, M. K., & Baker, D. (2006). *What Do You Know?: A therapeutic card game about child sexual, physical abuse, and domestic violence.* Stratford, NJ: CARES Institute.

Deblinger, E., & Runyon, M. K. (2005). Understanding and treating feelings of shame in children who have experienced maltreatment. *Child Maltreatment, 10*, 364–376.

Deblinger, E., Stauffer, L., & Steer, R. (2001). Comparative efficacies of supportive and cognitive behavioral group therapies for young children who have been sexually abused and their nonoffending mothers. *Child Maltreatment, 6*, 332–343.

Foa, E., Zoellner, L. A., & Feeny, N. C. (2006). An evaluation of three brief programs for facilitating recovery after assault. *Journal of Traumatic Stress, 19*, 29–43.

Hoagwood, K. E., Vogel, J. M., Levitt, J. M., D'Amico, P. J., Paisner, W. I., & Kaplan S. J. (2007). Implementing an evidence-based trauma treatment in a state system after September 11th: The CATS project. *Journal of the American Academy of Child and Adolescent Psychiatry, 46*, 773–779.

Jaycox, L. H., Cohen, J. A., Mannarino, A. P., Langley, A., Walker, D. W., et al. (2010). Children's mental health care following Hurricane Katrina: A field trial of trauma-focused psychotherapies. *Journal of Traumatic Stress, 23*(2), 223–231.

Koeppen, A. S. (1974). Relaxation training for children. *Journals of Elementary School Guidance and Counseling, 9*, 14–21.

Mannarino, A. P., & Cohen, J. A. (2001). Integrating cognitive behavioral and humanistic approaches for sexually abused children. *Journal of Cognitive Behavioral Practice, 7,* 361–367.

Moore, M., & Russ, S. W. (2006). Pretend play as a resource for children: Implications for pediatricians and health professionals. *Developmental and Behavioral Pediatrics, 27*(3), 237–248.

Morris, R. J., & Kratochwill, T. R. (1983). *Treating children's fears and phobias: A behavioral approach.* New York: Pergamon Press.

O'Connor, K. J. (1983). Color your life technique. In C. E. Schaefer & K. J. O'Connor (Eds.), *Handbook of play therapy* (pp. 251–258). New York: Wiley.

Runyon, M., Basilio, I., Van Hasselt, V. B., & Hersen, M. (1998). Child witnesses of interparental violence: A manual for child and family treatment. In V. B. Van Hasselt & M. Hersen (Eds.), *Sourcebook of psychological treatment manuals for children and adolescents* (pp. 203–278). Hillsdale, NJ: Erlbaum.

U.S. Department of Health and Human Services Substance Abuse and Mental Health Services Administration. (2001). *National registry of evidence-based programs and practices.* Available at *nrepp.samhsa.gov/index.asp.*

Weiner, D. A., Schneider, A., & Lyons. J. S. (2009). Evidence-based treatments for trauma among culturally diverse foster care youth: Treatment retention and outcomes. *Children and Youth Services Review, 31,* 1199–1205.

Wolpe, J. (1985). Systematic desensitization. In A. S. Bellack & M. Hersen (Eds.), *Dictionary of behavior therapy techniques* (pp. 215–222). New York: Pergamon Press.

APPENDIX 7.1. Games and Books Used in TF-CBT

Title	Author/developer	Publisher
	Games	
What Do You Know? (available in Spanish)	Esther Deblinger, Felicia Neubauer, Melissa Runyon, & Donyale Baker	CARES Institute: 856-566-7036
Angry Animals	Katelyn Mariah	Kidsrights: 1-800-892-KIDS
Dealing with Feelings Card Game	Eric Plugokinski	*www.feelingsfactory.com*
Dr. Playwell's Worry-Less Game	Karen Schader	Childswork/Childsplay, LLC
Emotional Bingo (available in Spanish)	Marjorie Mitlin	
Feelings Cards	Michele Kiblar	Kidsrights: 1-800-892-KIDS
FACE IT!		Childswork/Childsplay, LLC
Let's Talk About Touching	Toni Cavanaugh-Johnson	
Survivor's Journey	Catherine Rohlfs Burke	Kidsrights: 1-800-892-KIDS
The Peace Path Game	Lisa Marie Barden	WPS Creative Therapy Stores

(*continued*)

Title	Author/developer	Publisher
	Games	
Thoughts & Feelings Card Game	Lisa Marie Arneson	*www.BrightSpotsGames. com*
Play it Safe with SASA	Etti Hader & Susan Brown	
Safetyville		Kidz-idz: 1-856-234-5439 or *www.kidzidz.com*
	Children's books	
Helping Families Heal	Melissa K. Runyon, Beth Cooper, & Alissa R. Glickman	CARES Institute: 856-566-7036
Please Tell!	Jessie (Sandra Hewitt)	Hazelden Foundation
My Body Is Private	Linda Walvoord Girard	Albert Whitman & Co
Gilbert the Gilfish Races for the Rainbow (coloring book)	The New Jersey Task Force on Child Abuse and Neglect.	N.J. Division of Youth and Family Services (DYFS)
Spider-man and Power Pack	Stan Lee with Prevent Child Abuse America	Marvel Comics: 1-800-477-4776 or *www. channing-bete.com*
	Emotional expression and identification	
All Feelings Are OK—It's What You Do with Them That Counts	Lawrence E. Shapiro	
Double-Dip Feelings		APA Magination Press
Josh's Smiley Faces		APA Magination Press
Let's Talk about Feelings: Ellie's Day	Susan Conlin & Susan Levine Friedman	Parenting Press, Inc.
The Feelings Book: The Care & Keeping of Your Emotions	Lynda Madison	Pleasant Company Publications
The Way I Feel	Janin Cain	Parenting Press
Today I Feel Silly	Jamie Lee Curtis	HarperCollins

Title	Author/developer	Publisher
	Coping	
A Volcano in My Tummy	Elaine Whitehouse & Warwick Pudney	New Society Publishers
Blue Cheese Breath and Stinky Feet: How to Deal with Bullies	Catherine DePino	APA Magination Press
Don't Be a Menace on Sundays: The Children's Anti-Violence Book	Adolph Moser	Landmark Editions, Inc.
Don't Pop Your Cork on Mondays: The Children's Anti-Stress Book	Adolph Moser	Landmark Editions, Inc.
Don't Feed the Monsters on Tuesdays: The Children's Self-Esteem Book	Adolph Moser	Landmark Editions, Inc.
Don't Rant and Rave on Wednesdays: The Children's Anger-Control Book	Adolph Moser	Landmark Editions, Inc.
Don't Tell a Whopper on Fridays: The Children's Truth-Control Book	Adolph Moser	Landmark Editions, Inc.
4 Downs to Anger Control	Tom Letson	Finish Line Press
Eggbert, the Slightly Cracked Egg	Tom Ross	
How to Take the Grrrr Out of Anger	Elizabeth Verdick & Marjorie Lisovskis	Free Spirit Publishing
The Little Engine That Could	Watty Piper, George Hauman, & Doris Hauman	
I Want Your Moo		APA Magination Press
The Bear Who Lost His Sleep: A Story about Worrying Too Much	Jessica Lamb-Shapiro	Childswork/Childsplay, LLC

(*continued*)

Title	Author/developer	Publisher
The Hyena Who Lost Her Laugh: A Story about Changing Your Negative Thinking	Denise Gilgannon	Childswork/Childsplay, LLC
The Koala Who Wouldn't Cooperate: A Story about Responsible Behavior	Lawrence Shapiro	Childswork/Childsplay, LLC
The Lion Who Lost His Roar: A Story about Facing Your Fears	Marcia Shoshana Nass	Childswork/Childsplay, LLC
The Penguin Who Lost Her Cool: A Story about Controlling Your Anger	Marla Sobel	Childswork/Childsplay, LLC
The Rabbit Who Lost His Hop: A Story about Self-Control	Marcia Shoshanna Nass	Childswork/Childsplay, LLC
Words Are Not for Hurting	Elizabeth Verdick	Free Spirit Publishing

Therapy/psychoeducation/gradual exposure

A Guide for Teen Survivors	Barbara Bean & Shari Bennett	Jossey-Bass Publishers
A Place for Starr	Howard Schor	Kidsrights: 1-800-892-5437
A Safe Place to Live (available in Spanish)	Michelle A. Harrison	Kidsrights: 1-800-892-5437
A Terrible Thing Happened	Margaret M. Holmes	APA Magination Press
Back on Track: Boys Dealing with Sexual Abuse	Leslie Bailey Wright & Mindy B. Loiselle	
Brave Bart: A Story for Traumatized and Grieving Children	Caroline Sheppard	The Institute for Trauma and Loss in Children: 313-885-0390
I Can't Talk about It: A Child's Book about Sexual Abuse	Doris Sanford	Gold'n Honey

Title	Author/developer	Publisher
In Their Own Words: A Sexual Abuse Workbook for Teenage Girls	Lulie Munson & Karen Riskin	
It Happened to Me: A Teen's Guide to Overcoming Sexual Abuse	Wm. Lee Carter	
No More Secrets for Me	Orly Wachter	
The Trouble with Secrets	Karen Johnson	
Personal Safety		
Let's Talk about Taking Care of You!	Lori Stauffer & Esther Deblinger	Hope for Families, Inc.: 215-280-5369
It's My Body	Lory Freeman	Parenting Press Inc.
Your Body Belongs to You	Cornelia Spelman	
My Body Is Private	Linda Walvoord Girard	
The Teen Relationship Workbook	Kerry Moles	Wellness Reproductions and Publishing, Inc.: 1-800-669-9208
Uncle Willy's Tickles		APA Magination Press
No Body's Perfect: Stories by Teens about Body Image	Kimberly Kirberger	
Sex/relationship education		
Where Did I Come From?	Peter Mayle	Kensington Publishing Corp.
Spanish language resources		
Amor y Limites	Elizabeth Crary	Parenting Press, Inc.
Bright Spots—Thoughts and Feelings Card Game	Lisa Marie Arneson	Bright Spots Games
Self-Calming Cards/ Tarjetas para calmarse	Elizabeth Crary & Mits Katayama	Parenting Press, Inc.

(continued)

Title	Author/developer	Publisher
Everybody Has Feelings/ Todos Tenemos Sentimientos. The Moods of Children	Sandra Marulanda	Gryphon House, Inc.
Fernando Furioso	Hiawyn Oram	Ediciones Ekare
Gana la Guerra de los Berrinches y Otras Contiendas: Un plan de paz familiar	Cynthia Whitman	Perspective Publishing
La guia de los niños a quien tu puedes confiar: Protegete en la casa, en la escuela y el Internet	Catalina Herrerías	Kidsrights: 1-800-892-5437
Las Palabras Dulces	Carl Norac	Editorial Corimbo
Luisa dice palabrotas	Chirstian Lamblin	Luis Vives Editorial
Palabras Sabias Acerca de la Disciplina video (DVD)	James Sayre	University Distibutor: Active Parenting Publishers
Somos un Arcoiris/We Are a Rainbow	Nancy Maria Grande Tabor	Charlesbridge
Tanya y el Hombre Tobo	Lesley Koplow	Magination Press

8

Play Interventions for Children with Autism

Connie Kasari, Linh Huynh, and Amanda C. Gulsrud

P_{lay} is recognized as a critical aspect of child development. The ability to play with toys and with others contributes to early social, cognitive, language and representational/symbolic development, as well as to physical and emotional well-being (Casby, 2008). Play is often referred to as a reflection of cognitive development, and play skills occur in a sequential order, beginning from simple manipulative play, to functional play, to symbolic or representational play (Naber et al., 2008). In typically developing children, the progression of play skills arises without explicit instructions (Garvey, 1991). However, in children with autism, play has been described as absent or rigid and nonsymbolic. Developmental differences in play have been attributed to delays or deficits in cognitive and/or social development (Jarrold, Boucher, & Smith, 1996).

DEVELOPMENT OF PLAY
IN TYPICALLY DEVELOPING CHILDREN

Much work has been done on the developmental sequences of play in typically developing infants and toddlers. These sequences become important to consider, as children with autism show specific patterns of development in which some aspects of play are more difficult to acquire than are others (Minor, 2003). In this chapter we will focus on three categories of play: functional play with toys, symbolic play with toys, and social play with others around play routines.

Functional play develops at around 14 months of age in typically developing children and is characterized when the child assigns a function to an object. Functional play is defined as "the appropriate use of an object or the conventional association of two or more objects, such as a spoon to feed a doll, or placing a teacup on a saucer" (Ungerer & Sigman, 1981). Generally speaking, functional play involves the act of manipulating an object as a means for practice and eventual mastery of action schemas.

Symbolic/pretend play develops around 18–24 months of age and is considered a higher level or more sophisticated type of play than functional play. Symbolic/pretend play requires the ability to transform objects and actions symbolically; involves role taking, script knowledge, and improvisation; and is accompanied by social dialogue and negotiation (Jarrold, Boucher, & Smith, 1993; McCune-Nicolich, 1981). For play to be considered symbolic, the child has to manipulate objects to represent real-world interpretations, generate new ideas, and shift attention from one interpretation of toys to another. Symbolic/pretend play also provides opportunities to practice and understand the events occurring in daily life and the social world (Piaget, 1952). It can also be characterized as involving simulative or nonliteral behaviors (Fein, 1981), such as acting as if something is the case when in reality it is not (Leslie, 1987). Symbolic/pretend play takes three forms: object substitution, the attribution of false properties, and the attribution of presence to imaginary objects (Leslie, 1987). What separates symbolic play from functional play is the concept of pretense. *Pretense* is the involvement of first-order representation and a metarepresentation, a second-order representation about the first representation (Leslie, 1987). In other words, in pretend play a child must be aware of the primary representation of an object while being aware of the pretend identity of the same object.

Social Play shifts developmentally from play that begins as object-focused without the acknowledgment of others to social interaction that involves at least one other individual (Jordon, 2003). Through socialization children become aware of play by other children. They may play alongside other children, be aware of them, and even mirror their play. This type of play often leads to play that becomes more coordinated with others, and involves both cooperative and competitive social play (Jordon, 2003). Ultimately, socially engaged play leads to the development of more selective playmates and even friendships (Hartup & Sancilio, 1986). Social pretend play can serve as a basis for learning about relationships, trust, compromise, and negotiation (Howes & Matheson, 1992).

PLAY AND AUTISM

Recent reviews of the research on play in children with autism point to several major themes. First, many researchers have studied the development of object-based play and particularly the emergence of functional and symbolic play in children with autism. Although functional play may be delayed in emergence and/or may be repetitive in nature, it is relatively intact when compared to the marked deficits in the acquisition of symbolic or pretend play (e.g., Baron-Cohen, 1987; Jarrold et al., 1993). Compared to children with developmental delays and to typically developing children, several replications have shown that children with autism show reduced frequency, complexity, novelty, and spontaneity in pretend play with objects and particularly dolls (Baron-Cohen, 1987; Bernabei, Camaioni, & Levi, 1999; Doherty & Rosenfeld, 1984; Gould, 1986).

An issue has been the degree to which the difficulties in pretend play are due to performance or competence issues. Many studies have highlighted the limited spontaneous initiation of pretend play in children with autism (Riguet, Taylor, Benaroya, & Klein, 1981; Ungerer & Sigman, 1981; Rutherford, Young, Hepburn, & Rogers, 2007). Children with autism when left unstructured or on their own produce very little spontaneously initiated examples of pretend play; thus, they demonstrate a significant deficit in performance. In contrast, when children with autism are given prompts to perform, studies indicate that these children can engage in pretend play, and often are not different from matched nonautistic children. These results suggest that the difficulties children are experiencing may be related to performance more than competence (Charman & Baron-Cohen, 1997; Jarrold et al., 1996; Lewis & Boucher, 1995; Rutherford et al., 2007). However, Jarrold (2003) and Charman & Baron-Cohen (1997) noted that children might be using the items logically (in pretend fashion but not truly using pretense). Thus, the child might figure out how to use items in ways that are "expected pretend acts" given the limited items available and by using his or her best guess.

Second, and more recently, there has been a shift to emphasize the social aspects of play. Interpersonal and affective aspects of play have not been emphasized in research studies, and yet children generally learn play routines through interactions with more skilled partners, such as the parent (Vygotsky, 1967). These play routines are marked by shared positive affect and attention, joint engagement, and enjoyment. Hobson, Lee, and Hobson (2009) have recently examined performance and competence of pretend play in children with autism by examining the qualitative aspects of their representations. Children with autism did as well as comparison children with developmental delays on the mechanics of play, including substitutions and attributing pretend properties. However, they showed less playful pretend acts during both modeled and spontaneous play conditions. Children with autism did not show creativity and fun in pretending. This is an area that requires further study, particularly with younger children, as the children in this study were between 7 and 13 years of age.

Moving play interactions from a parent or other adult to peers requires greater flexibility and awareness on the part of the child. McGee, Feldman, and Morrier (1997) found that children with autism demonstrated fewer peer-related social behaviors, neither initiating nor responding to social bids made by their peers. They also exhibited higher rates of inappropriate and rigid toy use, had restricted interests in toy play, demonstrated less shared attention and affect, and engaged in more repetitive and stereotyped behaviors. These children may be missing the playful, creative, and flexible nature of play that is necessary in order to gain peers' attention. As a result, typically developing children may not be readily responsive to children with autism. Indeed, studies often find that typically developing children tend to play with other typically developing children (Strain, 1984).

Theoretical Explanations of Deficits in Pretend Play

There are several proposed theories for the deficits in pretend play found in children with autism. Leslie (1987) suggests that pretend play requires the same type of cognitive metarepresentational capacity found in the concept of theory of mind (ToM). ToM is the capacity to develop understanding of other people as subjective beings, with their own experiences and perspectives (Baron-Cohen, Leslie, & Frith, 1985). Although there has been some empirical support linking pretend play skills and ToM abilities, the view that pretend play requires the capacity of metarepresentation similar to ToM has not been widely accepted (Charman et al., 2003).

Other theories suggest that deficits in pretend play are linked to impairments in executive function. *Executive function* includes the idea of generativity, the ability to plan ahead in a sequence of action, the formulation and initiation of goal-directed behaviors, working memory, and the ability to generate novel behaviors (Jarrold et al., 1996). Children with autism show deficits in a variety of executive function tasks (Hughes & Russell, 1993), and these impairments may affect the child's ability to organize and execute play. However, deficits in play cannot be solely explained by deficits in executive functioning. Rutherford et al. (2007) found that play deficits in children with autism affected both spontaneous play where novel ideas could be generated by the child and scaffolded play that involved engagement in play with others with social support and modeling (Rutherford et al., 2007). Thus, although executive functioning has been related to impairments of organization and execution of play, it has not been shown to be solely responsible for impairments in play.

Despite several theories about deficits in pretend play in children with autism, none has satisfactorily explained the wide range and expansive deficits seen. Instead, researchers have begun to explore the correlates or relationships of play to other areas of development such as language, attachment style, and joint attention.

The Relationship of Play to Other Developmental Constructs

Studies of typically developing children have suggested that the emergence of symbolic play facilitates language development (Lewis, 2003; McCune, 1995; Tamis-LeMonda & Bornstein, 1994). Studies of children with autism find associations between language development and play skills both concurrently and over time. Children with autism who had poor language comprehension spontaneously produced less object-directed and self-directed functional play than children with autism with better language comprehension (Ungerer & Sigman, 1981). In addition, children with autism who had better language comprehension produced more symbolic play with the help of additional instructions and modeling. Another study reported significant associations between the number of symbolic play acts and both expressive and receptive language using the Reynell Developmental Language Scales (Mundy, Sigman, Ungerer, & Sherman, 1987). Most studies do not test the relationship of play skills to later language development; thus, the relationship between play and language development in children is not fully understood.

Studies have also pointed to attachment style as a construct related to the development of play behaviors in children with autism. In a study investigating manipulative, functional, and symbolic play behaviors of toddlers with and without autism, the type of attachment style predicted play behaviors (Naber et al., 2008). In the study, the children with autism who displayed secure attachment had better play behaviors, showed higher levels of play, displayed more symbolic play, and spent more time playing compared to children without secure attachment. Although children with autism displaying secure attachment engaged in more instances of pretend play, pretend play skills were still developmentally delayed.

The development of pretend play also appears to be linked to joint attention. *Joint attention* is the triadic coordination of attention between the child, another person, and an object or event (Bakeman & Adamson,

1984), and reflects the children's awareness of another's attention, intention, and affect (Charman, 2003). Children with autism are known to be impaired in the production and comprehension of joint attention gestures and the ability to follow or monitor someone's gaze (Mundy, Sigman, Ungerer, & Sherman, 1986; Mundy, Sigman, & Kasari, 1990). Moreover, children with autism who spend a relatively large proportion of time engaged in restricted object use appear less aware of adult attentional directives, prompts, and models to imitate (Brucker & Yoder, 2007). The correlational nature of this study makes it difficult to determine if limitations in joint attention lead to more object-focused play or vice versa. Restricted object use that is more stereotyped and repetitive also likely interferes with play development to a greater extent than restricted object use due to other developmental considerations (Stahmer & Schreibman, 1992).

However, the relationship between joint attention and play for children with autism is not clear. First, there is little data on the relation between these two constructs, particularly in longitudinal or experimental studies. In one longitudinal study on the correlates of play development in children with autism, a number of developmental constructs were examined including executive functions, joint attention, imitation, and cognitive abilities. While children with autism were profoundly delayed in both competence (prompted) measures and performance (spontaneous) measures of pretend play, only joint attention predicted changes in pretend play from 2 to 3 years of age (Rutherford et al., 2007). Thus, these data suggest that joint attention skills should be further examined for their role in the development of pretend play acts.

There is also some data to suggest that changes in joint attention skills are associated with changes in lower levels of functional play but not higher levels of pretend play (Kasari et al., 2006; Kasari et al., 2010). In a randomized controlled trial, children who were taught to engage in more joint attention gestures also improved in functional play acts, although these were not directly targeted (Kasari et al., 2006). Changes in pretend play did not occur unless these skills were specifically taught. In another experimental intervention study, mothers who were able to engage their children in joint engagement and play routines had children who improved in functional play skills and joint attention responding skills. Because these children were very young (between 2 and 3 years of age) and the intervention was short term (24 sessions), these data suggest that some aspects of joint attention and play are interrelated but that skills remain developmentally delayed in children with autism (Kasari et al., 2010). Future studies may want to examine these constructs and their interrelationships more closely.

PLAY INTERVENTIONS

Despite the documented difficulties children with autism have in playing symbolically with toys, intervention programs rarely target symbolic or pretend play. In practice, particularly in programs that utilize applied behavior analysis (ABA) as a teaching methodology, play is most often addressed in one of two ways. First, a child is taught to use toys appropriately. Thus, an adult may demonstrate the functional use of a toy, such as pushing a truck. The child correctly responds when he or she imitates the actions of the adult. Second, play is often offered as reinforcement (a break from work times) in which the child is allowed time to play without adult intervention. An issue is whether these behavioral approaches to teaching play yield generative play routines for the child with autism that are marked by flexibility, creativity, and fun.

Play intervention studies are rare. These studies are characterized by single-subject designs that are mostly behavioral in approach, and focus on discrete play acts. The behavioral approach relies on a wide range of ABA techniques (e.g., discrete trial training, differential reinforcement, reciprocal imitation, pivotal response training, self-management training, video modeling, and play scripts) and participants are reported to improve with intervention (Stahmer, Ingersoll, & Carter, 2003). The focus of most studies is on teaching children with autism to engage appropriately with toys or to demonstrate the functional use of objects (e.g. Santarcangelo, Dyer, & Luce, 1987; Stahmer & Schreibman, 1992; Nuzzolo-Gomez, Leonard, Ortiz, Rivera, & Greer, 2002). Although generalization to different settings or across different people is sometimes programmed, maintenance and generalization of taught skills remains problematic (Santarcangelo et al., 1987; Stahmer & Schreibman, 1992).

Fewer studies have focused on "pretend" or symbolic play in children with autism. These studies tend to blend methods of ABA and developmental approaches for more naturalistic teaching opportunities. Lifter, Sulzer-Azaroff, Anderson, and Cowdery (1993) demonstrated the importance of considering the developmental level of the child in teaching play skills. These authors used principles of discrete trial training to teach children with autism to play at an emerging level of play in their developmental repertoire or at a higher level of play consistent with their chronological age. Results of this single-subject design study demonstrated that the three children involved learned the play skills better when they showed developmental readiness for the skills, rather than assuming the skills should match their chronological age. In a later study, Lifter, Ellis, Cannon, and Anderson (2005) used a single-subject design to examine the acquisition of a wide variety of play skills in children with autism, and again found that targeting skills that were emerging in a child's repertoire was a more successful strategy than teaching skills that were more advanced but absent from his or her repertoire. Thus, children were better able to maintain and generalize skills that were taught to their developmental level.

The importance of teaching at the child's developmental level has not often been implemented in studies of symbolic play. Several studies have used naturalistic behavioral methods to teach symbolic play skills but rarely specify the play abilities of children prior to interventions. While these studies note success in teaching children the targeted skills, they often identify limited maintenance and generalization of the taught skills. One reason may be that the targeted skills are not within the child's current developmental frame.

Studies have focused less on the developmental appropriateness or the "what to teach" and more on the teaching technique, or the "how" of intervening with children with autism. Pivotal response training (PRT) is an intervention approach that utilizes both behavioral (e.g., contingent reinforcement, prompting) and naturalistic (e.g., following the child's lead) techniques within the child's natural play environment. Stahmer (1995) used PRT techniques and reported that all seven participants improved in the complexity and creativity of their symbolic play acts. Similarly, Thorpe, Stahmer, and Schreibman (1995) found that PRT was effective in teaching three boys sociodramatic play. While both of these studies reported positive effects, it is not clear the extent to which changes resulted in the *spontaneous initiation* of a range of play routines that could be characterized as playful, symbolic, and flexible.

Another issue that has received less attention in teaching children with autism is the availability of the play partner. In a study by Stahmer (1995), children played better with the therapist than with peers or with their mother. In addition, Thorpe et al. (1995) also found poorer generalization from therapist to mother. It is likely that peers and parents need to be brought into the teaching activities in order for the skills to generalize more smoothly. On the other hand, it is unclear if all of the children were showing developmental readiness to learn the play skills that were targeted.

Another issue is the familiarity and social nature of the play partners. Children often develop more playful, symbolic, and flexible play when interacting with others. Several studies have attempted to teach children with autism to engage in social play with others. Jahr, Eldrvik, and Eikeseth (2000) used *in vivo* modeling and imitation to teach social play. All six participants improved to the criteria of "mastery" of cooperative play and also improved in social validity measures of play rated by their teachers. Baker (2000) reported positive effects of a social play intervention for three siblings with autism by encouraging social play and positive affect and decreasing repetitive behaviors. Recently Liber, Frea, and Symon (2008) utilized a time-delay procedure to teach social play to three children with autism in a school setting. Results showed improvements in children learning the play sequence and becoming less dependent on adult prompts. Skill generalization occurred for two of the three children. These studies suggest that children with autism can learn to play with toys either functionally or symbolically and engage in social play with age mates when directly taught using principles of ABA.

Using ABA principles to teach play have met its share of criticism. On the whole, the structure, repetition, and marked hierarchical sequencing of tasks seem to defy the very nature of play that is characterized by flexibility, spontaneity, and little to no structure (Luckett, Bundy, & Roberts, 2007). One might argue that more naturalistic methods based upon the child's motivations and free from the constraints of the imposed structure of ABA would be a better fit for encouraging play (e.g., techniques of PRT, or developmental approaches such as Floortime). Teaching at the child's developmental level may be another factor as opposed to a set hierarchical structure that is predetermined in an ABA curriculum (Lifter et al., 1993). One issue that is unclear from most studies of play is whether the play repertoires of children with autism have changed to reflect truly integrated, generative play that is marked by flexibility and fun in playing.

In a recent review of teaching pretend play to children with disabilities, Barton and Wolery (2008) identified 10 studies that focused on children with autism (constituting 91 subjects altogether). All of the studies were single-subject designs involving two to seven subjects with the exception of one group design involving 58 children. While most studies utilized a multiple-baseline design, not all studies demonstrated good experimental control. Thus, some studies did not evidence a stable baseline before implementing an intervention and therefore could not rule out maturation. Other studies had overlapping data across conditions that was greater than 10% of data observed in a condition or lack of consistency in level or trend in order to establish experimental control (i.e., proof that the intervention caused the change in child behavior). This review of published data highlights problems with our current knowledge of play interventions for children with autism. Most concerning is the lack of experimental control in studies where authors concluded that significant changes occurred. The few subjects in each study are also a concern if data do not clearly demonstrate the efficacy of the intervention.

Studies of Play Interventions at the University of California, Los Angeles

To date there has only been one randomized controlled intervention study of play skills in children with autism. This group design involved teaching children with autism play skills with follow up assessments 6 and 12 months postintervention. The intervention itself was carried out daily for approximately 30 minutes for 5–6 weeks. Participants were 3- and 4-year-old children with autism who were enrolled in the same hospital-based early intervention program. This program provided 6 hours per day of intensive ABA-based services to children with autism 5 days per week. Average stays in this outpatient program were typically 5–6 weeks. The ABA program did not teach joint attention or symbolic play skills in keeping with typical ABA curricula at the time. Children with autism ($N = 58$) were randomized to an intervention focused on teaching joint attention skills, symbolic play skills, or the control condition that was the regular ABA program only.

The approach used in teaching children involved behavioral strategies of modeling and prompting along with developmental procedures of responsive and facilitative teaching (Kasari, Freeman, & Paparella, 2006). Each session began with a brief, 5-minute table-based episode of ABA, discrete trial training in order to prime children for the targeted goal. Thus, a child learning to use substitutions would be presented multiple trials across three different toy sets that involved substituting one item to stand in for another. After working at the table, the child would transfer play to the floor where there were many different toys available along with the ones used at the table. During the floor play, lasting approximately 20 minutes, the therapist would use developmental strategies of following the child's lead, expanding play routines, and language targets, as well as behavioral strategies of contingent and natural reinforcement, modeling, and prompting. Each child's play targets were individually and developmentally determined, and a variety of play routines were developed.

Similar to the work by Lifter et al. (2005), we chose teaching targets based on the child's current level of play development. Most often those targets were emerging in the child's repertoire. We began with functional play targets if that is where the child was functioning. We then moved through the play sequence developmentally as children mastered each play level. We paid particular attention to counting only spontaneous initiations of play acts, and helped children to develop generalized and novel acts of play.

Results of this first study demonstrate that play skills can be taught to a varied group of children with autism, and that these skills generalize to their mothers who were not involved in the intervention. Several features of the intervention are noteworthy. First, beginning treatment at the child's current developmental level of play led to increases in play level on an independently administered play assessment, and in diversity of their play acts when interacting with their mothers (also see Lifter et al., 1993). *Diversity of play acts* refers to the number of different types of play children used within a single level of play. Thus, if a child learned to substitute one item to stand in for another, he or she needed to spontaneously (unprompted) demonstrate a substitution across three different play sets for three consecutive sessions. For example, the child might use a block to make a slide, a pencil as a toothbrush for the doll, and a piece of sponge to represent a cracker for the doll to eat. All of these acts would be carried out within play routines with the goal of being marked by flexibility, creativity, and fun.

Second, the children generalized skills that they learned with the therapist to their mothers who were not involved in the treatment of their children. These data represent a far generalization of the intervention, and suggest that the skills were solidly in the child's repertoire in order for him or her to demonstrate them with a new partner.

Third, while children participating in the play intervention made greater gains in play than children in the other two groups (joint attention and control ABA), all of the children improved in their functional use of toys as a result of early intervention (a time effect). Only the children in the playgroup significantly improved in symbolic play, suggesting that changes can be made only when children are directly taught how to play (Stahmer,1995). Moreover, both play level and diversity of play acts significantly improved only for children in the play group.

Finally, in following up on these children 1 year later, both the joint attention and play group improved significantly more in expressive language than the control group (Kasari, Paparella, Freeman, & Jahromi, 2008). One reason for the similarity in outcome for both experimental groups may be that joint engagement (i.e., social play) was enhanced in the interventions. Thus in both the joint attention and the play interventions, the child played with a responsive adult who was sensitive to his or her developmental level and abilities, and he or she was better able to engage socially with others as a result.

In the 1970s, Bruner (1974–1975; Ninio & Bruner, 1978; Ratner & Bruner, 1978) described how mothers scaffold their children's early development of language through nonlinguistic, object-mediated social interaction routines. These routines (e.g., book reading, repetitive baby games) become an important context for mother and child to jointly attend to the same topic, and for the baby to identify the referential context of mother's language. These interactions, structured around a mutual topic, are referred to as "joint engagement" and can be thought of as a state of being as opposed to a particular discrete skill. Adamson, Bakeman, and Deckner (2004) have closely examined these engagement states and find that mutually attending to the same object/event is associated with early language skills in typically developing infants in the age range of 18 to 30 months. In particular, mother–infant dyads spend the most time in periods where mother and child attend to the same focus or topic and the child is not required to communicate with obvious communication intent (e.g., looking to mother, showing toys). The amount of time children spend in this "supported joint engagement" state is associated with later language development. Similarly Tomasello and Farrar (1986) found that young children who engaged in longer episodes of joint engagement with their mothers had larger vocabularies. Thus, mothers who maintain a focus of attention on the same play topic with their child leads to a number of important child development outcomes.

Theoretically, then, increasing joint engagement between the child with autism and others could provide an important platform for the development of skills, such as communication and play. In a subsequent study, we taught caregivers to jointly engage their children with autism. The goal of this intervention was to teach caregivers strategies to improve their children's focus of attention, and increase engagement, joint attention and play skills (Kasari et al., 2010). Children were randomly assigned to one of the two conditions, immediate active treatment or wait-list control condition.

Compared to the wait-list group, the active treatment dyads improved in the duration of time jointly engaged in play interactions and children decreased the amount of isolative object-based play. These children expanded the variety of toy play with their mothers by engaging in more varied play acts after the intervention. Treatment children also responded more to their mother's joint attention bids. These skills maintained at a follow-up visit 1 year later. Thus, these data highlight the importance of social play, or engagement with others, as a foundation upon which other developmental skills can be taught, including joint attention and play skills.

The Future of Play Interventions for Children with Autism

The studies reviewed in this chapter point to several areas of research that need expansion in order for us to confidently recommend effective practices. First, there are few studies of interventions for teaching play to children with autism. Current studies tend to be behavioral in approach, limited in their focus on play skills (i.e., often discrete single skills), and mostly single-subject designs that are often reported with inadequate experimental control (Barton & Wolery, 2008). The field clearly needs more rigorously designed studies that demonstrate efficacy for teaching play to children with autism.

Second, while one randomized controlled trial has been published of a symbolic play intervention for children with autism, replications are needed before one can safely recommend changes to current early intervention practices. The results of this study suggest that diversity of play acts and play level can be improved in children with autism, and that when children are taught at their developmental level they also can generalize improved joint engagement and play with their mothers. A number of elements of this study deserve further investigation. One is whether the separate priming and naturalistic play elements are both necessary for teaching play to children with autism. It may be that particular children may benefit more or less from each approach. Our understanding of fitting a particular intervention to individual children requires further study. Another element concerns the social nature of the play intervention in which a responsive adult engages the child in developmentally targeted play routines that are marked by joint engagement and playful interactions (Sherratt, 2002). Future studies will need to determine the importance of joint engagement in play routines as foundational for improving discrete skills of joint attention, or the diversity of play acts.

Finally, more attention needs to be paid to the agent of change for children with autism. Most studies use an expert therapist or a teacher to intervene on play skills with the child with autism. Studies are just beginning to use parents to mediate change in their children with autism, but the approaches used vary widely from parent education to direct coaching of parents with their children. The content of these coaching sessions is also important to consider, with some focused on attention-eliciting aspects of interaction, and others on communication strategies. Few focus on play or social play routines. Social play relies heavily on the social partner; more attention needs to be paid to how this partner helps the child create socially meaningful and fun play routines that are generative. Methodologically rigorous studies are needed to compare these different methods of working with parents and/or other social partners.

Ultimately children will need to transfer these play skills to peers who will be less expert social partners than the therapist or parent. Social pretend play becomes important for the further development of healthy peer interactions and friendships for young children (Howes & Matheson, 1992). Thus, helping children with autism develop peer play that is jointly engaged and playful will likely help them to continue to develop their play skills, and to ultimately to fit into the social networks of their classrooms (Chamberlain, Kasari, & Rotheram-Fuller, 2007).

REFERENCES

Adamson, L. B., Bakeman, R., & Deckner, D. F. (2004). The development of symbol-infused joint engagement. *Child Development, 75*(4), 1171–1187.

Bakeman, R., & Adamson, L. B. (1984). Coordinating attention to people and objects in mother infant and peer infant interaction. *Child Development, 55,* 1278–1289.

Baker, M. J. (2000). Incorporating the thematic ritualistic behaviors of children with autism into games: Increasing social play interactions with siblings. *Journal of Positive Behavior Interventions, 2*(2), 66–84.

Baron-Cohen, S. (1987). Autism and symbolic play. *British Journal of Developmental Psychology, 5,* 139–148.

Baron-Cohen, S., Leslie, A. M., & Frith, U. (1985). Does the autistic child have a "theory of mind"? *Cognition, 21,* 37–46.

Barton, E. E., Wolery, M. (2008). Teaching pretend play to children with disabilities: A review of the literature. *Topics in Early Childhood Special Education, 28*(2), 109–125.

Bernabei, P., Camaioni, L., & Levi, G. (1999). An evaluation of early development in children with autism and pervasive developmental disorders from home movies: Preliminary findings. *Autism, 2,* 243–258.

Brucker, C. T., & Yoder, P. (2007). Restricted object use in young children with autism: Definition and construct validity. *Autism, 11,* 161–171.

Bruner, J. S. (1974–1975). From communication to language: A psychological perspective. *Cognition, 3*(3), 255–287.

Casby, M. W. (2008). The development of play in infants, toddlers, and young children. *Communication Disorders Quarterly, 24*(4), 163–174.

Chamberlain, B., Kasari, C., & Rotheram-Fuller, E. (2007). Involvement or isolation?: The social networks of children with autism in regular classrooms. *Journal of Autism and Developmental Disorders, 37*(2), 230–242.

Charman, T. (2003). Why is Joint Attention a pivotal skill in autism? In U. Frith & E. Hill (Eds.), *Autism: Mind and brain* (pp. 67–87). New York: Oxford University Press.

Charman, T., & Baron-Cohen, S. (1997). Brief report: Prompted pretend play in autism. *Journal of Autism and Developmental Disorders, 27*(3), 325–332.

Charman, T., Baron-Cohen, S., Swettenham, J., Baird, G., Drew, A., & Cox, A. (2003). Predicting language outcome in infants with autism and pervasive developmental disorder. *International Journal of Language and Communication Disorders, 38*(3), 265–285.

Charman, T., Swettenham, J., Baron-Cohen, S., Cox, A., Baird, G., & Drew, A. (1997). Infants with autism: An investigation of empathy, pretend play, joint attention, and imitation. *Developmental Psychology, 33*(5), 781–789.

Doherty, M. B., & Rosenfeld, A. A (1984). Play assessment in the differential diagnosis of autism and other causes of severe language disorder. *Journal of Developmental and Behavioral Pediatrics, 5,* 26–29.

Fein, G. G. (1981). Pretend play in childhood: An integrative review. *Child Development, 52,* 1095–1118.

Garvey, C. (1991). *Play* (2nd ed.). London: Fontana Press.

Gould, J. (1986). The Lowe and Costello Symbolic Play Test in socially impaired children. *Journal of Autism and Developmental Disorders, 16*, 199–213.

Hobson, R. P., Lee, A., & Hobson, J. A. (2009). Qualities of symbolic play among children with autism: A social-developmental prospective. *Journal of Autism and Developmental Disorders, 39*, 12–22.

Howes, C., & Matheson, C. (1992). Sequences in the development of competent play with peers: Social and social pretend play. *Developmental Psychology, 28*(5), 961–974.

Hughes, C., & Russell, J. (1993). Autistic children's difficulty with mental disengagement from an object: Its implication for theories of autism. *Developmental Psychology, 29*, 498–510.

Hartup, W. W., & Sancilio, M. F. (1986). Children's friendships. In E. Schopler & G. B. Mesibov (Eds.), *Social behaviour in autism* (pp. 61–79). New York: Plenum Press.

Jahr, E., Eldevik, S., & Eikeseth, S. (2000). Teaching children with autism to initiate and sustain cooperative play. *Research in Developmental Disabilities, 21*(2), 151–169.

Jarrold, C. (2003). A review of research into pretend play in autism. *Autism, 7*(4), 379–390.

Jarrold, C., Boucher, J., & Smith, P. (1993). Symbolic play in autism: A review. *Journal of Autism and Development Disorders, 23*, 281–308.

Jarrold, C., Boucher, J., & Smith, P. (1996). Generativity defects in pretend play in autism. *British Journal of Developmental Psychology, 14*(3), 275–300.

Jordon, R. (2003). Social play and autistic spectrum disorders: A perspective on theory, implications and educational approaches. *Autism, 7*(4), 347–360.

Kasari, C., Gulsrud, A., Wong, C., Kwon, S., & Locke, J. (2010). Randomized controlled caregiver mediated joint engagement intervention for toddlers with autism. *Journal of Autism and Developmental Disorders.*

Kasari, C., Paparella, T., Freeman, S., & Jahromi, L. (2008). Language outcome in autism: Randomized comparison of joint attention and play interventions. *Journal of Consulting and Clinical Psychology, 76*(1), 125–137.

Kasari, C., Freeman, S., & Paparella, T. (2006). Joint attention and symbolic play in young children with autism: A randomized controlled intervention study. *Journal of Child Psychology and Psychiatry, 47*(6), 611–620.

Leslie, A. (1987). Pretense and representation: The origins of "theory of mind." *Psychological Review, 94*(4), 412–426.

Lewis, V. (2003). Play and language in children with autism. *Autism, 7*(4), 391–399.

Lewis, V., & Boucher, J. (1995). Generativity in the play of young people with autism. *Journal of Autism and Developmental Disorders, 25*(2), 105–121.

Liber, D. B., Frea, W. D., & Symon, J. B. G. (2008). Using time-delay to improve social play skills with peers for children with autism. *Journal of Autism and Developmental Disorders, 38*(2), 312–323.

Lifter, K., Ellis, J., Cannon, B., & Anderson, S. (2005). Developmental specificity in targeting and teaching play activities to children with pervasive developmental disorders. *Journal of Early Intervention, 27*(4), 247–267.

Lifter, K., Sulzer-Azaroff, B., Anderson, S. R., & Cowdery, G. E. (1993). Teaching play activities to preschool children with disabilities: The importance of developmental considerations. *Journal of Early Intervention, 17*(2), 139–159.

Luckett, T., Bundy, A., & Roberts, J. (2007). Do behavioural approaches teach children with autism to play or are they pretending? *Autism, 11*(4), 365–388.

McCune, L. (1995). A normative study of representational play in the transition to language. *Developmental Psychology, 31*(2), 198–206.

McCune-Nicolich, L. (1981). Toward symbolic functioning: Structure of early pretend games and potential parallels with language. *Child Development, 52*(3), 785–793.

McGee, G., Feldman, R., & Morrier, M. (1997). Benchmarks of social treatment for children with autism. *Journal of Autism and Developmental Disorders, 27*, 353–364.

Minor, L. A. (2003). The developmental progression of play in children with autism. *Dissertation Abstracts International Section A: Humanities and Social Sciences, 64*(2-A), 462.

Mundy, P., Sigman, M., & Kasari, C. (1990). A longitudinal study of joint attention and language development in autistic children. *Journal of Autism and Developmental Disorders, 20*(1), 115–128.

Mundy, P., Sigman, M., Ungerer, J., & Sherman, T. (1986). Defining the social deficits of autism: The contribution of non-verbal communication measures. *Journal of Child Psychology and Psychiatry and Allied Disciplines, 27*, 657–669.

Mundy, P., Sigman, M., Ungerer, J., & Sherman, T. (1987). Nonverbal communication and play correlates of language development in autistic children. *Journal of Autism and Developmental Disorders, 17*(3), 349–364.

Naber, F. B., Bakermans-Kranenburg, M. J., van IJzendoorn, M. H., Swinkels, S. H. N., Buitelaar, J. K., Dietz, C., et al. (2008). Play behavior and attachment in toddlers with autism. *Journal Autism Developmental Disorders, 38*, 857–866.

Ninio, A., & Bruner, J. (1978). The achievement and antecedents of labeling. *Journal of Child Language, 5*(1), 1–15.

Nuzzolo-Gomez, R., Leonard, M. A., Ortiz, E., Rivera, C. M., & Greer, R. D. (2002). Teaching children with autism to prefer books or toys over stereotypy or passivity. *Journal of Positive Behavior Intervention, 4*(2), 80–87.

Piaget, J. (1952). *Play, dreams, and imitation in childhood*. New York: Norton.

Ratner, N., & Bruner, J. (1978). Games, social exchange and the acquisition of language. *Journal of Child Language, 5*(3), 391–401.

Riguet, C. B., Taylor, N. D., Benaroya, S., & Klein, L. S. (1981). Symbolic play in autistic, Down's, and normal children of equivalent mental age. *Journal of Autism and Developmental Disorders, 11*(4), 439–448.

Rutherford, M. D., Young, G. S., Hepburn, S., & Rogers, S. J. (2007). A longitudinal study of pretend play in autism. *Journal of Autism and Developmental Disorders, 37*(6), 1024–1039.

Santarcangelo, S., Dyer, K., & Luce, S. C. (1987). Generalized reduction of disruptive behavior in unsupervised settings through specific toy training. *Journal of the Association for Persons with Severe Handicaps, 12*(1), 38–44.

Sherratt, D. (2002). Developing pretend play in children with autism: A case study. *Autism, 6*(2), 169–179.

Stahmer, A. C. (1995). Teaching symbolic play skills to children with autism using pivotal response training. *Journal of Autism and Developmental Disorders, 25*(2), 123–141.

Stahmer, A. C., Ingersoll, B., & Carter, C. (2003). Behavioral approaches to promoting play. *Autism, 7*(4), 401–413.

Stahmer, A. C., & Schreibman, L. (1992). Teaching children with autism appropriate play in unsupervised environments using a self-management treatment package. *Journal of Applied Behavior Analysis, 25*(2), 447–459.

Strain, P. S. (1984). Social behavior patterns of nonhandicapped and developmentally disabled friend pairs in mainstream preschools. *Analysis and Intervention in Developmental Disabilities, 4*, 15–28.

Tamis-LeMonda, C. S., & Bornstein, M. H. (1994). Specificity in mother–toddler language–play relations across the second year. *Developmental Psychology, 30*(2), 283–292.

Thorpe, D., Stahmer, A., & Schreibman, L. (1995). Effects of socio-dramatic play training on children with autism. *Journal of Autism and Developmental Disorders, 25*, 265–282.

Tomasello, M., & Farrar, M. J. (1986). Joint attention and early language. *Child Development, 57*, 1454–1463.

Ungerer, J. A., & Sigman, M. (1981). Symbolic play and language comprehension in autistic children. *Journal of the American Academy of Child Psychiatry, 20*, 318–337.

Vygotsky, L. S. (1967). Play and its role in the mental development of the child. *Soviet Psychology, 5*(3), 6–18.

9

Integrating Play into Cognitive-Behavioral Therapy for Child Anxiety Disorders

Donna B. Pincus, Rhea M. Chase, Candice Chow, Courtney L. Weiner, & Jessica Pian

> Play is the beginning of knowledge.
> —GEORGE DORSEY

Child clinicians who treat psychological disorders are acutely aware of the importance of finding ways to make treatment palatable to each individual child, to ensure that the treatment is presented in a way that is developmentally appropriate, and to employ methods that increase the child's motivation to engage in treatment. The use of play in therapy can address these issues within the context of evidence-based treatments for child psychological disturbances. This chapter focuses on the use of play to increase the effectiveness of treatment for childhood anxiety disorders. More specifically, the chapter explores how play can be used to facilitate the synthesis of concepts presented in the framework of cognitive-behavioral therapy (CBT), the most empirically supported treatment for child anxiety disorders. The purpose of this chapter is to introduce the theory, components, and structure of CBT; to discuss the role of play within the intervention; to illustrate the effectiveness of play in CBT; and to highlight future directions for research in this area.

CBT FOR CHILD ANXIETY DISORDERS

The foundation of CBT rests on the notion that an individual's maladaptive thoughts, learned behaviors, and negative environmental influences are what ultimately contribute to psychological disturbances. The primary goals of CBT, therefore, are to identify maladaptive thoughts and replace them with more adaptive ones, to teach the use of both cognitive and behavioral coping strategies in various situations, and to help the individual learn to regulate his or her own behaviors.

Currently, CBT is the most efficacious treatment for childhood anxiety disorders (Kazdin & Weisz, 1998; Velting, Setzer, & Albano, 2004). Several controlled studies have demonstrated the efficacy of CBT for anxiety disorders in youth (Barrett, Dadds, & Rapee, 1996; Kendall, 1994; Kendall et al., 1997). The cognitive-behavioral therapeutic process for children typically involves psychoeducation, problem-solving skills, and behavioral and cognitive coping strategies. These techniques teach children about the nature of anxiety; the ways in which anxious thoughts, emotions, physical sensations, and behaviors are linked; and adaptive coping methods to decrease the frequency and intensity of negative responses to the feared stimulus. These procedures increase positive behaviors such as assertiveness, social skills, focused attention, and relaxation, while decreasing more problematic behaviors such as anxiety and disruptive behavior.

Rather than focus on the historical antecedents of anxiety-related disturbances, CBT is directed at altering the factors that *maintain* anxiety and targets specific symptoms and behaviors. Because there are many common symptoms across different anxiety disorders, treatment strategies are fairly similar within this spectrum of psychological disturbance. CBT targets a child's thoughts, physical symptoms, and avoidance behaviors. The child is provided with skills to think about his or her fears in a more realistic way, to confront his or her fears and test their validity, and to react to his or her anxious sensations in a more adaptive way (Wagner, 2002).

The interventions employed in CBT protocols for child anxiety can be divided into fairly distinct behavioral and cognitive categories. Cognitive interventions within CBT include increasing realistic thinking, problem-solving skills training, and self-instruction training. Teaching children to increase their *realistic thinking* involves instructing them on how to identify and evaluate unrealistic thoughts and replace them with more realistic cognitions. *Problem-solving skills training* helps the child recognize that there are a number of possible solutions to any given problem. Often when in an anxiety-producing situation, children are unable to recognize solutions to a problem because they are overwhelmed by their emotions. Providing the child with problem-solving skills encourages the child to break down tasks into a series of steps, learn how to systematically test a variety of solutions to a given problem, and view stressful situations as more manageable. *Self-instruction training* is a technique that is particularly useful for a younger child, whose abstract cognitive abilities may not be as developed as those of an older child. Self-instruction encourages children to replace their anxious self-talk with calming self-talk. Rather than look for evidence in the situation to determine whether thoughts are realistic, children are encouraged to replace their worried thought with a calm thought.

The behavioral interventions within CBT seek to increase desired behaviors and decrease undesired behaviors. These interventions can include exposure, exposure and ritual prevention, and modeling. In *exposure*, the child approaches avoided situations and tests the reality of the fear. The goal of exposure is to help the child realize that the feared outcome usually does not occur in the given situation, and even if it does happen, the anxiety will dissipate over time. Thus, the experience allows the child to change his or her beliefs about the feared situation. *Exposure and ritual prevention* (ERP) is a type of exposure that is usually used to treat obsessive–compulsive disorder (OCD). While exposure involves confronting the situations or objects that trigger obsessions, ritual prevention involves refraining from engaging in the rituals that relieve the anxiety caused by the obsessions. In *interoceptive exposure*, a child purposely elicits the physical sensations associated with anxiety. For example, a child with panic disorder who fears symptoms of dizziness, nausea, and shortness of breath may be asked to spin in a chair or breathe through a small straw in order to induce those symptoms. Through repeated exposure to these physical sensations, the child learns that the somatic symptoms are not dangerous and that he or she can cope with the feelings in his or her body when they occur in real-life situations. *Modeling* involves watching an adult or another child approach and successfully cope with a feared situation. Modeling can be particularly useful for younger children who require some demonstration around how to employ the skills they learned through CBT.

CBT additionally introduces relaxation training to manage anxiety outside of exposure situations. For both children and adults, anxiety often manifests in physical sensations such as nausea/stomach upset, headache, tension, heart palpitations, trouble breathing, and muscle soreness. Through relaxation training, which typically involves deep breathing in conjunction with thinking of calming images or coping statements, children can begin to control their body's automatic reactions to anxiety-provoking events and objects. *Progressive muscle relaxation* (PMR) teaches a child to target specific muscle groups and notice and identify feelings of tension in order to contrast those feelings with relaxation. Learning to relax muscle groups allows the child to prevent the escalation of physical symptoms while in a stressful situation. It also provides the child with a way of exhibiting control over a situation that does not seem controllable. With practice, the child learns to elicit feelings of relaxation with minimal effort.

CONTEXTUAL FACTORS WITHIN CBT

An important component of the therapeutic process is child involvement in a collaborative process. The therapist and the child are both active participants in establishing treatment goals, the most effective coping strategies for the particular child, and the behavioral techniques that might maximize desired behaviors (Ehrenreich, Kyle-Linkovich, & Rojas-Vilches, 2005). In this way, the child is not merely a recipient of information but is instead able to apply the acquired skills in a way that allows him or her to eventually implement the cognitive-behavioral strategies on his or her own. As will be seen later in the chapter, incorporating play techniques into therapy can help consolidate presented information and provide more concrete, developmentally appropriate ways to think about the concepts taught in treatment.

CBT protocols also account for the child's family, friends, and school environment through the inclusion of additional treatment components that focus on environmental contingencies. Individuals in a child's environment may reinforce the child's maladaptive responses to feared stimuli or stressful situations. Young children often look to their parents or other caregivers for signals that inform them about emotional and behavioral regulation. When caregivers are not able to assist with providing their child with necessary coping skills or to model adaptive responses, the child is less likely to cope effectively with negative events. The younger the child, the more treatment should involve instructing parents on ways in which to teach their children self-control strategies. Even with older children, it is often beneficial to involve parents in session to maximize the effects of therapy in the home environment. The therapist needs to consider the child's family systems, relationships, and dynamics to develop the most effective treatment plan. To this end, it is helpful for the therapist to involve the parents, school, and child so that all players share in the responsibility of treatment.

While CBT incorporates specific behavioral, cognitive, and physical components, treatment is flexible, and the therapist has the opportunity to present information in a way that seems appropriate given a specific child's age, interests, and communication style. The working alliance with the child is as important in CBT as in any other treatment modality, and the therapist can be creative and playful to promote child engagement in treatment. Establishing rapport and maintaining child interest can increase communication and yield more rapid, positive results throughout the course of treatment.

The implementation of CBT with anxious children requires the clinician to be developmentally sensitive, and to consistently review concepts with concrete examples. A number of approaches that may be useful in CBT with adults might need to be tailored to reflect a child's age and developmental level. The therapist should provide tangible and appropriate examples, visual aids, images, memory aids, and age-appropriate language with the child. Play can be an important component in delivering the intervention in a way that is palatable to a child. The incorporation of play can solidify concepts, facilitate memorization and internalization of CBT skills, and increase rapport and the working alliance with the therapist.

TREATMENT PROTOCOLS FOR CHILD ANXIETY

The *Coping Cat Workbook* (Kendall, Kane, Howard, & Siqueland, 1990; Kendall & Hedtke, 2006) is the most widely disseminated manualized CBT protocol for anxiety developed specifically for children and adolescents. Due to its broad distribution, the protocol has been adapted for use in various geographical regions (e.g., the Coping Koala in Australia). The Coping Cat protocol is a time-limited intervention that is typically administered in 16–20 sessions and delivers traditional CBT strategies to youth in a developmentally appropriate manner. The protocol is broken down into two parts, with the first part focusing on skills training and the second on applying the newly acquired skills to anxiety-provoking situations.

During the first stage of treatment, patients are provided with psychoeducation about anxiety. Anxiety is broken down into three parts—cognitions, physiological sensations, and behaviors—which interact to maintain the cycle of anxiety. In the next stage of treatment, patients are introduced to the "FEAR" acronym, which stands for the four-step plan for coping with anxiety: "F—Feeling frightened?", "E—Expecting bad things to happen?", "A—Actions and attitudes that help", and "R—Rate and reward." In the first step, patients are taught to recognize the physiological sensations that they experience in anxiety-provoking situations. Once awareness of somatic responses to anxiety is increased, patients are provided with relaxation techniques, such as PMR, to reduce physiological arousal. The next step focuses on evaluating and correcting the cognitive distortions that characterize anxiety. Patients are playfully taught to become "detectives" and to seek out evidence for and against their anxious thoughts. Additionally, patients are encouraged to generate calm, coping thoughts to counter their worried thoughts. During the third step of the FEAR plan, children develop an anxiety management plan by learning how to produce alternative solutions for dealing with a situation and choosing a more appropriate plan of action. In the fourth and final step of the plan, patients are encouraged to monitor and rate their level of anxiety before and after implementing their coping skills and to reward themselves for their efforts.

Once patients are familiar with the FEAR plan, the last phase of treatment involves systematic, gradual exposure to feared and/or avoided situations. Together, the patient and clinician construct a "fear ladder". Several anxiety-provoking situations are operationally defined and exposures are approached in a graduated format, progressively targeting more difficult situations. Throughout treatment, patients are also given homework tasks to perform outside of session: "Show That I Can" (STIC) tasks. A distinguishing feature of CBT protocols developed for children, such as Coping Cat, is the inclusion of rewards to motivate patients to engage in challenging tasks. The inclusion of rewards is often an effective strategy to increase child motivation and engagement in treatment. Upon completion of the Coping Cat program, patients are encouraged to continuously practice the FEAR plan in their daily lives to increase the generalization of learning and maintain treatment gains.

Aside from the Coping Cat program and other CBT protocols designed to treat a broad spectrum of anxiety disorders, specialized cognitive-behavioral treatments for children and adolescents are available to target various problems, including depression, school refusal, and social anxiety. For instance, March and Mulle (1998) developed a manualized protocol for OCD in youth that includes psychoeducation, cognitive training, and systematic exposure. Similar to traditional CBT, ERP is a short-term, problem-focused intervention. However, the treatment specifically addresses the obsessive thoughts and compulsive behaviors characterizing OCD. During the first stage of treatment, children are educated about their disorder in a developmentally sensitive manner. OCD is described as a neurological disorder caused by "brain hiccups." The protocol suggests framing OCD treatment as the child "bossing back" or "talking back" to the disorder. OCD is presented as an antagonistic entity, and the child, parents, and therapist create a battle plan to challenge OCD. Children are encouraged to name their OCD (e.g., "Germy") to further externalize the disorder. Patients might even draw a caricature of their OCD to make therapy playful and provide a concrete representation of their OCD to "boss back." Clinicians are encouraged to continually use metaphors and examples to make the treatment more compelling and accessible to children.

In the beginning of treatment, patients map out their disorder. This process involves creating a visual representation of their experience and the aspects of their lives that are controlled by OCD. Patients are then informed that they will begin bossing back OCD to "win" against the disorder. The next stage of treatment focuses on cognitive training and involves teaching the patient strategies, such as constructive self-talk and cognitive restructuring, for coping with anxiety and resisting obsessions and compulsions. Finally, the exposure phase requires that the patient approach anxiety-provoking stimuli and refrain from engaging in subsequent anxiety-reducing rituals or avoidance behaviors. Due to the stressful nature of ERP, therapists are encouraged to include playful techniques, humorous story metaphors, and rewards with younger patients.

More recently, researchers have investigated the use of intensive forms of treatment for anxious youth. For instance, a 1-week "summer camp" intervention is currently being evaluated for treating girls ages 8–12 with separation anxiety disorder (SAD); (Santucci & Ehrenreich, 2007; Santucci, Ehrenreich, Bennett, Trasper, & Pincus, 2009). In this treatment, traditional cognitive-behavioral skills are delivered in an enjoyable camp setting that includes group activities, field trips, and a sleepover. Providing the treatment in a group format enables naturalistic exposure to separation situations while engaging in developmentally appropriate peer interactions. Throughout the week, parent involvement is gradually decreased to expose children to increasingly challenging separation situations. In addition to exposure, several other CBT techniques are incorporated into the camp, including relaxation exercises, cognitive restructuring, and developing coping statements and positive self-talk. The camp culminates in a sleepover on the final night, which is an activity that most of the patients have been fearful about and/or avoiding in their daily lives. The camp ends with a reward ceremony in front of parents in order to recognize and applaud treatment progress.

Thus, many existing CBT protocols for child anxiety disorders incorporate play techniques to increase their developmental sensitivity for younger populations. Current treatments for youth present the essential components of CBT through playful and engaging methods. The *Coping*

Cat Workbook presents the concept of realistic thinking as "detective work." March and Mulle's (1998) OCD treatment encourages children to externalize the disorder into an antagonistic character they can "boss back." An innovative treatment approach for SAD provides an intensive weeklong "camp," which naturally allows for exposure exercises in a fun and developmentally appropriate manner. The field has recognized the need to tailor CBT techniques with play when treating anxious youth. Indeed, infusing play within the CBT framework is likely an instinctual process that occurs naturally for clinicians.

THE ROLE OF PLAY IN CBT FOR CHILD ANXIETY DISORDERS

In our clinical work at the Center for Anxiety and Related Disorders, we have integrated play techniques into many aspects of our cognitive and behavioral treatment programs for youth with anxiety disorders. Anecdotally, we have found that play can facilitate many aspects of the treatment process, including helping therapists glean information in evidence-based assessment, assisting children as they learn cognitive and behavioral concepts, helping to increase patients' motivation, and improving patient and family engagement in the treatment. The following section provides brief case examples to illustrate specific ways that play can be used in evidence-based treatments for anxiety disorders in youth. The children described in this section are of varying ages, underscoring the ways that play may be used across development during childhood and adolescence.

Therapist-Created Games

Several therapists have created "games" for their school-age child patients to enhance comprehension of cognitive-behavioral concepts. For example, children with generalized anxiety disorder (GAD) often have difficulty making decisions quickly. Children describe belaboring over decisions and wondering whether they have made the "right" one. Many therapists at the center play "Quick Decision Catch" with these patients. The therapist identifies a problem and asks, "What are all the things you could do or think about to make things better in this situation?" The therapist throws the ball to the child, who must name one possible solution. The child then throws the ball back to the therapist, who models quick thinking of a healthy coping response. The game of catch continues until there are no more ideas from either party. The therapist ends the game by asking, "Which solution would you use if this really happened to you?" and throws the ball to the patient. The patient chooses a response, and the therapist praises the child for quick responding and refraining from ruminating over the decision. This game illustrates to the child that there are many possible solutions to a situation, and the child is capable of making a decision. Using the ball keeps children engaged in the process and teaches problem-solving skills in a fun, active way.

Many therapists have designed board games to teach a particular CBT skill. One such unpublished board game was created to teach children about the behavioral, physical and cognitive components of anxiety, called the "Think–Feel–Do Game." Using play pieces and dice, the game was tailored specifically for school-age children. Another therapist-created game is "Bravery Bingo." The therapist lists situations from the child's fear and avoidance hierarchy on a bingo card. For a child with social phobia, situations might include: "Say hi to somebody I know," "Order a pizza on the phone," and "Talk to a new friend at school." Each time the child completes an item from the bingo card, he or she receives a star or sticker on that bingo square. When children fill five consecutive squares, they have won "BINGO" and receive a treat from their reward list. In this way, the fear avoidance hierarchy that is typically used in cognitive-behavioral therapy can be transformed to a more "playful" format.

The game of "scavenger hunt" has also been used to motivate children to complete situations from their fear avoidance hierarchy. The therapist hides messages with tasks that correspond with situations on his or her hierarchy. For example, a child with social anxiety might be asked to ask someone a question about his or her favorite movie, and after doing this, he or she must then follow the clues to find the next card. By the end of the scavenger hunt, the child is rewarded for his or her efforts.

Sometimes therapists find ways to use existing, published games to teach and illustrate a CBT skill. For example, prior to introducing relaxation techniques, therapists will sometimes play a game of Jenga with their child patients. During the game, the player's hands typically shake slightly as he or she tries to remove a wooden block from a tall tower of blocks. The aim of the game is to not let the tower fall down. Therapists use this game to illustrate the difference between muscle tension and relaxation.

Another game that has been utilized is the game Topple, in which colored plastic pieces are placed on a plastic tray so that the tray is balanced and does not "topple." Therapists ask the child to name a thought, feeling, or behavior as he or she puts the plastic piece on the tray to help children learn how to "break down" anxiety into its three components. Thus, if a child picks up a pink piece, he or she names a thought, a blue piece he or she names a behavior, or a green piece he or she names a physical feeling associated with anxiety. This game helps therapist build rapport while also providing psychoeducation about anxiety.

Sometimes therapy can be made more "playful" by tailoring treatment techniques to the child's specific interests. In treating a 10-year-old boy with severe OCD, he and the therapist externalized the disorder by naming it his favorite cartoon "villain". He chose the Joker from the cartoon *Batman*. He reported that imagining himself talking back to the Joker helped him resist his obsessions and compulsions. He showed almost immediate improvement, and his reported time spent on performing compulsions went from 4 hours to 30 minutes per day in just 2 weeks.

Use of Puppets

Puppets can be particularly helpful with younger children to model CBT skills. For example, one therapist used a puppet called "Mr. OCD" to help a child externalize the disorder. The child was taught how to "talk back" to Mr. OCD, rather than being bossed around by him. The child became highly engaged in these cognitive restructuring exercises, and would frequently comment on how he was going to "win" against Mr. OCD. We have also used turtle puppets with patients ages 4–6 with SAD and social phobia. The puppet tucks its head into its shell when the turtle is feeling "shy." The puppet often helps children express their own emotions, as they indicate feeling the "same as the turtle" when at school or away from their parents.

Coloring/Drawing/Art

We frequently encourage children to "name" their anxiety and draw a representation of their emotional experience. Children have produced a range of creative responses, including "Mr. Spineyhead," the "Anxiety Monster," and "The Big A." They can draw pictures of themselves winning against their opponent (anxiety), by using their "toolbox" of coping skills. Children who enjoy art seem to respond well when integrating this medium into therapy. They have also drawn "before" pictures of their emotions and experiences pretreatment, and then "after" pictures of their feelings posttreatment. One child, after learning PMR, drew a picture of her most relaxing place; she then reported that she imagined the picture to remind her to use the skill. Another adolescent with OCD used art to incorporate his love of basketball into treatment. He drew a detailed scoreboard and basketball court and then engaged in an "icky scavenger hunt" (touching a series of things that he deemed "dirty"). He awarded himself a point each time he was able to successfully touch something without performing a compulsion. He was delighted at the end of treatment when his team beat "Team OCD." He was highly engaged in treatment, and reported that he enjoyed modifying the scoreboard each time he "scored," as it made him feel like he was "winning" against his anxiety.

Art techniques are often helpful when working with children with attention problems, as younger children may be incapable of sitting for an hour session that consists solely of talking. Drawing and writing techniques can help children focus and concentrate on the material, especially when provided with tasks to illustrate the specific cognitive-behavioral "tools."

Using Play Techniques to Improve Family Relationships

Play techniques can also help promote change outside the therapy room. In one case, the therapist created a game to increase positive reinforcement in the home environment. Each family member received five animal figurines, and was instructed to give their animals to one another throughout the week, along with a labeled praise. The goal was to have given all of the animals away by the next session. The family described the game as a fun and enjoyable way to increase positive interactions, as well as providing a concrete reminder of therapeutic goals. Even after treatment, the family continued to use this game to promote positive reinforcement in the home.

Role Playing

Role playing is another technique frequently used in our work with children and adolescents. This can also be seen as a form of play, as we might instruct children to take on a role other than themselves during the role play. The therapist acts out the role of the child, and thus models adaptive coping strategies and positive self-talk. Role plays can help prepare a child for an anxiety-provoking situation or an exposure exercise scheduled for homework outside of the therapy session. For example, the therapist and the child might act out a challenging situation, such as attending a party and approaching a group of peers. Role play can also help teach social skills and model the use of CBT skills in a range of different situations.

EMPIRICAL SUPPORT FOR CBT
FOR CHILD ANXIETY DISORDERS

Several controlled studies have demonstrated the efficacy of CBT for anxiety disorders in youth (Barrett et al., 1996; Kendall, 1994; Kendall et al., 1997), and research has demonstrated that CBT outcomes are superior to alternative interventions, including a psychological placebo intervention (Muris, Meesters, & Melick, 2003). In a between-group study conducted by Kendall et al. (1997), the Coping Cat program was compared to a wait-list control condition. Forty seven children ages 9–13 years were diagnosed with overanxious disorder ($n = 30$), avoidant disorder ($n = 9$), or SAD ($n = 8$) and were assigned to either a wait list ($n = 20$) or treatment condition ($n = 27$). Posttreatment, 64% of the children in the treatment condition no longer met diagnostic criteria for any anxiety disorder, in contrast to 5% of children from the wait-list condition. Kendall and Southam-Gerow (1996) found that treatment gains for this group were maintained at 1 and 3 years posttreatment. In a subsequent study, Kendall and colleagues (1997) showed in a group of 9- to 13-year-old anxious children ($n = 94$) that 71% of the CBT treated children ($n = 60$) did not meet diagnostic criteria at the end of treatment, in comparison to 5.8% for the wait-list condition ($n = 34$). Barrett and colleagues (1996) also found that the Coping Cat was more effective in treating anxiety than the wait-list control group.

Research also suggests that different formats of CBT are effective in treating anxiety disorders, including CBT administered in a group setting (e.g., Barrett, 1998; Flannery-Schroeder & Kendall, 2000; Muris, Mayer, Bartelds, Tierney, & Bogie, 2001) and CBT that incorporates parent training (e.g., Barrett et al., 1996; Spence, Donovan, & Brechman-Toussaint, 2000). In a study of 37 children with anxiety, individuals were conditioned to individual CBT, group CBT, and a wait-list control condition. Researchers found no difference in outcome between individual CBT and group CBT, both of which were more effective than the wait-list control group (Flannery-Schroeder & Kendall, 2000). In addition to examining the efficacy of Kendall's manualized CBT, Barrett and colleagues (1996) compared individual CBT, CBT with a parent training component, and a wait-list control in 79 children ages 7–14 years. While outcomes for both individual CBT and CBT with parent training were superior to the wait-list control, the parent training condition resulted in significantly greater improvements than CBT alone, with these differences maintained at 6- and 12-month follow-up.

Many empirically validated treatments exist for child anxiety disorders, and as discussed above, most incorporate some form of play to increase developmental sensitivity for children and adolescents. However, limited research specifically examines the use of play within the CBT framework. The need to increase the accessibility and applicability of CBT, particularly for younger children, has led to the proposal of cognitive-behavioral play therapy (CBPT; Knell, 1998; Knell & Moore, 1990; Knell & Ruma, 1996). CBPT maintains the key elements of CBT, but uses play to provide developmentally appropriate adaptations to traditional cognitive therapy, thereby increasing its applicability to younger children. For example, by using a puppet or stuffed animal, the therapist models cognitive strategies taught in CBT, such as countering maladaptive beliefs and the use of positive statements and problem-solving skills (Knell, 1994). Thus, the core skill of thought countering remains, but the presentation is modified to increase developmental sensitivity. However, the efficacy of CBPT has not been established through randomized clinical trials.

Play techniques can also be used in different formats of CBT in the treatment of child anxiety. For example, clinicians may use play techniques in group treatment of children with social anxiety, fostering social skill development and encouraging interaction between young patients through play. Play in the context of CBT for anxiety can also facilitate parents' implementation of therapy skills in the home. Parent training has been shown to be an important aspect of CBT treatment, especially for younger children (Velting et al., 2004; Ginsburg, Silverman, & Kurtines, 1995; Dadds, Heard, & Rapee, 1992). Parents may implement a token or reward system to provide positive reinforcement for brave or assertive behaviors. Play can also provide a naturally occurring and rewarding context in which parents can model appropriate coping strategies and emotion regulation. Concerns about the applicability of traditional CBT to very young children, along with the importance of parent involvement in treatment, has led to an adaptation of parent–child interaction therapy (PCIT; Brinkmeyer & Eyberg, 2003) for children with SAD. Families are first introduced to the child-directed interaction skills according to the standard PCIT protocol (please see Chapter 6, this volume, on PCIT for a detailed description). Thus, parents are taught to play with their child using skills specifically designed to encourage adaptive child behavior. The CDI phase is followed by a CBT component that includes psychoeducation about anxiety and graduated exposure to feared situations (Brinkmeyer & Eyberg, 2003; Pincus, Eyberg, & Choate, 2005). Thus, parents are provided with skills to help promote positive child behavior before they enter into difficult exposure situations. The CDI phase also enhances the parent–child relationship, thereby increasing a child's sense of security. This innovative treatment approach combines the use of parent-led play and traditional CBT techniques to create a developmentally sensitive treatment for separation-anxious youth.

SUMMARY AND FUTURE DIRECTIONS

Few would dispute that CBT is the standard of care in the treatment of child anxiety. However, a significant number of children continue to demonstrate clinically significant levels of anxiety after a trial of CBT. Notably, the majority of existing research supports the use of CBT in a university setting with predominantly Caucasian school-age children and adolescents. Research is needed on adaptations to CBT that may increase its effectiveness with a range of populations. Now that a solid evidence base supports the use of CBT in children with anxiety, the field can examine specific techniques that allow clinicians to appropriately tailor treatment to best meet the needs of each child. Play, which is naturally occurring event for children that promotes learning, may increase the accessibility and efficacy of CBT. Research specifically examining the use of play in CBT treatment for anxiety is limited, although research has begun to examine innovative treatment approaches that incorporate play techniques. Additionally, most therapists would likely agree that play is a valuable clinical tool that is naturally woven into the implementation of CBT with children.

This chapter outlines various ways to use play in CBT treatment for child anxiety. Notably, many of the current treatment manuals for child anxiety disorders incorporate playful techniques to increase the accessibility and applicability of CBT principles to child and adolescent populations. Specifically, many treatment manuals use child-appropriate language, introduce CBT concepts with the use of fictional characters, and include fun activities to promote child comprehension and engagement in treatment. In addition, there is an endless array of more informal play and games that clinicians can use when implementing CBT interventions. We provided some common activities used in our clinic; however, the possibilities for the use of play are endless. Clinicians use play to increase a child's understanding of CBT principles and his or her engagement in the therapeutic process. Developmental research suggests that play is an important communication tool for children, and allows them to actively process information (Youngblade & Dunn, 1995). Future research should therefore systematically evaluate the benefits of incorporating play into CBT, and specifically its effect on child comprehension of treatment material, treatment outcome, and overall engagement in therapy. It may be that different types of play are clinically indicated depending on the developmental level and needs of the individual child and family.

Certainly, clinicians are constantly seeking to increase the applicability and accessibility of treatment for each patient. Incorporating play is likely an instinctual process for many clinicians, particularly when working with younger children. Very little evidence supports the use of CBT specifically with a preschool population, and some have suggested that young children may not be appropriate candidates for this treatment approach. However, recent research has examined treatment programs that maintain fundamental CBT principles, but introduce developmentally appropriate modifications to increase its applicability to preschool-age children. Whether it involves the more formal inclusion of play techniques, such as in cognitive-behavioral play therapy (CBPT; Knell, 1998), or the delivery of CBT procedures in an intensive "camp" setting, there are several new programs that seek to increase the applicability of CBT to children through the use of play. More research is needed on these innovative treatment approaches. Does the more formal inclusion of play truly improve the efficacy of standard CBT? What populations are most likely to benefit from this approach? How might we standardize the play techniques within an intervention without robbing clinicians of therapeutic creativity? What types of play activities are most effective with different populations? Does the use of play truly lead to greater cognitive change? These all represent important directions for future research.

Perhaps one of the most appealing aspects of integrating play into any treatment program is its positive effect on the therapeutic relationship and overall rapport. Play is inherently rewarding for children, families, and therapists, and is an important activity that allows an adult to build a relationship with a child (Russell, Petit, & Mize, 1998). Incorporating play into traditional CBT therapy may affect a range of process variables, such as the strength of the therapeutic alliance and client engagement in therapy. To the extent that play increases engagement and accessibility for children and families, it may also improve treatment satisfaction and attrition rates. Research has yet to systematically evaluate the influence of play on these variables, particularly within CBT or CBPT. The positive affects of incorporating play techniques into traditional CBT may appear obvious. However, it may be that a delicate balance exists between using play to increase the accessibility of CBT techniques while maintaining the integrity and effectiveness of the intervention. For example, if the therapist uses a game to teach cognitive restructuring techniques, it is important that the child truly be able to extract the cognitive skills necessary, and not only focus on winning the game. A better understanding of the crucial components of CBT treatment and true mechanisms of change will help inform our use of play, so that any adaptations or modifications are empirically based, and we are sure to maintain key elements of the CBT treatment program.

An important focus in CBT treatment programs for anxiety is the maintenance of treatment gains and relapse prevention. Researchers and clinicians alike increasingly recognize the importance of parent involvement in treatment, particularly for younger children (Velting et al., 2004). Parent involvement likely encourages the generalization of skills outside the therapy session, and may also help prevent relapse once treatment has ended. Play is a naturally occurring and rewarding context that can be used to encourage parent involvement in treatment. Much as a therapist might do in session, parents can use play activities at home to model appropriate coping and reinforce positive child behaviors. Thus, future research should also examine the use of parent-led play in treatment to determine its affects on treatment outcome and the maintenance of treatment gains.

Future research should focus on the implementation of play techniques within the CBT framework to fully appreciate the role of play in maximizing the effectiveness of CBT for anxious children. This chapter has discussed several ways in which play might be infused into current evidence-based practices. Systematic evaluation of specific play techniques will allow the field to better understand their use in the treatment of anxious youth. Play can be a powerful tool that allows clinicians to tailor treatment to the needs of each individual child and family.

REFERENCES

Albano, A. M., & DiBartolo, P. M. (2007). *Cognitive-behavioral therapy for social phobia in adolescents: Therapist guide.* New York: Oxford University Press.

Barrett, P. M. (1998). An evaluation of cognitive-behavioral group treatments for childhood anxiety disorders. *Journal of Clinical Child Psychology, 27,* 459–468.

Barrett, P. M., Dadds, M., & Rapee, R. (1996). Family treatment of childhood anxiety: A controlled trial. *Journal of Consulting and Clinical Psychology, 64,* 333–342.

Brinkmeyer, M. Y., & Eyberg, S. M. (2003). Parent–child interaction therapy for oppositional children. In A. E. Kazdin & J. R. Weisz (Eds.) *Evidence-based psychotherapies for children and adolescents* (pp. 204–223). New York: Guilford Press.

Dadds, M. R., Heard, P. M., & Rapee, R. M. (1992). The role of family intervention in the treatment of child anxiety disorders: Some preliminary findings. *Behavior Change, 9,* 171–177.

Ehrenreich, J. T., Kyle-Linkovich, T., & Rojas-Vilches, A. (2005). Cognitive behavior therapy: Child clinical applications. In M. Hersen, A. M. Gross, & R. S. Drabman (Eds.), *Encyclopedia of behavior modification and cognitive behavior therapy Vol. 2. Child clinical applications* (pp. 767–775). Thousand Oaks, CA: Sage.

Flannery-Schroeder, E. C., & Kendall, P. C. (2000). Group and individual cognitive-behavioral treatments for youth with anxiety disorders: A randomized clinical trial. *Cognitive Therapy and Research, 24*, 251–278.

Ginsberg, G. S., Silverman, W. K., & Kurtines, W. K. (1995). Family involvement in treating children with phobic and anxiety disorders: A look ahead. *Clinical Psychology Review, 15*, 457–473.

Kazdin, A. E., & Weisz, J. R. (1998). Identifying and developing empirically supported child and adolescent treatments. *Journal of Consulting and Clinical Psychology, 66*, 19–36.

Kendall, P. C. (1994). Treating anxiety disorders in children: Results of a randomized clinical trial. *Journal of Consulting and Clinical Psychology, 62*, 100–110.

Kendall, P. C., Chansky, T. E., Kane, M. T., Kim, R. S., Kortlander, E., & Ronan, K. R. (1992). *Anxiety disorders in youth: Cognitive-behavioral interventions.* Needham Heights, MA: Allyn & Bacon.

Kendall, P. C., Flannery-Schroeder, E., Panichelli-Mindel, S. M., Southam-Gerow, M. A., Henin, A., & Warman, M. (1997). Therapy for youths with anxiety disorders: A second randomized clinical trial. *Journal of Consulting and Clinical Psychology, 65*, 366–380.

Kendall, P. C., & Hedtke, K. A. (2006). *Cognitive-behavioral treatment for anxious children: Therapist's manual* (3rd ed.). Ardmore, PA: Workbook.

Kendall, P. C., Kane, M., Howard, B., & Siqueland, L. (1990). *Cognitive-behavioral treatment of anxious children: Treatment manual.* Ardmore, PA: Workbook.

Kendall, P. C., & Southam-Gerow, M. A. (1996). Long-term follow-up of a cognitive-behavioral therapy for anxiety-disordered youth. *Journal of Consulting and Clinical Psychology, 64*, 724–730.

Knell, S. M. (1994). Cognitive-behavioral play therapy. In K. O'Connor & C. Schaefer (Eds.), *Handbook of play therapy: Vol. 2. Advances and innovations* (pp. 111–142). New York: Wiley.

Knell, S. M. (1998). Cognitive-behavioral play therapy. *Journal of Clinical Child Psychology, 27*, 28–33.

Knell, S. M., & Moore, D. J. (1990). Cognitive-behavioral play therapy in the treatment of encopresis. *Journal of Clinical Child Psychology, 19*, 55–60.

Knell, S. M., & Ruma, C. D. (1996). Play therapy with a sexually abused child. In M. Reinecke, F. M. Dattilio, & A. Freeman (Eds.), *Cognitive therapy with children and adolescents: A casebook for clinical practice* (pp. 367–393). New York: Guilford Press.

March, J. S., & Mulle, K. (1998). *OCD in children and adolescents: A cognitive behavioral treatment manual.* New York: Guilford Press.

Muris, P., Mayer, B., Bartelds, E., Tierney, S., & Bogie, N. (2001). The revised versionof the Screen for Child Anxiety Related Emotion Disorders (SCARED-

R): Treatment sensitivity in an early intervention trial for childhood anxiety disorders. *British Journal of Clinical Psychology, 40,* 323–336.

Muris, P., Meesters, C., & Melick, M. (2003). Treatment of childhood anxiety disorders: A preliminary comparison between cognitive-behavioral group therapy and a psychological placebo intervention. *Journal of Behavior and Experimental Psychiatry, 33,* 143–158.

Pincus, D.B., Eyberg, S.M., & Choate, M.L. (2005). Adapting parent–child interaction therapy for young children with separation anxiety disorder. *Education and Treatment of Children, 28,* 163–181.

Russell, A., Petit, G. S., & Mize, J. (1998). Horizontal qualities in parent–child relationships: Parallels with and possible consequences for children's peer relationships. *Developmental Review, 18,* 313–352.

Santucci, L. C., & Ehrenreich, J. T. (2007). *Summer treatment program for separation anxiety disorder: Therapist guide.* Unpublished manual. Center for Anxiety and Related Disorders, Boston University, Boston.

Santucci, L. C., Ehrenreich, J. T., Bennett, S. M., Trosper, S., & Pincus, D. P. (2009). *Development and preliminary evaluation of a one-week summer treatment program for separation anxiety disorder.* [Special Issue] *Cognitive and Behavioral Practice, 16*(3), 345–358.

Spence, S. H., Donovan, C., & Brechman-Toussaint, M. (2000). The treatment of childhood social phobia: The effectiveness of a social skills training-based, cognitive-behavioural intervention, with and without parental involvement. *Journal of Child Psychology and Psychiatry, 41,* 713–726.

Velting, O. N., Setzer, N. J., & Albano, A. M. (2004). Update on and advances in assessment and cognitive-behavioral treatment of anxiety disorders in children and adolescents. *Professional Psychology: Research and Practice, 35,* 42–54.

Wagner, A. P. (2002). *Worried no more: Help and hope for anxious children.* Rochester, NY: Lighthouse Press.

Youngblade, L. M., & Dunn, J. (1995). Individual differences in young children's pretend play with mother and sibling: Links to relationships and understanding of other people's feelings and beliefs. *Child Development, 66,* 1472–1492.

10

Cognitive-Behavioral Play Therapy

Susan M. Knell and Meena Dasari

Cognitive-behavioral therapy (CBT), a form of psychotherapy developed for adults, aims to identify and modifying negative thinking styles that cause negative emotions and the maladaptive behaviors associated with those thinking styles. CBT has been shown to be effective in individuals ages 8 and above for a variety of disorders. Cognitive-behavioral play therapy (CBPT) is a developmentally sensitive adaptation of CBT. With CBPT, play is used as a medium to deliver empirically supported techniques to young children ages 3–8 years. Through the use of play activities, techniques can be communicated and taught to children indirectly and in an engaging way (Knell, 1993a, 1993b, 1994, 1998, 1999, 2000; Knell & Dasari, 2006, 2009). For example, puppets and stuffed animals can be used to teach cognitive strategies such as challenging negative thinking styles and creating positive self-statements.

CBPT has been used to treat children presenting with a variety of disorders. Children with specific diagnoses such as selective mutism (Knell, 1993a, 1993b), encopresis (Knell & Moore, 1990; Knell, 1993a), and anxiety/phobias (Knell, 1993a; Knell & Dasari, 2009) have been successfully treated with CBPT. In addition, CBPT has been used with children with multiple diagnoses or who have experienced life events/traumas such as divorce (Knell, 1993a; Knell & Dasari, 2009) and sexual abuse (Ruma, 1993; Knell & Ruma, 1996, 2003).

DEVELOPMENTAL ISSUES/ADAPTING CBT FOR USE WITH YOUNG CHILDREN

Since the inception of CBT over 50 years ago, adaptations of CBT for use with increasingly younger populations have emerged (e.g., adolescents—Emery, Bedrosian, & Garber, 1983; school-age children—Kendall & Braswell, 1985), largely due to the documented effectiveness in adult populations. However, many doubted that CBT could be adapted for preschool and very young school-age children. This doubt came in large measure from the developmental literature, which noted that preoperational-stage children (i.e., approximately 2–7 years) do not have the cognitive sophistication and flexibility to benefit from CBT. Given that CBT with adults requires the ability to follow a rational, logical sequence, such cognitive sophistication is typically not present in young children. Further, for CBT to be effective, individuals must have the capacity to differentiate between rational and irrational/logical and illogical thinking

Young children, however, may not understand the differences between irrational, illogical thinking and more rational, logical thought. The application of CBT with young children is thus fraught with difficulties. Consequently, most of the work with youth and CBT has focused on adolescents and older school-age children. The preoperational-stage child's egocentrism, concrete thought processes, and seemingly irrational thinking would seem to preclude the kind of cognitive abilities necessary to participate in CBT. Adaptations for younger populations have changed the methods through which CBT is delivered, but not the theoretical underpinnings of the approach. Finding ways to deliver CBT without an emphasis on language that might be too complex for a young child represents one of the challenges faced in the development of CBPT.

Knell (1993a, 1993b, 1994, 1997, 1998) demonstrated that CBT could be modified for use with young children if presented in a more accessible way. For example, puppets, stuffed animals, books, and other toys could be used to model cognitive strategies. Using research (e.g., Bandura, 1969; Meichenbaum, 1971) that suggested that child behavior change occurs more successfully after observing a coping model, Knell developed CBPT, which used such models in a psychoeducational way. Coping models make "mistakes" along the way, and model learning from these mistakes. The child is then observing a model in its efforts to learn more appropriate behaviors. With a coping model approach, the model (e.g., a puppet) might verbalize problem-solving skills or solutions to problems that parallel the child's own difficulties.

Adapting CBT for preschoolers has received increasing attention over the last 10 years. CBPT, as conceptualized by Knell (Knell, 1993a,

1993b, 1994, 1997, 1998, 1999, 2000; Knell & Moore, 1990; Knell & Ruma, 1996, 2003; Knell & Beck, 2000, Knell & Dasari, 2006, 2009) was developed for use with children between 2½ and 6 years, and incorporates cognitive, behavioral, and traditional play therapies. CBPT is based on the cognitive theory of emotional disorders and cognitive principles of therapy, and adapts these in a developmentally appropriate way. It is sensitive to the developmental issues of children and emphasizes the empirical validation of effectiveness of interventions.

Cognitive distortions in very young children may be developmentally appropriate, yet maladaptive. For example, a child whose parents separate shortly after he misbehaves may believe that he was the cause of the separation. In most cases, children incorporate life experience into their thinking, and with the help of everyday parent–child discourse are able to integrate this learning into a more adaptive thought (e.g., "My mommy didn't leave me at preschool because I was bad. She loves me and wants me to go to school like all the other kids"). Given that maladaptive thoughts may be developmentally appropriate, the concept of cognitive distortions is problematic with young children. For this reason, it is more appropriate to label these thoughts "maladaptive," rather than "distorted."

Sometimes children do not attach any set of beliefs or meanings to an event. In these instances maladaptive cognitions may not be present. However, there still may be an absence of adaptive beliefs that would facilitate coping. In these instances, the child might need some assistance in creating functional, adaptive self-statements as a coping device, not to replace the maladaptive ones, but to boost more adaptive thinking and behavior. For example, a young child may have difficulty coping with the birth of a sibling. Maladaptive beliefs (e.g., "I'm not the baby anymore," "No one loves me") may not be present or they may not be expressed verbally. Helping the child cope with the new sibling by providing adaptive, positive coping statements can facilitate the child's functioning. Statements such as "We have a new baby but Mom and Dad still love me" can provide the child with a positive outlook on the experience. Such statements can replace maladaptive beliefs (either spoken or felt, but not verbalized) or be a new cognition replacing either neutral or nonexistent beliefs.

Thus, facilitating adaptive cognitive change is not only possible, but quite common with young children. Often, as mentioned, inducing such change takes place in the normal, every day life of parent–child interactions. When situations are brought to a therapist, the use of developmentally appropriate adaptations of CBT to facilitate such changes may be indicated. Bierman (1983) wrote about interviewing techniques, including the use of concrete examples and less open-ended questions as a means to facilitate the young child's understanding of complex problems. Through the use of play, cognitive change can be communicated indirectly (Shirk & Russell, 1996; Knell, 1998). Additionally, the therapist's ability to be flexible, reduce focus on verbalizations, and increase use of experiential approaches can contribute to the successful adaptation of CBT with young children (Knell & Ruma, 1996, 2003; Knell & Dasari, 2006).

THEORY

The development of CBPT was based on several well-established psychological theories of personality, cognition, behavior, and development. Mischel's (1968) theories provided a foundation for the cognitive-behaviorists, in focusing on traits and habits, and less on personality types, emphasizing the importance of situational factors in understanding behavior. As originally conceptualized, the cognitive-behavioral approaches were insight-oriented and used introspective techniques to change overt personality (e.g., Beck, 1967; Ellis, 1962). These approaches emphasized the changing of cognitive schemas (controlling beliefs) as well as behavioral symptoms. However, there is no personality theory, per se, that underlies cognitive-behavioral theory. Rather, the focus has been more on psychopathology, and the factors that contribute to normal developmental processes being disrupted, rather than on personality development and theory.

Cognitive therapy is based on the cognitive model of emotional disorders, which involves the interplay among cognition, emotion, behavior, and physiology (Beck & Emery, 1985). This model states that behavior is mediated through verbal processes. Disturbances in emotions and behavior are considered to be expressions of irrational thinking. There are three major premises of cognitive therapy: (1) thoughts influence the individual's emotions and behaviors in response to events, (2) perceptions and interpretations of events are shaped by the individual's beliefs and assumptions, and (3) errors in logic or cognitive distortions are prevalent in individuals who experience psychological difficulties (Beck, 1976). These cognitions are unspoken, often unrecognized, assumptions made by the individual.

While this model is not specifically a personality theory, it does address cognitive distortions as the basis of human behavior and thought, particularly as related to psychopathological development. For children, these distortions are often considered maladaptive, but not necessarily irrational. This is particularly true for very young children, whose thinking is, by definition, often illogical, egocentric, and concrete.

Cognitive therapy is based on the assumption that people's affect and behavior are determined in large part by the way they construe the world (Beck, 1967, 1972, 1976). Thus, it is one's *perceptions* of events—not the *circumstances* themselves—that determine how a person understands these events. Cognitions can be in the form of covert verbal statements or images and are based on the attitudes or assumptions (schemas) developed from earlier experiences. Cognitive theory asserts that these cognitions will determine to a large extent the individual's emotional experiences.

According to the cognitive model, by knowing the meaning that a person attaches to particular situations, we can predict his or her emotional reaction. The range of cognitive distortions is infinite, but certain types of errors in thinking seem to occur with regularity. A great deal of the cognitive literature has been focused on depressed individuals, who often exhibit automatic thoughts reflecting a negative view of present, past, and future experiences (Beck, 1976). In summary, cognitive therapy is concerned with both how individuals perceive events and the cognitions based on these perceptions.

Cognitive therapy is based on a broad theory of psychopathology that details the intricate reciprocal interaction among cognitions, emotions, behavior, and environment. Cognitive therapy consists of a set of treatment techniques that aim to relieve symptoms of psychological distress through the "direct modification of the dysfunctional ideation that accompanies them" (Bedrosian & Beck, 1980, p. 128). The cognitive therapist uses a phenomenological approach to identify, find patterns for, and then change dysfunctional thinking. In general, the patient's thoughts are revealed through focused questions and careful introspection. The cognitive therapist also uses questioning not only to produce symptom reduction, but to modify attitudes, beliefs, and expectations that maintain negative emotions and behaviors. The primary goal of cognitive therapy is to identify and modify maladaptive thoughts associated with the patient's symptoms (Bedrosian & Beck, 1980).

Behavioral theories often supplement cognitive theories and the combination results in effective techniques to help children cope with difficult events and emotions (for reviews, see Compton et al., 2004, and Velting, Setzer, & Albano, 2004). Whether the therapy is direct or delivered through the parents, the therapist identifies factors that reinforce and maintain problematic behaviors so that they can be altered. In general, the roots of behavior therapy are grounded in the principles of classical conditioning developed by Ivan Pavlov, operant conditioning developed by B. F. Skinner, and social learning theory developed by Albert Bandura. When applied to target behaviors in children, the goal of behavior therapy is to modify the relationships between an environmental trigger, a child's specific behavior response, and an environmental response (e.g., parent's discipline, teacher's reaction). The result is that the child learns new, adaptive behavioral responses.

The central techniques are (1) contingency management (e.g., reinforcement, consequences); (2) variations of systemic desensitization and exposure; and (3) learning and modeling. Contingency management programs, which are derived from operant conditioning research, consist of reward systems, positive reinforcement (e.g., praise), and consequences. Over time, these techniques have been shown to be highly successful for changing maladaptive behaviors in children. Systematic desensitization and exposure refer to the gradual introduction of feared or disliked stimuli paired with adaptive coping, which evolved from respondent conditioning. There is significant research to demonstrate its effectiveness with children, particularly with anxiety and phobias (King & Ollendick, 1997). Social learning theory can be considered a bridge or a transition between behaviorist learning theories and cognitive learning theories. The premise is that children's behaviors can be learned through modeling, such that children can learn by observing others' behavior and the outcomes of those behaviors. Therefore, modeling is integrated into CBPT in that the technique is used to teach new behaviors and decrease the frequency of maladaptive learned behaviors.

KEY VARIABLES

Child Involvement

CBPT places a strong emphasis on the child's involvement in treatment and on a framework for the child's participation by addressing issues of control, mastery, and responsibility for one's own behavior change. By incorporating the cognitive components, the child may become an active participant in change. For example, by helping children identify and modify their potentially maladaptive beliefs, they may experience a sense of personal understanding and empowerment. Integrating cognitive and behavioral interventions may offer effects of the combined properties of all approaches, which might not be available otherwise (Knell, 1993a).

Symptoms/Behavior

In CBPT, decreasing symptoms and/or specific behaviors is often the focus. CBT contends that behavior is mediated through verbal processes: the way individuals interpret their world in large measure determines how they feel and behave (Beck, 1967, 1972, 1976). Behavioral theories contend that behaviors are learned or acquired through conditioning. Taken together, CBPT incorporates both theories to reduce symptoms and develop more adaptive behaviors to replace current behavior.

Coping Skills

Because CBT is psychoeducational in nature, teaching the child more adaptive coping skills is a natural fit within therapy. Adaptive coping skills include learned behaviors that allow the child to effectively manage emotions or difficult situations. There are many ways that more adaptive coping skills can be taught through CBT. Among these are teaching the child (1) to verbalize emotions, rather than acting them out; (2) relaxation skills; and (3) effective problem-solving skills.

Processes

The primary processes in CBPT with young children are (1) cognitive flexibility/shift and (2) learning and practicing. Over the course of therapy, children's irrational or maladaptive thoughts about an event or object shift from negative to either neutral or positive (Kendall, 2006). As these negative thoughts are diminished and replaced during therapy, children's symptoms decrease. With adults, Bedrosian and Beck (1980) explain that cognitive change as producing a "quieting down" (Rachman, 1968), which might be the result of such therapy components as the therapist's empathy and acceptance (Truax & Carkhuff, 1967), specific relaxation techniques (e.g., Wolpe & Lazarus, 1966), or verbal approval (Wagner & Cauthen, 1968). Therapy also gives patients the chance to experience and test the reality of verbal or pictorial cognitions that are connected to their affect. Individuals can examine distorted ideas, learn to discriminate between rational and irrational ideas, and see the irrational nature of some of their thoughts. One critical mechanism of CBT is the modification or shift of the ideational system; as irrational concepts are deactivated, psychopathology may recede.

The other critical process is learning and practicing behaviors. Within the context of CBPT, children are taught new coping skills and adaptive behaviors to replace maladaptive ones. Over the course of therapy, children practice the new behaviors in different scenarios. Reinforcement, either visual (e.g., stickers) or verbal (e.g., praise), is used to increase the frequency of the new behaviors. Parent involvement allows for new behaviors to be practiced at home and in other settings with the addition of reinforcement. Thus, the critical mechanisms of CBPT are the modification or shift of the child's thinking style and behavioral responses.

DESCRIPTION OF THE INTERVENTION

Setting/Materials

CBPT is usually conducted in a playroom with a wide array of play materials available. A typical play therapy room is well stocked with toys, art supplies, puppets, dolls, and other materials. The use of materials in play therapy has been written about extensively (e.g., Axline, 1947; Landreth, 2002; Giorano, Landreth, & Jones, 2005; O'Connor, 1991). In CBPT, play materials are a critical component of therapy, with both child and therapist choosing appropriate materials either collaboratively or independently. See Appendix 10.1 for a list of recommended play materials. In CBPT, toys are (1) visible and easily accessible to the child and (2) kept in the same place so that the child knows where they are from one session to the next. If the child is working on a project, or has papers (e.g., pictures, an individual, self-created book), it is important that the therapist and the child have a safe, consistent place to keep these materials. A locked drawer/place is recommended, so the child knows that his or her confidentiality is being respected.

Although play therapy is usually conducted in a playroom, the child may need to be seen in a setting that more closely resembles specific real-life situations. For instance, the child fearful of medical personnel may need to be seen at a physician's office or clinic.

Assessment

As part of the assessment, the therapist uses all possible data to understand the context of the presenting problems, get clarity about diagnostic issues, and develop a treatment plan. This typically begins with an interview of parent(s) to obtain background data and history. The more thorough the assessment, the better. Data regarding the child's developmental level of cognitive, emotional, social, and problem-solving skills should be included, in addition to information about the presenting problem. The child's self-report, therapist behavioral observations, and/or school evaluations are utilized to supplement parental report. In general, the purposes of the assessment are to determine (1) whether the child's skills are similar to same-age peers (Knell & Dasari, 2006) and (2) the best treatment plan. The therapist can supplement this information with behavioral observations of the child's ability to express and regulate emotions in a therapeutic setting. Understanding children's pretend play ability is important in determining whether CPBT is an appropriate intervention for a child. Research has shown that play therapy is more effective for children who already have good pretend play skills (Russ, 2004). But CBPT can be useful even with children with developmental delays, as the intervention can be adapted based on individual needs. Treatment can be flexible, individualized, and rely on more play and fewer verbalization.

More structured play assessments may be used in addition to other assessment methods. A number of such assessment measures, described in Gitlin-Weiner, Sandgrund, and Schaefer (2000), include scales for assessing therapeutic play, tapping both affective and thematic characteristics of play. The Puppet Sentence Completion Task (PSCT) is one example of a developmentally sensitive projective assessment measure appropriate for use in CBPT assessment with young children (Knell, 1992, 1993a; Knell & Beck, 2000).

Treatment

CBPT takes place as the child moves through several treatment stages, which have been described as the introductory/orientation, assessment, middle, and termination stages (see Knell, 1999, for more comprehensive descriptions). During the treatment, or middle, stage of CBPT, the therapist has developed a treatment plan, and the therapy begins to focus on increasing the child's self-control, promoting his or her, sense of accomplishment, and teaching him or her more adaptive responses to deal with specific situations. Depending on the presenting problem(s), the therapist will have a wide array of cognitive and behavioral interventions from which to chose. These are considered carefully, providing as much specificity as possible between the intervention and the child's specific problems/concerns. Generalization and relapse prevention will be incorporated into the middle stages of therapy so that the child can learn to utilize new skills across a broad range of settings, and to begin to develop skills that will decrease the chances of setbacks after therapy is completed.

One important question during the middle stage is the issue of structured versus unstructured play. According to Knell (1993a, 1999), both are important for change to occur in the child. By its nature, CBPT involves structured, goal-directed activities. Structured, goal-directed activities are important for working on problem solving and teaching more adaptive behaviors. This is a format for the psychoeducational aspects of the therapy. However, CBPT must also include unstructured time, during which the child brings spontaneous material to the session. Unstructured, spontaneously generated information is critical to treatment, for without it the therapist would lose a rich source of clinical information. The balance of spontaneously generated and more structured activities is a delicate one in CBPT. Through unstructured play, the therapist can gain a sense of the child's thoughts and perceptions by observing the child's spontaneous behavior and verbalizations.

It is usually helpful to structure the therapy sessions by using several puppets or toys with a variety of problems. Two or three puppets are chosen. The therapist names them (or if the child is willing, the child helps the therapist give them names). Finally, the therapist identifies the puppets' "problems." At least one of the puppets should have a "problem" that closely matches the child's problem (e.g., "This puppet gets angry when his dad drops him off at Mom's house. Sometimes, he hits and kicks, because he doesn't want his dad to leave").

Most cognitive-behavioral interventions with children of all ages include some form of modeling. This is particularly true of CBPT, where modeling is a critical component in the play. In CBPT, modeling is used to demonstrate adaptive coping skills to the child, with a toy, book, or puppet demonstrating the behavior that the therapist wants the child to learn. Role playing can also be used, although it is more appropriate for older, school-age children, but it is possible to role-play via modeling for younger children.

The specific interventions used in CBPT interventions can be categorized as either behavioral or cognitive. Although behavioral approaches have often been implemented via a significant adult, they can be used directly with the child in therapy. In either case, the therapist tries to identify factors that reinforce and maintain problematic behaviors so that they can be altered. Behavioral methods usually involve an alteration in activity, whereas cognitive methods deal with changes in thinking. Because maladaptive thoughts lead to maladaptive behaviors, changes in thinking should produce changes in behavior. Through cognitive interventions, children learn to identify maladaptive thoughts, replace them with more adaptive ones, and ultimately change maladaptive behaviors. Because of the verbal nature of cognitive interventions, both behavioral and cognitive interventions are delivered in CBPT in a more "child-friendly" way. In general, research suggests that the combination of cognitive and behavioral interventions are effective in helping children cope with difficult events and emotions (for reviews, see Compton et al., 2004, and Velting, Setzer, & Albano, 2004). For a more comprehensive discussion of how behavioral and cognitive techniques can be integrated into play therapy, see Knell and Dasari (2009).

There is no specific formula for deciding on which interventions to use in CBPT, beyond integrating evidenced-based practice into the treatment. Any of a vast number of empirically supported techniques from the CBT literature can be incorporated into the play and used to help children build skills. Clinicians are urged first to determine what the most important interventions would be for a particular problem, and then to decide how to integrate and deliver these in a developmentally sensitive manner. For example, treatment of separation anxiety usually involves management of specific anxiety symptoms (e.g., contingency management, shaping, extinction, systematic desensitization and cognitive techniques). The CBP therapist would integrate these techniques into the play therapy paradigm in delivering the most developmentally sensitive treatment.

One aspect of the treatment planning is considering treatments that will promote generalization and guard, as much as possible, against relapse (relapse prevention). There has been much attention in CBT regarding the need for therapists to help children generalize what is learned in therapy to be able to apply these skills to the home and other environments (e.g., Braswell & Kendall, 1988). CBT interventions that promote self-control of behavior will help the child generalize, so that his or her behavior is not completely "other-driven." It is critical to teach parents, teachers, and other important adults in the child's life to help the child maintain gains from therapy. Children will be more likely to maintain gains if adults support these skills, and therapy should be designed to promote and facilitate generalization, rather than assuming it will occur naturally (Stallard, 2006).

In therapy, the cognitive-behavioral play therapist can promote generalization directly by creating play scenarios with settings and people similar to the ones in the child's life. Also, the significant adults in the child's life should be trained to use appropriate reinforcement and extinction techniques. Finally, by promoting generalization and transfer of skills, the therapist begins to decrease reliance on the therapist (Velting et al., 2004) and promote relapse prevention. One technique cognitive-behavioral play therapists use is a book of "lessons learned" that the child and the therapist can work on together.

Termination

During the termination phase, the child and family are prepared for the end of therapy. As the treatment nears an end, the child deals with the reality of termination, as well as his or her feelings about ending treatment. Additionally, because setbacks are part of learning any new skill, children and parents should be helped to understand how they can cope when such setbacks occur. Treatment should prepare the child and family for setbacks by addressing this issue directly and discussing what to expect and what strategies to use in certain situations. High-risk situations are identified as things that might present a "threat" to the child's sense of control and ability to manage.

Ideally, it is recommended that therapy termination is a gradual process, so that preparation for completion of therapy takes place over several sessions. The child should be prepared for the concrete reality of termination (e.g., "You will only be coming in for two more sessions and then we will be saying good-bye"), as well as for the feelings that may accompany the end of treatment. It is common for children to have conflicting feelings about the end of treatment. Such feelings may be addressed directly by the therapist (e.g., " It seems like you may be a little sad that we won't be meeting anymore") or indirectly (e.g., "Some kids tell me that they feel sad when they stop coming to therapy"). Some children may benefit from hearing the therapist model an appropriate emotion related to the end of therapy (e.g., "I will miss seeing you, but I will feel happy knowing that you are doing so well"). The cognitive-behavioral play therapist can confirm for the child that he or she is important and it is okay to have feelings about termination (e.g., "I will miss you too"; "The puppets will miss you, but we're all happy to know you are doing so well").

Younger children often benefit from some type of concrete representation of the end of treatment (e.g., a construction paper chain with each link representing a therapy session until the last one). Older children may understand a calendar, marked with the final therapy sessions. These concrete reminders may also provide visual aides that help the child talk about affect related to the end of therapy. Some children are also helped by a concrete "transitional" object, such as the therapist's business card, or a picture the child draws for the therapist, that he or she sees is being kept in a special place in the therapist's office.

Often times, the final sessions are tapered, so that the therapist may meet the child biweekly or monthly for a period of time. These intermittent appointments may serve to communicate to the child that he or she can manage without the therapist. This is often supplemented with positive reinforcement from the therapist regarding how well the child is doing between sessions. Sometimes, these appointments are scheduled over a period of time, as part of the phasing-out period. Other times, they are intermittently scheduled with a particular event in mind (e.g., the beginning of the school year, a family move, parent remarriage). For example, a child who is doing well, but has some concerns about starting a new school, may be seen intermittently until after he or she has begun in the new setting.

It is important for the child to understand the end of therapy as a positive, rather than a negative, event. The therapist should identify and praise the child's accomplishments in therapy (e.g., working hard, talking about difficult feeling). If he or she feels that "bad" behavior or problems will prompt a return to therapy, the child may act out to see the therapist again. In addition, the therapist should normalize the experience of saying good-bye to significant relationships by talking about examples in the child's life (e.g., friends at the end of camp, teachers at the end of the school year). Reassurances and suggestions for "keeping in touch" can be helpful. Children often like to hear that the parents will keep in touch with the therapist, or that the child can send the therapist a picture or card. Describing an open-door policy, particularly that it is acceptable to return to see the therapist even if things are good, may help the child understand that the therapist still cares, even if the child is not coming in regularly.

Finally, a termination "party" or celebration scheduled for the final session provides a concrete bridge between therapy and termination. It can be useful to involve the child in specific plans about the celebration. The main purpose of this event is to highlight the positive gains made in therapy, emphasizing the child's self-control and mastery of self-help skills. It is appropriate to provide the child with a small, symbolic token of these gains (e.g., a certificate, or small puppet like one that helped the child most in treatment).

FREQUENCY AND DURATION OF TREATMENT

Based on the research, CBPT is most likely to be effective when the session frequency is weekly and the length is approximately 45–50 minutes. However, as treatment progresses and symptoms are reduced, weekly sessions may gradually be more spaced out (e.g., twice a month, then monthly) as movement toward termination is established. Although a 45- to 50-minute session length is preferred, this can be flexible if parents meet with the therapist before or after the play session. However, the time with the child should be at least 25–30 minutes. Duration of CBPT is considered short term, approximately 6 months to a year. But, no specific time frame applies to all cases because the treatment progress depends on multiple variables (e.g., diagnosis, child's motivation, developmental stage).

THE ROLE OF PLAY IN THE INTERVENTION

Play has a critical role in CBPT, as it provides an appropriate, accessible, developmentally specific context for children to participate in therapy. Since play has been shown to improve problem solving, creativity, and emotional expression (e.g., Russ, 2004), it makes sense that play would be the modality for a psychoeducational therapy like CBPT. In order to deliver more complex concepts and techniques, play allows the cognitive-behavioral play therapist to translate these interventions into a modality of play that is understandable to the child and by which the child can communicate. Without play, it is unlikely that the cognitive and behavioral interventions could be communicated to the young child, or that the child could communicate his or her beliefs, emotions, assumptions, and other thoughts.

RESEARCH SUPPORT

Since its emergence as an effective treatment for adult psychological disorders, CBT has consumed the spotlight for childhood treatments. In reviews using either expert criteria or statistical summaries of these numerous studies, CBT has been classified as efficacious for anxiety (Compton et al., 2004; Ishikawa, Okajima, Matsuoko, & Sakano, 2007; King, Heyne, & Ollendick, 2005; Silverman et al., 2008), posttraumatic stress disorder (PTSD)/trauma (Feeny et al., 2004; Silverman et al., 2008), obsessive–compulsive disorder (OCD; Barrett, Farrell, Pina, Peris, & Piacentini, 2008), and depression (David-Ferdon & Kaslow, 2008). For example, Barrett and colleagues (2008) evaluated treatment studies comparing CBT to other treatments for OCD. The authors found that, of the children participating in the CBT treatment group, 40–85% were in remission or no longer met criteria for OCD. Clinical trials, though on a smaller scale than reviews, have shown that CBT is successful for anger management and for reduction of conduct problems (Koegl, Farrington, Augimeri, & Day, 2008). Overall, a large body of research exists to suggest that CBT is a powerful treatment for childhood psychological disorders.

Furthermore, CBT has been effective in treating complex cases involving developmental deficits and comorbity (Hudson, Krain, & Kendall, 2001), improving children's social skills (Lopata, Thomeer, Volker, & Nida, 2006), promoting emotion regulation (Hannesdottir & Ollendick, 2007; Suveg, Kendall, Comer, & Robin, 2006). Also, a few studies suggest that CBT works for anxiety in children with autism spectrum disorders (ASD; Chalfant, Rapee, & Carroll, 2007; Sofronoff, Attwood, & Hinton, 2005). For instance, one study compared group CBT versus wait-list control to treat anxiety in children with ASD (Chalfant et al., 2007). Results indicated that 71.4% of the CBT group no longer met criteria for anxiety.

Although the effectiveness of CBT with school-age children has been well documented, less is known about the effectiveness of CBT, or CBPT, with young children (i.e., ages 3–8). Previous research has been limited to samples of children between the ages of 8 and 15, with the findings being extrapolated to younger populations (i.e., ages 3–8). Kingery and colleagues (2006) propose that, while developmental differences are present in younger children, manualized treatments can be successfully modified for child's cognitive, social, and emotional skills. Several case studies have supported this theory, particularly when children are treated for one disorder. Hirschfeld-Becker et al. (2008) adapted a manualized treatment for children ages 4–7 and piloted the protocol with children who presented with risk factors for an anxiety disorder. Of the nine children treated, eight were judged as improved after receiving the CBT treatment. Additionally, case reports have described effective adaptations of CBT for PTSD (Sheeringa et al., 2007) and a phobia (Miller & Feeny, 2003). CBT seems to show promise for treating complex youth cases, with one case study showing symptom improvement for a child with specific phobia, behavior problems, and developmental delays (Davis, Kurtz, Gardner, & Carman, 2007) and another for trauma related to sexual abuse (Neubauer, Deblinger, & Sieger, 2007). Thus, preliminary evidence suggests that adapting existing CBT protocols works with young children. However, these studies have not specifically included a play component in the interventions.

Two recent studies look at CBT as a preventive intervention. In the first study, fables were used to deliver CBT to elementary schoolchildren in a developmentally sensitive medium. Allain and Lemieux (2007) evaluated the use of a coping skills program in which metaphorical fables were used to teach children about the connections among thoughts, feelings, and behaviors and how to change the connections when behaviors were problematic. This study with approximately 2,000 second to fourth graders showed participation in the intervention was associated with increases in measures of rational thinking after the intervention, as well as improvement in independent teacher ratings on measures of problem behaviors, social skills, and academic competence, as well as self-reported student satisfaction with curriculum.

In the second study, Pearson (2007) used a sample of young children and included the play component inherent in CBPT. In this study, typically developing preschoolers, with school adjustment as the target problem, participated in a study comparing the effects of a cognitive-behavioral play intervention group to two control groups (free-play control, puzzles/coloring control) In the cognitive-behavioral intervention group, dolls and toys were used for modeling and delivery of praise to teach hopeful thinking skills. Self-instruction and practicing positive self-statements were modeled while the children were engaged in pretend play. Pearson found that teachers reported significantly higher hope, higher social competence, and fewer anxiety-withdrawal symptoms for preschoolers in the cognitive-behavioral play intervention group than those in the matched free-play and puzzles/coloring control groups. The children in the cognitive-behavioral play intervention group were seen individually for three sessions incorporating cognitive-behavioral interventions, though this was not technically CBPT. This study represents the first to empirically support CBPT interventions.

CASE STUDIES OF CBPT

CBPT has been shown to be successful in several clinical cases. Approximately 20 case studies of CBPT have been cited in the literature. These cases specifically use play as a means of delivering CBT and are thus considered to be distinctly different from the previously mentioned CBT cases with younger children. Table 10.1 breaks down these studies, based on age, presenting problem, and citation source. (The given name in the citation is listed for ease of locating these case examples.)

Case 1: Elissa

Elissa is a 5-year-old female diagnosed with selective mutism and seen for CBPT for a total of 28 sessions over a 17-month period. The treatment goal was to overcome anxiety in order to talk in the presence of a nonfamily member. Therefore, treatment variables were brave talking behavior and independent coping skills. Process-oriented techniques were learning (i.e., emotional education, modeling) and repeated practice.

A comprehensive intake assessment was conducted through an outpatient clinic at a university medical center. A clinical interview was conducted with parents and behavioral rating scales were obtained. Parents described Elissa's temperament since infancy as shy and slow to warm up. She spoke with her immediate family and peers outside of the classroom, and after a warm-up period of an hour spoke with extended family and some close peers. She had never spoken to teachers or to new adults. However, at age 4, Elissa attended a summer camp where she did not know anyone. Though parents describe her affect as happy, they noted a significant decrease in her talking. After that experience, Elissa stopped talking to extended family and peers. Since age 4, she has not spoken to anyone outside of the family or in the school setting. On the Child Behavior Checklist, her scores for withdrawn and depressed fell in the above-average range (i.e., 84th percentile), while her anxiety score fell in the normal range. Despite her silence with nonfamily members, parents reported that she was happy at home, very connected with her family, and liked by peers at school. After evaluation was com-

TABLE 10.1. Case Studies of CBPT

Presenting problem(s)	Child's age/gender	Name	Citation
Asperger syndrome with features of ADHD and OCD	7 years/female	Samantha	Knell (2003)
Disruptive acting out, secondary to mother's cancer treatment	8 years/female	Tina	Knell (2000)
Divorce	6 years/male	Kenny	Knell (1993a)
Divorce, traumatic observation of domestic violence	6 years/female	Cassandra	Knell (2003)
Encopresis	5 years/male	Terry	Knell & Moore (1990); Knell (1993a)
Fear and phobia-specific fear (fire trucks, sirens)	2 years/male	Billy	Knell (1993a)
Fear and phobia (sleeping in own room)	4 years/female	Laura	Knell (2000); Knell & Dasari (2006)
Fear and phobia (closed spaces)	5 years/male	Jim	Knell (1993a)
Fear and phobia (specific phobia of animals) and adjustment issues	8 years/female	Lisa	Knell & Dasari (2009)
Selective mutism	6 years/female	Chrissy	Knell (1993a, 1993b)
Separation anxiety	4 years/female	Cara	Knell (1999, 2000); Knell & Dasari (2006)
Sexual abuse	3 years/female	Elaine	Ruma (1993)
Sexual abuse	3 years/female	Lisa	Ruma (1993)
Sexual abuse	4 years/male	Richard	Ruma (1993)
Sexual abuse	5 years/ female	Casey	Ruma (1993)
Sexual abuse	6 years/female	Carol	Ruma (1993)

TABLE 10.1. (continued)

Presenting problem(s)	Child's age/gender	Name	Citation
Sexual abuse	6 years/female	Diane	Ruma (1993)
Sexual abuse	7 years/female	Debbie	Ruma (1993)
Sexual abuse	5 years/female	Julie	Knell & Ruma (1996, 2003)
Shyness, inattention, anxiety	6 years/male	Evan	(Knell, 2000)

pleted the parents received feedback and education about the therapy process.

After meeting the therapist initially, an exposure plan was developed in which Elissa was to remain in the presence of the therapist while her mother was gradually faded from the room. A psychoeducational component, provided to Elissa and her mother, involved the goal of "brave talking," which was rewarded with stickers and prizes. In general, for the exposure plan, the steps were (1) mother and child to play in the presence of the therapist, with no interaction from therapist; (2) mother and child to play in the presence of the therapist, therapist plays with mother and child; (3) therapist and child play in the presence of mother, mother gradually moves toward the door. In the past, when placed in a situation with expectation to talk, Elissa either cried or threw a tantrum. Therefore, Elissa's play was considered as a coping skill, as well as a distraction, for which she received stickers as she was learning. Elissa did not talk during this exposure but was able to remain in the room alone with the therapist.

The middle stage of therapy began once the mother was faded out of the room and the exposure plan #2 was explained. The next exposure plan was for Elissa to engage in "brave talking" in the presence of the therapist. Each session started with Elissa and her mother to explain the session agenda. The therapist first introduced a small dog puppet who was also afraid of brave talking. While her mother was still in the room, Elissa named it "Puppy Puppet" by whispering in her mother's ear. Over the course of several months, the therapist modeled how Puppy Puppet approached talking tasks (exposure), used positive self-statements to be brave (coping), and received stickers and praise (reinforcement) from a mommy puppet. For instance, the therapist would have Puppy Puppet describe liking the color red and asking "What is your favorite color?" The process of Puppy Puppet telling facts about himself and asking Elissa the same question continued for several sessions. Finally, after the therapist had Puppy Puppet state that he had one brother (i.e., like Elissa) and then ask Elissa "Do you have any brothers or sisters?" Elissa answered yes in a quiet, barely audible whisper. The therapist remained calm and praised Elissa. She was a given a reward for brave talking.

Initially, Elissa only talked to the puppet, avoiding eye contact with the therapist. Then Elissa was rewarded for talking in a progressively louder voice, talking directly to the therapist, and then making eye contact with therapist. By the end of the middle phase, Elissa talked directly to the therapist in the presence of Puppy Puppet.

Generalization was the primary challenge in this case. Elissa was verbal in session with the therapist, responding to questions in long sentences and in a clear voice at an audible volume. The exposure plan #3 was to work on Elissa talking to adults and peers at both home and school. Each week, Elissa, parents, and therapist developed specific practice tasks for home initially (which was a safer setting) and then for school. For home tasks, parents were asked to organize play dates in their home and have the expectation that Elissa talk to her friends. Rewards were determined and provided consistently for talking. Over the course of a few weeks, Elissa was talking to friends on her own, as well as at other's homes. For school, the therapist worked with the school psychologist and teachers to develop a task list for Elissa. The teacher met independently with Elissa for 15 minutes during lunch time and provided stickers for brave talking. In addition, Elissa was encouraged to do one task from this list each day:

> Say hi to my teacher.
> Say hi to my teacher's aide.
> Talk to friend near the school.
> Say hi to a friend in the classroom loud enough so another child can hear.
> Talk with Mom and group of friends in afterschool room.

With praise, encouragement, and gentle coaching from therapist and family, Elissa spoke to children in the classroom and finally spoke a few words to her teacher.

Elissa was talking at home and at school with both peers and adults. Therefore, at this point, Elissa was seen biweekly for therapy and tentative plans were set for termination. Relapse prevention was developed with the parents on (1) strategies to maintain and continue generalization of skills to home and school, (2) "warning signs" for relapse (e.g., refusing to talk for a period of time), and (3) an open-door policy for returning to therapy. Parents reported that, overall, Elissa was better able to manage her anxiety and approach previously avoided situations. As plans were being made for her therapy graduation party, Elissa expressed much excitement. Her parents and younger brother attended. The parents were asked to discuss Elissa's progress in therapy. Both gave brief speeches. The therapist presented Elissa with a graduation certificate. Afterward, Elissa and parents enjoyed cookies and snacks in session.

Six weeks after termination, Elissa's mother sent an e-mail to the therapist, with the heading, "ELISSA SPOKE IN FRONT OF THE WHOLE CLASS TODAY!!" In the e-mail, the mother noted that Elissa had "bravely" spoken to each boy in the class, and whispered to the last three students, after having a discussion with the teacher about needing to speak with each child in the class individually. After speaking to all the children, she then spontaneously answered a question during circle time by standing up and answering out loud (as opposed to coming up to the teacher and whispering the answer in her ear as she usually did). One year after termination, Elissa's mother sent another e-mail describing that Elissa had maintained treatment progress of brave talking in all settings. Furthermore, she had received a main role in the school play, which she accepted, and was looking forward to the performance.

Case 2: Robert

Robert is a 6-year-old male who was referred by a school psychologist who had completed a recent neuropsychological assessment. The results of the assessment indicated that anxiety tended to interfere with Robert's school performance and social interactions. His symptoms were consistent with generalized anxiety disorder and mild oppositional defiant disorder. At present, Robert has been seen for CBPT for a total of eight sessions, with treatment ongoing. The key treatment variable was child involvement. Process-oriented techniques were learning (i.e., emotional education, modeling) and cognitive restructuring.

Robert and his mother came to the initial session together. First, a clinical interview with the mother was conducted to supplement the neuropsychological assessment. Mother noted that the following behaviors were observed at home and school: expressing worries about school performance and pleasing parents, seeking reassurance, "freezing up" in new situations, frequent headaches, and not wanting to speak in class. When Robert was seen alone, he separated from his mother to enter the therapy room. He presented as a friendly, talkative child who responded appropriately to the therapist's questions. When asked about his anxiety and related symptoms, Robert seemed uncertain of how to respond and repeatedly asked the therapist, "What do you mean?" or "Why do you want to know that?" in a very calm inquisitive way. Furthermore, when asked to participate in pretend play, he was reluctant to engage. For instance, when the therapist introduced a dog stuffed animal that was anxious, Robert responded with "What do I say?" and "I don't really understand." The therapist described pretend play and used analogies with TV shows (e.g., *Sesame Street*) and childhood games like school. Although Robert understood the context, he said that he did not want to pretend play and that he was unsure how to answer. As a result, the therapist decided to use games and drawings as the play medium for psychoeducation.

In the initial stage of treatment, the goal was to prepare Robert for CBPT with the broader context of anxiety management. During behavioral observations in the initial sessions, the therapist noted that Robert was able to label other's, but not his own, emotions. The therapist used modeling and shaping to increase Robert's comfort with play and emotional expression. Robert and the therapist played the Emotions Game (Johnson, 2003). This is a developmentally appropriate board game in which children are given points for guessing matches between an event and 12 different emotions (e.g., "You are not invited to a friend's party" matches with sad). Also, Robert was asked to play "feeling charades," a game in which people take turns acting out an event and matching emotion while the other person guesses. Robert wanted to play but asked the therapist to act out the events. He stated that he was "not good at acting out things." The therapist agreed to act out three events to model the strategy. Then Robert was asked to try acting out some that the therapist selected as easy (e.g., "You get a bad grade on a math test"). He agreed to try one and therapist praised him for his efforts. At this point, Robert was better able to identify his own emotions. When asked about his week, Robert described feelings that accompanied certain events such as a time when he worried about meeting his parent's friend.

Next, in order for Robert to increase comfort with play, the therapist used books to normalize negative emotional experiences. Robert was asked to read children's books on emotions such as *Today I Feel Silly* (i.e., for all emotional experiences) and *Don't Rant and Rave on Wednesday* (i.e., for anger). Through the use of the books, the therapist was able to validate and provide a model for emotional experiences. In addition, Robert and the therapist selected "helpful phrases" from the books, which were written down and were similar to positive coping statements (e.g., "all kids feel negative emotions," "emotion are not right or wrong but behaviors can be right or wrong"). To continue a step further, the playful strategy for modeling anxiety as an emotion was watching You Tube clips of cartoons or children experiencing anxiety. Overall, the purpose was to help shift Robert to an accurate, realistic view of emotions as universal human experience.

In a recent session, Robert demonstrated the skills to begin the middle stages of CBPT. He was reintroduced to the dog stuffed animal (e.g., now named Pooch) with anxiety problems. Robert agreed to answer questions for Pooch and chose to be an elephant stuffed animal. Yet he was reluctant to select a name for the elephant. When the therapist suggested "Floppy," he smiled and said "Okay." He repeatedly checked in with the therapist about how to answer questions, but was pleased when praised for his efforts. At the end of the session, the therapist asked Robert if he wanted to "hang out" with the characters and play, and Robert was very agreeable to such structured play.

Play has served a number of roles in the psychotherapeutic work with Robert. Initially, Roberts' difficulty with pretend play and his problems with emotional expression made the play component of CBPT problematic. Mann and McDermott (1983) noted that some children who experienced a trauma have not learned how to play, and must be taught to play and trust the therapist before any form of play therapy can take place. Although Robert had been neither abused nor neglected, he reported that his parents were highly critical and used harsh discipline techniques, possibly contributing to his difficulty in initially engaging in a trusting therapeutic relationship and being spontaneous. In modeling pretend play for Robert, the therapist began at a point where he was comfortable and engaged, showing him how to play. Thus, as with all CPBT, play was used as a means of modeling. In this case, a more basic level of teaching Robert to play was needed, whereas many children have these basic skills before beginning CBPT. As Robert's ability to engage in this play increased, the therapist introduced more modeling of positive coping self-statements and problem solving. In regard to Robert's ability to communicate, play was his indirect method of talking about his emotional experiences in ways that he could not do with words. Finally, play served to normalize emotions, a difficult arena for Robert, and showed ways to express emotions (again via modeling) through puppets.

RECOMMENDATIONS FOR NEXT STEPS IN RESEARCH

CBPT is a significant contribution to the child psychotherapy literature. It offers a developmentally appropriate approach while using empirically supported techniques. However, based on the present review of the research, several recommendations for future studies arise. First, more case studies with outcome assessment are needed. Of the published case studies, many have not completed pre- and post-assessment. Despite clinical impressions of improvement, showing empirical support for such improvement is an important step in establishing the efficacy of CBPT. Also, it is recommended that reviews of current clinical case studies be conducted. This is because an evaluation of the research in a systematic fashion will allow more concrete conclusions about the existing literature.

Another recommendation is for the development of a manualized CBPT treatment using modification from existing CBT manuals. Such a manual would incorporate the significant play component added to CBT, so that treatment is developmentally appropriate for younger children. Clearly, there is a significant need to use effective CBT protocols to inform the implementation of manualized treatments based on developmental factors (Kingery et al., 2006). The challenge is for the manual to be structured but also to allow flexibility. Such flexibility would be important for individual children to be able to bring spontaneous therapeutic material to treatment, as well as for applications to a variety of childhood psychological disorders. Lastly, although ambitious given the infancy of CBPT research, randomized, clinical intervention studies comparing CBPT to wait list controls should be developed.

REFERENCES

Allain, G. B., & Lemieux, C. M. (2007). The use of metaphorical fables with children: Application of cognitive behavior therapy to prevention interventions. In T. Ronen, & A. Freeman (Eds.), *Cognitive behavior therapy in clinical social work practice* (pp. 213–233). New York: Springer.

Axline, V. (1947). *Play therapy.* New York: Houghton-Mifflin.

Bandura, A. (1969). *Principles of behavior modification.* New York: Holt, Rinehart and Winston.

Barrett, P. M., Farrell, L., Pina, A. A., Peris, T. S., & Piacentini, J. (2008). Evidence-based psychosocial treatments for child and adolescent obsessive–compulsive disorder. *Journal of Clinical Child and Adolescent Psychology,* 37(1), 131–155.

Beck, A. T. (1967). *Depression: Clinical, experimental, and theoretical aspects.* New York: Harper & Row.

Beck, A. T. (1972) *Depression: Causes and treatment.* Philadelphia: University of Pennsylvania Press.

Beck, A. T. (1976). *Cognitive therapy and the emotional disorders.* New York: International Universities Press.

Beck, A. T., & Emery, G. (1985). *Anxiety disorders and phobias: A cognitive perspective.* New York: Basic Books.

Bedrosian, R., & Beck, A. T. (1980). Principles of cognitive therapy. In M. J. Mahoney (Ed.), *Psychotherapy process: Current issues and future directions* (pp. 127–152). New York: Plenum Press.

Bierman, K. L. (1983). Cognitive development and clinical interviews with children. In B. B. Lahey & A. Kazdin (Eds.), *Advances in clinical child psychology* (Vol 6, pp. 217–250). New York: Plenum Press.

Braswell, L., & Kendall, P. C. (1988). Cognitive-behavioral methods with children. In K. S. Dobson (Ed.), *Handbook of cognitive behavioral therapy* (pp. 167–213). New York: Guilford Press.

Chalfant, A. M., Rapee, R., & Carroll, L. (2007). Treating anxiety disorders in children with high functioning autism spectrum disorders: A controlled trial. *Journal of Autism and Developmental Disorders, 37*(10), 1842–1857.

Compton, S. N., March, J. S., Brent, D., Albano, A. M., Weersing, V. R., & Curry, J. (2004). Cognitive-behavioral psychotherapy for anxiety and depressive disorders in children and adolescents: An evidence-based medicine review. *Journal of the American Academy of Child and Adolescent Psychiatry, 43*, 930–959.

David-Ferdon, C., & Kaslow, N. J. (2008). Evidence-based psychosocial treatments for child and adolescent depression. *Journal of Clinical Child and Adolescent Psychology, 37*(1), 62–104.

Davis, T. E., Kurtz, P. F., Gardner, A. W., & Carman, N. B. (2007). Cognitive-behavioral treatment for specific phobias with a child demonstrating severe problem behavior and developmental delays. *Research in Developmental Disabilities, 28*(6), 546–558.

Ellis, A. (1962). *Reason and emotion in psychotherapy*. New York: Lyle Stuart.

Emery, G., Bedrosian, R., & Garber, J. (1983). Cognitive therapy with depressed children and adolescents. In D. P. Cantwell & G. A. Carlson (Eds.), *Affective disorders in childhood and adolescence—An update* (pp. 445–471). New York: Spectrum.

Feeny, N. C., Foa, E. B., Treadwell, K. R. H., & March, J. S. (2004). Posttraumatic stress disorder in youth: A critical review of the cognitive and behavioral treatment outcome literature. *Professional Psychology: Research and Practice, 35*, 466–476.

Giorano, M., Landreth, G., & Jones, L. (2005). *A practical handbook for building the play therapy relationship*. Lanham, MD: Aronson.

Gitlin-Weiner, K., Sandgrund, A., & Schaefer, C. (2000). *Play diagnosis and assessment* (2nd ed.). New York: Wiley.

Hannesdottir, D. K., & Ollendick, T. H. (2007). The role of emotion regulation in the treatment of child anxiety disorders. *Clinical Child and Family Psychology Review, 10*(3), 275–293.

Hirshfeld-Becker, D. R., Masek, B., Henin, A., Blakely, L. R., Rettew, D. C., Dufton, L., et al. (2008). Cognitive-behavioral intervention with young anxious children. *Harvard Review of Psychiatry, 16*(2), 113–125.

Hudson, J. L., Krain, A. L., & Kendall, P. C. (2001). Expanding horizons: Adapting manual-based treatments for anxious children with comorbid diagnoses. *Cognitive and Behavioral Practice, 8*(4), 338–345.

Ishikawa, S., Okajima, I., Matsuoka, H., & Sakano, Y. (2007). Cognitive behavioural therapy for anxiety disorders in children and adolescents: A meta-analysis. *Child and Adolescent Mental Health, 12*(4), 164–172.

Johnson, P. F. (2003). *The emotions game*. East Moline, IL: LinguiSystems.

Kendall, P. C. (Ed.). (2006). *Child and adolescent therapy: Cognitive-behavioral procedures* (3rd ed.). New York: Guilford Press.

Kendall, P. C., & Braswell, L. (1985). *Cognitive-behavioral therapy for impulsive children*. New York: Guilford Press.

King, N. J., Heyne, D., & Ollendick, T. H. (2005). Cognitive-behavioral treatments for anxiety and phobic disorders in children and adolescents: A review. *Behavioral Disorders, 30*(3), 241–257.

King, N. J., & Ollendick, T. H. (1997). Annotation: Treatment of childhood phobias. *Journal of Child Psychology and Psychiatry and Allied Disciplines, 38*, 349–400.

Kingery, J. N., Roblek, T. L., Suveg, C., Grover, R. L., Sherrill, J. T., & Bergman, R. L. (2006). They're not just "little adults": Developmental considerations for implementing cognitive-behavioral therapy with anxious youth. *Journal of Cognitive Psychotherapy, 20*(3), 263–273.

Knell, S. M. (1992). *Puppet sentence completion task*. Unpublished manuscript.

Knell, S. M. (1993a). *Cognitive-behavioral play therapy*. Northvale, NJ: Aronson.

Knell, S. M. (1993b). To show and not tell: Cognitive-behavioral play therapy in the treatment of elective mutism. In T. Kottman & C. Schaefer (Eds.), *Play therapy in action: A casebook for practitioners* (pp. 169–208). Northvale, NJ: Aronson.

Knell, S. M. (1994). Cognitive-behavioral play therapy. In K. O'Connor & C. Schaefer (Eds.), *Handbook of play therapy: Vol. 2. Advances and innovations.* (pp. 111–142). New York: Wiley.

Knell, S. M. (1997). Cognitive-behavioral play therapy. In K. O'Connor & L. Mages (Eds.), *Play therapy theory and practice: A comparative presentation* (pp. 79–99). New York: Wiley.

Knell, S. M. (1998). Cognitive-behavioral play therapy. *Journal of Clinical Child Psychology, 27*, 28–33.

Knell, S. M. (1999). Cognitive behavioral play therapy. In S. W. Russ & T. Ollendick (Eds.), *Handbook of psychotherapies with children and families* (pp. 385–404). New York: Plenum Press.

Knell, S. M. (2000). Cognitive-behavioral play therapy with children with fears and phobias. In H. G. Kaduson & C. E. Schaefer (Eds.), *Short term therapies with children* (pp. 3–27). New York: Guilford Press.

Knell, S. M. (2003). Cognitive-behavioral play therapy. In C. E. Schaefer (Ed.), *Foundations of play therapy* (pp. 175–191). New York: Wiley.

Knell, S. M., & Beck, K. W. (2000). Puppet sentence completion task. In C. E. Schaefer, K. Gitlin-Weiner, A. Sandgrund (Eds.), *Play diagnosis and assessment* (Vol. 2, pp. 704–721). New York: Wiley.

Knell, S. M., & Dasari, M. (2006). Cognitive-behavioral play therapies for children with anxiety and phobias. In H. G. Kaduson & C. E. Schaefer (Eds.), *Short-term play therapy for children* (2nd ed., pp. 22–50). New York: Guilford Press.

Knell, S. M., & Dasari, M. (2009). CBPT: Implementing and integrating CBPT into clinical practice. In A. Drewes (Ed.), *The effective blending of play therapy and cognitive behavioral therapy: A convergent approach* (pp. 321–352). New York: Wiley.

Knell, S. M., & Moore, D. J. (1990). Cognitive-behavioral play therapy in the treatment of encopresis. *Journal of Clinical Child Psychology, 19,* 55–60.

Knell, S. M., & Ruma, C. D. (1996). Play therapy with a sexually abused child. In M. Reinecke, F. M. Dattilio, & A. Freeman (Eds.), *Cognitive therapy with children and adolescents: A casebook for clinical practice* (pp. 367–393). New York: Guilford Press.

Knell, S. M., & Ruma, C. D. (2003). Play therapy with a sexually abused child. In M. Reinecke, F. M. Dattilio, & A. Freeman (Eds.), *Cognitive therapy with children and adolescents: A casebook for clinical practice* (2nd ed., pp. 338–368). New York: Guilford Press.

Koegl, C. J., Farrington, D. P., Augimeri, L. K., & Day, D. M. (2008). Title evaluation of a targeted cognitive-behavioral program for children with conduct problems—The SNAPReg. Under 12 Outreach Project: Service intensity, age and gender effects on short- and long-term outcomes. *Clinical Child Psychology and Psychiatry, 13*(3), 419–434.

Landreth, G. (2002). *Play therapy: The art of the relationship* (2nd ed.). New York: Brunner Routledge.

Lopata, C., Thomeer, M. L., Volker, M. A., & Nida, R. E. (2006). Effectiveness of a cognitive-behavioral treatment on the social behaviors of children with Asperger disorder. *Focus on Autism and Other Developmental Disabilities, 21*(4), 237–244.

Mann, E., & McDermott, J. F. Jr (1983). Play therapy for victims of child abuse and neglect. In C. E. Schaffer & K. J. O'Connor (Eds.), *Handbook of play therapy* (pp. 283–307). New York: Wiley.

Meichenbaum, D. (1971). Examination of model characteristics in reducing avoidance behavior. *Journal of Personality and Social Psychology, 17,* 298–307.

Miller, V. A., & Feeny, N. C. (2003). Modification of cognitive-behavioral techniques in the treatment of a five-year-old girl with social phobia. *Journal of Contemporary Psychotherapy, 33*(4), 303–319.

Neubauer, F., Deblinger, E., & Sieger, K. (2007). Trauma-focused cognitive-behavioral therapy for child sexual abuse and exposure to violence: Case of Mary, age 6. In F. Neubauer, E. Deblinger, K. Sieger, & N. Boyd Webb (Eds.), *Play therapy with children in crisis: Individual, group, and family treatment* (3rd ed., pp. 107–132). New York: Guilford Press.

O'Connor, K. (1991). *The play therapy primer.* New York: Wiley.

Pearson, B. (2007). *Effects of a Cognitive Behavioral Play Intervention on children's hope and school adjustment.* Unpublished doctoral dissertation, Case Western Reserve University.

Rachman, S. (1968). The role of muscular relaxation in desensitization therapy. *Behavior Research and Therapy, 6,* 159–166.

Ruma, C. (1993). Cognitive-Behavioral Play Therapy with sexually abused children. In S. M. Knell (Ed.), *Cognitive-behavioral play therapy* (pp. 197–230). Northvale, NJ: Aronson.

Russ, S. W. (2004). *Play in child development and psychotherapy: Toward empirically supported practice*. Mahwah, NJ: Erlbaum.

Scheeringa, M. S., Salloum, A., Arnberger, R. A., Weems, C. F., Amaya-Jackson, L., & Cohen, J. A. (2007). Feasibility and effectiveness of cognitive-behavioral therapy for posttraumatic stress disorder in preschool children: Two case reports. *Journal of Traumatic Stress, 20*(4), 631–636.

Shirk, S. R., & Russell, R. L. (1996). *Change processes in child psychotherapy: Revitalizing treatment and research*. New York: Guilford Press.

Silverman, W. K., Ortiz, C. D., Viswesvaran, C., Burns, B. J., Kolko, D. J., Putnam, F. W., et al. (2008). Evidence-based psychosocial treatments for children and adolescents exposed to traumatic events. *Journal of Clinical Child and Adolescent Psychology, 37*(1), 156–183.

Sofronoff, K., Attwood, T., & Hinton, S. (2005). A randomised controlled trial of a CBT intervention for anxiety in children with Asperger syndrome. *Journal of Child Psychology and Psychiatry, 46*(11), 1152–1160.

Stallard, P. (2006). The involvement of parents in child-focused cognitive behaviour therapy. *Hellenic Journal of Psychology, 3*, 23–38.

Suveg, C., Kendall, P. C., Comer, J. S., & Robin, J. (2006). Emotion-focused cognitive-behavioral therapy for anxious youth: A multiple-baseline evaluation. *Journal of Contemporary Psychotherapy, 36*(2), 77–85.

Truax, C. B., & Carkhuff, R. R. (1967). *Toward effective counseling and psychotherapy: Training and practice*. Chicago: Aldine.

Velting, O., Setzer, J., & Albano, A. (2004). Update on and advances in assessment and cognitive-behavioral treatment of anxiety disorders in children and adolescents. *Professional Psychology Research and Practice, 35*, 42–54.

Wagner, M. K., & Cauthen, N. R. (1968). Case histories and shorter communications. *Behaviour Research and Therapy, 6*, 225–227.

Wolpe, J., & Lazarus, A. (1966). *Behavior therapy techniques: A guide to the treatment of neuroses*. Oxford, UK: Pergamon Press.

APPENDIX 10.1. Play Materials

CBPT is usually conducted in a playroom or office equipped with appropriate play materials. To some extent, such materials can be chosen by the individual cognitive-behavioral play therapist. Ideally, the room has a variety of toys, art supplies, puppets, dolls, and other materials, such as the following suggested items:

- Puppets: dog (for children with dog phobias), alligator or shark (for use with children who bite, or have issues with the expression of aggression), turtle (for children who are shy or have social anxieties)
- Construction paper of different colors
- Markers/crayons
- Dollhouse—include toilet (for children with toilet issues); bed (for those with sleep problems)
- Family set of figures—includes mother, father, sibling-male, sibling-female, baby. Ideally there should be families representing different ethnic/racial groups
- Books on many different topics, including those related to moods/feelings, anxiety/fear, divorce, going to a new school, etc.
- Toy cars
- Games to build therapeutic alliance—*Checkers, CandyLand, Connect Four*
- Therapeutic games—*Talking, Feeling, Doing Game; Ungame*
- Clay or Play-Doh
- Legos or other building supplies
- Feeling faces, posters, and feeling blocks
- Stickers—particular ones that tie in with therapy themes (e.g., sign language "I love you stickers" from *The Kissing Hand*, trains from the *Little Engine That Could*, positive reinforcement themes)
- Dry erase board
- Worksheets with pictures of people or animals with thought bubbles above their heads

11

The Importance of Play in Both the Assessment and Treatment of Young Children

Elizabeth J. Short, Maia Noeder, Suzanne Gorovoy, Michael J. Manos, and Barbara Lewis

Play is a central aspect of the lives of young children. The world of play serves not only as a relaxation and enjoyment function for children, but also serves adults as an important window into children's skills in the cognitive, motor, social, and emotional domains (Linder, 1993; Johnson-Martin, Attermeir, & Hacher, 2004). Additionally, play is an ideal developmental medium for directly and indirectly teaching children critical cognitive, linguistic, behavioral, and emotional skills (Piaget, 1962; Vygotsky, 1986; Linder, 1993). The purposes of this chapter are as follows: First, we delineate evidence that documents the importance of play as an essential assessment tool for young children, particularly those with special needs. Second, we discuss individual differences in the play skills of children diagnosed with language disabilities, attention-deficit/hyperactivity disorder (ADHD) and Asperger syndrome. Third, we present an overview of the therapeutic interventions typically used with each of these populations and the important role that play can serve in the intervention process. Finally, we identify important future directions in both assessment and intervention using play as an essential vehicle.

PLAY AS AN ESSENTIAL ASSESSMENT TOOL

Assessment of young children with special needs is done for a variety of reasons including screening, diagnostic assessment, program planning, and evaluation (Linder, 1993). Initial screenings are conducted by educators and clinicians alike as an expeditious way to determine which children are in need of further evaluation and which children appear to be developing in a typical or accelerated manner. When screeners identify children at risk, further diagnostic assessment is undertaken in order to identify patterns of strengths and weaknesses that can be targeted for intervention. Comprehensive assessment can lead to more accurate diagnoses and ultimately to increasingly effective treatments (Sattler, 2001). Diagnostic assessment tends to utilize a traditional, individualistic approach that rarely addresses the important environmental factors that play a crucial role in problematic behaviors. According to Linder (1993), program planning adopts a broader approach to assessment by examining not only the specific skills and processes within the child that are in need of remediation but also the environmental modifications necessary to optimize the child's growth and development. Thus, traditional diagnostic assessment is more consistent with the static assessment model that is designed to assess a child's current state of knowledge, whereas program planning is more consistent with the dynamic assessment model that is designed to assess not only what the child has learned, but also his or her rate of learning and environmental modifications that can optimize learning (Haywood & Lidz, 2006; Feurstein, 1979, 1980). Finally, the purpose of assessment should be tied less to identifying defects in the individual and more toward ascertaining what treatment is likely to be effective and whether an implemented treatment is efficacious. This evaluation component has become of paramount importance to the fields of clinical psychology and education as both fields attempt to establish the cost-effectiveness and the reliability of psychosocial, educational, and psychopharmacological treatments.

Calls for accountability and efficacy of treatment have pressed for the creation of new ways to chart individual growth through the comparison of baseline skill sets to outcome measures in order to determine the effects of short-term and long-term interventions. Since the passing of the 2001 No Child Left Behind Act, billions of dollars have been funneled into the creation of new, increasingly refined, precise, and dynamic tests to assess not only a child's current state of knowledge but also his or her rate of learning. Teacher-training programs have emphasized the need to understand the "whole child," with a new emphasis placed on employing a diverse set of measures designed to assess development in a variety of domains including the physical (gross and fine motor), cognitive, communicative (expressive, receptive, and pragmatic), social–emotional, and functionally adaptive. As with all new tests, the importance of standardization, reliability, validity, and age-normed comparisons have been stressed (Sattler & Hoge, 2006).

Despite the acknowledged importance of dynamic assessment tailored to the individual child within a broader social context and social network, most psychological tests employ standardized instructions that do not allow the examiner to modify procedures and as such appear to be primarily designed to meet the needs of typically functioning middle-class children (Li, Walton, & Nuttal, 1999). Unfortunately, "standardized, norm-referenced assessment approaches are not appropriate or desirable for all young children with disabilities" (Bucy, Smith, & Landau, 1999, p. 319). The need to adapt traditional norm-referenced tests to accommodate the special abilities of children with developmental disabilities has become common practice, with the information gleaned from "limits testing" often presenting a more accurate picture of the young child's profile of strengths and weaknesses. According to Sattler (2001), assessments of the skills of young children should ideally first begin with a complete static, standardized presentation of the measure, followed by a nonstandardized, dynamic administration of select subtests. During the dynamic or "limits-testing" reassessment, educators and clinicians may choose to modify the testing procedure through a variety of means including but not limited to the following: (1) provision of additional time, (2) allowing pointing responses in place of verbal naming, (3) reformatting open-ended responses to multiple-choice questions, (4) changing the modality of the task (multimodal presentation instead of overreliance on auditory presentation), and (5) altering the format of the task presentation (use of play as an important medium; Salvia & Ysseldyke, 2001). Careful assessment of the young child should be multidimensional and elicit information from a variety of sources including family members, teachers, and professionals. In addition, the assessment should carefully examine the young child's environment, with an eye for how the environment may facilitate or adversely impact the child's developmental outcomes.

Does the inclusion of both static and dynamic approaches in assessment procedures address the problem of authentic assessment for educators and clinicians who work with young children diagnosed with developmental disabilities? According to Linder (1993), traditional assessment is often inappropriate for young children with developmental disabilities for several reasons:

1. It may penalize children with special needs (e.g., high verbal requirements of a test can adversely impact the performance of a child with language delays).
2. It may be used inappropriately with children with disabilities (e.g., children with cerebral palsy can be given motor subtests).
3. It often omits functional assessments.
4. It lacks a direct relationship between the result and the intervention required.
5. It has limited predictive validity.
6. It is quite costly in terms of both time and money.

Additionally, because traditional assessment materials are presented in a decontextualized fashion, they rarely capitalize on the important role that hands-on interactive play assessments serve in enabling young children to demonstrate cognitive competence.

Frustrated by the limitations of standardized measures and responsive to the unique demands posed by young children, the field of assessment has turned away from the exclusive use of standardized tests and instead relies on a combination of standardized tests and observational approaches. A close examination of these alternatives reveals that "play-based assessment" is the assessment measure most commonly used with young children (Bagnato & Neisworth, 1994). By employing play as the assessment medium from which to observe cognitive competence, preschoolers have been shown to demonstrate greater cognitive competence than they otherwise would in a less interactive assessment venue (Short & Miller, 1981). Play-based assessments seem ideally suited for young children, particularly because play is a central element in the lives of young children. According to Lerner and his colleagues (Lerner, Mardell-Czudnowski, & Goldberg, 1987), play-based assessments are important for children with disabilities for several reasons: First, play provides a perfect medium for facilitating growth and development in motor, cognitive, language, and social skills domains. Second, the arena of play provides a perfect method with which to reinforce newly and previously acquired skills, while simultaneously extinguishing inappropriate behaviors. Finally, the world of play is pleasurable, safe, and nonthreatening, with the mastery of skills enhancing the pleasurability of the play. It is not surprising that the interest of educators and clinicians in play as a key assessment tool has risen. Furthermore, it is understandable that increasingly numerous measures have been created using play as an assessment medium and that research has been designed to address the utility of this approach.

PLAY-BASED ASSESSMENT

Although all play-based methods of assessment differ from traditional assessment, they are also quite diverse in scope and specificity. First, specificity of item content may vary in play-based assessment, with some play assessments employing standardized instructions, items, procedures, and scoring (Affect in Play Scale [APS]; Russ, 1987) and other measures (Transdisciplinary Play-Based Assessment [TPBA]; Linder, 1993) adopting a more flexible approach allowing for different sets of materials, instructions, and procedures that can be tailored to the needs of individual children. Thus, play assessments can fall on a continuum from formal to informal, with formal assessments using a series of standardized toys and explicit directions while informal assessments use a less standardized sequence of toys and may rely on data gleaned from informants (i.e., parents and teachers) who are privy to information gained outside of the actual assessment. Second, the role of the clinician varies in play-based assessments, with the clinician serving as an observer in some instances and as an active participant/facilitator in other cases. Third, play-based measures differ in the scores they produce. Some measures yield descriptive profiles of strengths and weaknesses, while others yield categorical scores (e.g., organization, positive affect), and still others produce a standard "play age" score. Fourth, play-based methods of assessment differ in whether they utilize free play or structured elicitation (Linder, Holm, & Walsh, 1999). Free-play assessments typically take place with the child unaware of the evaluation component and can occur in a variety of settings (e.g., home, school, office) and under little or no guidance by adults. In contrast, the structured elicitation assessment model of play is designed to optimize the level of play exhibited by the child through the guidance afforded by a skilled adult model. As noted by Linder et al. (1999), comparisons can be made between play performance exhibited in the static (i.e., independent) free-play situation and play performance exhibited under the more dynamic structured elicitation model (i.e., adult-facilitated play), with these comparisons often yielding important insights into developmental competencies in a wide variety of domains. Finally, play-based assessments can be short in duration (APS-PR: 10 minutes) or quite lengthy (TPBA: 60 minutes). When used in conjunction with other standardized assessments, play assessments should be short and focused. When used in isolation, play assessments can be lengthier. Regardless of your assessment strategy, play-based assessments are becoming a critical component of comprehensive assessments because they afford educators and clinicians a rich database of information on young children's skills in the motor, cognitive, linguistic, and social–emotional domains. Play-based assessments appear to be particularly advantageous when young children with developmental disabilities are unable to or refuse to complete standardized, decontextualized assessment instruments. Play-based assessments open a window into the young child's skills that had been temporarily closed by the more decontextualized, standardized techniques. In subsequent sections of this chapter, we attempt to highlight what is known about play in each diagnostic category and how play has allowed us to find out more about children with developmental disabilities than was previously gleaned from traditional assessment instruments.

CHILDREN WITH LANGUAGE DISABILITIES

Communication disorders are common during early childhood and are typically identified early in the preschool period due to an absence of speech or an atypical pattern of language development. Communication disorders are classified into three broad categories: speech sound disorder (SSD), speech–language impairment (SLI), and combined SSD + SLI. The most common childhood language disorder is SSD, with prevalence rates as high as 15.6% in children under age 3. Rates of SSD decline during the preschool period quite rapidly, with 3.8% of children still classified at 6 years of age (Campbell et al., 2003; Shriberg, Tomblin, & McSweeny, 1999). SSD is the most easily identified speech disorder, with parents and teachers readily identifying it due to its impact on the intelligibility of speech in young language users (Short, Freebairn, Hansen, & Lewis, 2008). SSD includes both motoric errors of articulation or phonetic structure as well as phonological errors caused by a misapplication of linguistic rules required to combine sounds. Children with SSD may therefore present with specific speech-production difficulties, phonological-processing difficulties, or both.

SLI is less frequently diagnosed in the preschool period than SSD but is more commonly seen in kindergarten-age children (males 8%, females 6%; Tomblin et al., 1997). Diagnosed later than SSD, SLI tends to be independent of speech sound production and instead is primarily rooted in the comprehension and production of spoken language. SLI encompasses a broad range of difficulties in language skills, including those that are receptive, expressive, or both. Deficits are common in semantics, syntax, and pragmatics, as well as phonological processing and memory. According to the SLI Consortium (2002, 2004), SLI and SSD appear to be genetically independent language disorders. Despite this perceived independence, the two language disorders tend to coexist in a small subgroup of children, with approximately 7% of children experiencing combined SSD + SLI (Johnson et al., 1999).

Identifying speech and language deficits appears to be the most straightforward of all preschool assessments. Despite the ease of early diagnosis, language disabilities (SSD, SLI, and the combined SSD + SLI) resolve slowly and increase the probability of academic, behavioral, and psychological difficulties (Reilly et al., 1999). Given the importance of preschool language status in predicting later academic outcomes (Bishop & Adams, 1990), efforts have been directed at refining assessment and intervention strategies for young language users. While standardized, linguistically based methods of assessment have been the norm in the field, play assessments offer hope for understanding language in context. Additionally, theoretical links between the symbolic processing skills required by both play and language provide further evidence for the utility of play-based assessment measures for understanding the needs of young language users.

Hypothesized Link between Play Skills and Language Disabilities

Debate continues regarding the underlying causes of language deficits in young children. Perhaps the most widely accepted hypothesis is that children with language delays have an "impaired development of more general representational abilities" (Casby, 1997, p. 2). The assumption is that failure to develop linguistic skills in children with language delays is not an isolated disability but rather part of a larger package of under-developed representational skills. Support for the representational deficit theory in children with communication disorders was derived in part from an examination of their play skills. Rescorla and Goossens (1992) argued that symbolic play skills and expressive language skills may follow a similar developmental trajectory during the early childhood period, with a delay in expressive language paralleling a delay in symbolic play.

Although there is general consensus regarding the presence of a representational deficit, less agreement exists as to why these deficits occur. Three hypotheses are currently being entertained as possible explanations for delayed representational play in children with communication disorders: First, the *stylistic hypothesis* argues that delays in symbolic play stem from a stylistic inclination toward repetitive, patterned, and kinesthetic types of play (Rescorla & Goossens, 1992). Rather than adopting a more symbolic or "dramatist" orientation to play, children with communication disorders appear to take great comfort in a repetitive, simplistic, or "patterner" approach to play. Second, the *developmental delay hypothesis* argues that play differences stem from the slower maturation of the symbol-making system of children with language delays as compared to children with normally developing language abilities. The primary assumption underlying the developmental delay hypothesis is that, with time, children with communication delays will develop appropriate play schemes, eventually achieving the flexibility, complexity, and richness in play of typical language learners. The final hypothesis regarding play differences between children with and without language problems focuses on a *retrieval hypothesis*. The argument posits that children with delayed language often experience difficulty accessing words and ideas. They consequently appear to adopt a helpless stance and also appear unmotivated to speak. Fear of failure and lack of practice spirals the child with language disabilities into a passive position. This passive approach to learning and interacting with people and objects transcends their world of play, thus coloring everyday interactions.

Differences in Play Skills between Children with and without Language Impairment

Individual differences in toddlers' and preschoolers' play skills as a function of language competence have been consistently reported, with group differences increasing in magnitude with developmental age (Rescorla & Goossens, 1992). In an early study by Lovell, Hoyle, and Siddal (1968), preschoolers with expressive language delays demonstrated less well-developed sequential play, fewer occurrences of symbolic play, less sophisticated simultaneous play, and less overall complexity in their play patterns when compared to same-age peers without language delays. More specifically, Lovell et al. (1968) found that older and younger preschoolers demonstrated comparable rates of sensorimotor (i.e., functional) play regardless of their language status. In contrast, although no differences emerged between 3-year-old children on symbolic play, dramatic differences emerged between 5-year-old children with and without language impairment. While symbolic play was the most prevalent form of play in all the preschoolers regardless of language status, its frequency appeared to decline in children with language impairments whereas it increased in children without impairments. According to Casby (1997), these findings do not support a developmental delay hypothesis but instead lend credence to both the stylistic and retrieval hypotheses that explain why language delays affect the symbolic performance of children with language impairments.

A similar pattern of findings was obtained by Brown and his colleagues (Brown, Redmond, Bass, Liebergott, & Swope, 1975) when they compared language-impaired (LI) and normally developing language (NL) groups on complexity of play at 3, 4, and 5 years of age. Consistent with the results of Lovel et al. (1968), only the 5-year-old LI and NL groups differed in complexity of play, with older LI children's play rated less complex due to an inability to incorporate language into play scripts. Attempts to disentangle language skills from play skills in children with LI and NL were examined by comparing mean length-of-play sequences (MLPS) to mean length of utterance (MLU; Lombardino, Stein, Kricos, & Wolf, 1986). As expected, MLPS were always superior to MLU in the children with LI, whereas MLU was always superior to MLPS in NL children. Interestingly, when MLU was controlled in this sample, no difference between complexity of play emerged between children with and without language impairment.

In the most comprehensive review of symbolic play and language literature, Casby (1997) summarized the findings as follows: (1) children with LI spend less time than children with NL engaged in symbolic play and (2) children with LI use materials less appropriately (adaptivity) and are more disorganized in their play than children without LI. Casby contended that support for the general symbolic competence and developmental delay hypotheses seemed to be lacking at present. Early differences in symbolic play were absent when comparing LI and NL groups, with minor differences emerging in the presence of more advanced language skills. He further argued that small sample size and heterogeneity (the presence of three diverse language subtypes) precludes a definitive statement about the relationship between language processing and play skills. Additionally, he cautioned clinicians and researchers regarding the possibility that assessment of symbolic play skills may be confounded by the presence of language in the verbal instructions and in the behavioral output. Rather than argue for a general representational hypothesis, Casby contends that children with LI are less able to incorporate language into their symbolic play than NL children. The importance of verbal mediation not only in play, but in other cognitive and behavioral domains as well, appears to increase with development. Future research on the relationship between language and play skills should more carefully examine whether differences in play skills persist on tasks in which the verbal load has been reduced on both the input (modeled task instructions) and the output (scoring play behavior independent of verbal output) side of the equation.

More recently, research has begun to look at the role of language ability in the play behaviors of children with language disabilities (Lewis, Boucher, Lupton, & Watson, 2000). Convinced that language plays a more prominent role in both the conceptual and the symbolic skills of young children than in their functional ability, Lewis and her colleagues assessed the play skills of 2- to 6-year-olds on the Test of Pretend Play (ToPP). Even after controlling for age, symbolic play was significantly correlated with both expressive and receptive language skills, whereas functional play and nonverbal ability were not. These results further support the maturational hypothesis that advancements in linguistic skills influence the quality of children's play.

Taken together, the results from these studies on children with language disabilities suggest strongly that language skills are intimately tied to symbolic play ability. Unanswered questions remain regarding the role that language serves in symbolic play. While it makes sense to contend that language and play skills may in fact be governed by the same symbolic or representational skills, it is also possible that the assessment of play skills are confounded by the presence/absence of language. Adults' ability to understand and score the play behaviors of young children are greatly facilitated by the presence of context, including linguistic context. The failure of the child with language disabilities to provide the examiner or peer with a well-articulated linguistic context might adversely affect his or her ability to demonstrate proficient play skills. Further research is needed to disentangle the verbal context from the play world in an effort to ascertain whether the deficits exhibited are pervasive.

Interventions for Children with Language Disabilities

In general, interventions for children with language impairments have focused on the semantic, syntactic, and phonological aspects of language. The therapy's focus has varied with the type of speech and language disorder that the child presents. For example, children with SSD have primarily been enrolled in therapy designed to enhance articulation as well as phonological processing, phonemic understanding, and grapheme–phoneme relationships (Gillon, 2004; Tallal & Gaab, 2006). Therapy is initiated in the early preschool period and typically continued through early elementary school. Therapy is typically comprised of both individual and group therapy, with the intended outcomes being improved speech articulation, as well as improved spoken and written language skills. The recognition that many children with speech and language disorders also have reading difficulties has led to the incorporation of reading instruction in therapy. Although numerous programs are currently available, the most commonly employed programs are Orton–Gillingham and Lindamood–Bell. These programs utilize a systematic and structured approach to reading and decoding. There is a particular emphasis on phonemic awareness and the programs often incorporate multisensory input.

In addition to phonological processing, many language interventions address deficits in pragmatics or the social use of language (Beilinson & Olswang, 2003; Brinton & Fujiki, 2006). The goal of most pragmatic interventions is to increase social communication, with particular attention paid to essential entry behaviors (i.e., greeting behaviors). Although not typically conceptualized as a play intervention, the clinical implementation of pragmatic interventions frequently relies heavily on role playing and modeling in the context of a small-group setting. The response elicitation model is often employed, as therapists and peers model appropriate social interactions for the child with language impairment. Experimental evidence supporting the feasibility of peer models for improving the language skills of children with language impairments has recently been obtained (DeKroon, Kyte, & Johnson, 2002). In an effort to enhance the conversational competence and play behaviors of children with SLI, dyadic play partnerships were formed between a target child with SLI and either a child without SLI or a child with SLI. Play interactions for children with SLI who had been partnered with a child without SLI were superior to children with SLI who had been paired with another impaired speaker. Greater communicative behaviors, higher conversational success, and higher quality of play were evidenced in the dyads with one typical speaker. Peer partnerships in which one of the participants is more skilled may enable linguistic scaffolding and provide a more optimal learning environment for the less skilled language learner. More research investigating the value of play intervention for improving both the linguistic and the play skills of the young child with language impairments needs to be conducted, however, before solid conclusions can be reached. Nonetheless, contextualized assessments couched in a play context may minimize the passivity and anxiety evidenced by children with language impairments and instead provide them with a rich, supportive environment that encourages active participation and supports their linguistic competence.

CHILDREN WITH ADHD

The diagnosis and treatment of ADHD in preschool children has traditionally been guided by clinical experience, as there is little empirical data available to inform practice. Definitively arriving at a diagnosis of ADHD in preschoolers is problematic since high activity level, impulsivity, and a short attention span are age-appropriate characteristics for most children (Blackman, 1999). Daily variability of behavior, situational responses to environment, and inaccurate adult interpretations of behavior further complicate the diagnostic process. In addition, inappropriate behavioral responses caused by environmental stressors, inadequate parenting skills, and other disorders can mimic ADHD symptoms. Despite diagnostic difficulties, it is clear that ADHD symptoms can impede successful socialization, optimal learning, and goodness-of-fit in parent–child and teacher–child interactions (Barkley, Cooke, Diamond, Zametkin, Thapar, et al., 2002).

Much of the research on children with ADHD focuses on diagnostic precision when utilizing cross-informant interviews. Proper diagnosis requires evidence directly obtained from parents or caregivers regarding the core symptoms of ADHD in various settings, the age of onset, the duration of symptoms, and the degree of functional impairment. Evaluation of a child who may have ADHD should also include assessment for coexisting conditions such as learning disabilities and other psychiatric disorders. In order to meet DSM-IV-TR criteria for ADHD, an assessment of ADHD must determine whether the core behavior symptoms of inattention, hyperactivity, and impulsivity are present in two or more settings. Multi-informant assessment (e.g., parents, preschool teachers, and other professionals) includes an examination of the core symptoms, duration of symptoms, and degree of functional impairment. Largely comprised of clinical interviews, ADHD questionnaires, and rating scales, multi-informant assessments have been shown to successfully differentiate children with ADHD from children without the disorder (Wolraich et al., 2004).

The importance of early diagnosis of ADHD in the preschool period was first noted by Alessandri (1992). He argued that it is imperative to identify ADHD early in order to circumvent the influence of negative interaction with a child's environment, as well as other commonly occurring comorbidities (e.g., conduct disorders, learning disabilities). Furthermore, he contended that early diagnosis is critical when looking at the essential behavioral characteristics associated with the disorder, the developmental trajectory, and the development of "prevention-oriented interventions." Unfortunately, despite Alessandri's recommendations (1992), the field still relies largely on parent/teacher reports of symptoms and no gold behavioral standard exists for evaluating preschoolers independent of adult report. In 1999, Rappley and his colleagues reaffirmed the lack of uniformity in questionnaires employed in assessments of preschoolers with ADHD and further suggested that more than half of preschoolers in the Michigan Medicaid system already exhibited problems that coexisted with ADHD (i.e., psychiatric problems, health issues, or injuries). Within Rappley's sample, it was also found that no standard treatment was consistently being employed, with 57% receiving psychotropic medication (22 different medications employed) and only 27% receiving psychological services. The authors contend that the scarcity of information concerning the diagnosis of ADHD in preschoolers and the limited data pertaining to the efficacy and safety of psychotropic medications for this age group leads to the great variability seen in individual medication regimens.

ADHD and Play

Although play-based assessment has largely been overlooked in the field of ADHD, it may be an especially important tool in understanding the behavioral issues that define ADHD, including inattention, hyperactivity, impulsivity, noncompliance, and antisocial behaviors. Symptoms that define ADHD may affect play behaviors adversely, especially interactive play. First, attentional impairments thought to characterize ADHD have been linked to problematic behaviors in preschoolers, such as excessive shifting of activities during free-play activities and loss of sustained attention during structured tasks (Alessandri & Schramm, 1991; Schleifer et al., 1975; Campbell, 1987). Based on these findings, Alessandri (1992) developed two hypotheses: Children with ADHD would engage in less sustained play behaviors, with considerably more disruptive behaviors in response to requests for transitions than children not previously diagnosed. Also, deficits in attentional control would predispose children with ADHD to immature play behaviors.

In one of the only comprehensive studies of play in preschoolers diagnosed with ADHD and a matched control, Alessandri (1992) made explicit a link between ADHD symptomatology and aberrant play behaviors. Comparisons were made between 20 preschoolers with ADHD and 20 controls who attended a university-based preschool with groups matched for gender, race, and IQ. Free-play data were collected using a time-sampling approach and outcome data were based on a 60-minute sample of behavior for each child. As predicted, children with ADHD exhibited less overall play and greater off-task transition activity than preschoolers without ADHD. These differences in play behaviors are indicative of problems in sustained attention. Developmental delays emerged for children with ADHD in both cognitive and social play as compared to matched controls. The cognitive play of children with ADHD focused on functional or sensorimotor skills rather than symbolic play. The social play of children with ADHD was less parallel and less compliant than the social play exhibited by children without ADHD. These deficits in early play behaviors are concerning to teachers and parents alike as they place the child with ADHD at high risk for academic failure and peer rejection. Through the employment of a play-based assessment instrument, however, clinicians may be better able to identify weaknesses in need of targeted intervention.

Interventions for Children with ADHD

Typically, ADHD interventions are of three types: psychopharmacological, parent training, and behavior management (Barkley, 1990; Pelham et al., 2000). Although psychopharmacological approaches are the mainstay intervention for ADHD, they are more cautiously employed with preschoolers. Only about 1% of preschoolers are prescribed stimulant medication, with stimulants shown to improve behavioral compliance, decrease off-task behaviors, and decrease activity level in overactive preschoolers (Alessandri & Schramm, 1991; Faraone et al., 2002; Short, Manos, Findling, & Schubel, 2004; Zito et al., 2000). Despite the improvements noted in preschooler's behaviors, these improvements are often couched in a backdrop of adverse side effects. Side effects in preschoolers appeared more frequently than typically reported in school-age children; nonetheless, severe side effects were reported in less than 10% of the sample. Side effects most often noted in preschool samples include decreased social interaction, loss of appetite, and dysphoric mood. Recently, Short and her colleagues (2004) suggested that parents and teachers may mistakenly attribute behavioral problems to side effects of medication rather than viewing these problems as typical ADHD behaviors. For example, emotional lability expressed as tantrums may be misconstrued as a medication side effect, when in fact it is often associated with ADHD (Barkley, 1997). With the exception of appetite suppression, comparisons demonstrated that baseline symptoms prior to medication initiation were often more elevated than those present after the initiation of medication (Short et al., 2004). These findings provide further support for Connor's (2002) contention that preschoolers benefit from stimulants and side effects appear minimal; however, great care should be used in the treatment of young children.

To our knowledge, few studies have examined the impact of stimulant medication on the play skills of preschoolers (Alessandri & Schramm, 1991). Despite the paucity of research, findings are quite encouraging. Using a single-subject design, Alessandri and Schramm (1991) examined the effects of dextroamphetamine on attention and impulse control in the social and cognitive play of a 4-year-old child. Employing an A–B–A–B design allowed the authors to more precisely assess changes in play behavior as a function of medication. While on medication, the 4-year-old engaged in developmentally more advanced play behaviors (i.e., greater frequency of symbolic play as compared to functional play) than when he was not on medication. Not only did sustained attention increase during play and group activities under medical management, but play also became more sequentially organized and symbolic. The authors make a strong case for the continued use of play-based assessments as evaluations of the efficacy of psychostimulant treatments (Alessandri & Schramm, 1991), yet further work is needed. Unfortunately, assessments of play have received little formal attention in the field of ADHD since the work of Alessandri and Schramm (1991).

Behavioral interventions have also been found to reduce core symptoms of ADHD and associated problem behaviors (Abikoff et al., 2004; Pelham, Wheeler, & Chronis, 1998). According to Pelham and Fabiano (2008) in their comprehensive review of treatment outcome studies, behavioral parent training and behavioral classroom interventions are empirically supported treatments for ADHD. Additionally, Pelham and Fabiano (2008) found that intensive peer-focused behavioral treatments presented in a recreational setting were also quite effective, regardless of age. While not specifically using a play-like treatment, the implementation of a behavioral treatment in a play-like setting (e.g., recreational games) proved effective in improving peer interactions and social skills and offers hope that play-based interventions may be quite useful with children diagnosed with ADHD.

In summary, preschoolers diagnosed with ADHD are at high risk for future cognitive, behavioral, and socioemotional problems. Careful diagnosis and treatment can impact the course of development in order to avoid lifelong problems. At present, early diagnosis and treatment of the preschoolers presents a set of unique challenges as we try to understand the disorder in a changing developmental landscape. Although little is known about the efficacy of play-based assessment in diagnosing and treating ADHD, we argue that play is an important avenue to pursue to increase the ecological validity of our assessments.

CHILDREN WITH AUTISM AND ASPERGER SYNDROME

Asperger syndrome is a form of autism and as such the core deficit resides in a disturbance in social relatedness (Atwood, 1998). Although social deficits characterize both disorders, important differences must also be noted. First, language deficits plague the child with autism, whereas children with Asperger syndrome typically possess age-appropriate language skills. Second, cognitive differences are apparent such that children with Asperger syndrome exhibit normal or superior cognitive ability and children with autism display significant cognitive impairments. These disabilities tend to manifest differently in the social arena as well. Typically, children with autism are seen as socially indifferent and preferring contact with inanimate objects over humans. In contrast, children with Asperger syndrome are best classified as socially awkward. While they long for social connectedness, their lack of empathy and poor pragmatic skills destine them to social isolation. Finally, children with both autism and Asperger syndrome often have obsessions which they pursue relentlessly. Obsessions span the spectrum from inanimate objects (e.g., cars) to animate objects (e.g., animals/people). Individuals with Asperger syndrome tend to speak rigidly about their current obsession which can be detrimental in social interactions. Adults tend to be more accepting of and intrigued with children who have Asperger syndrome, whereas peers are less forgiving and often annoyed with these children who lack sensitivity to the rules required in initiating and maintaining normal social interactions (Fattig, 2008). This failure to engage in appropriate social reciprocity dooms the child diagnosed with Asperger syndrome to a world of social isolation.

The Play Skills of Children with Asperger Syndrome

The play skills of children diagnosed with either Asperger syndrome or autism has been the subject of careful scrutiny over the last 10 years (Holmes & Willoughby, 2005; Rutherford, Young, Hepburn, & Rogers, 2007; Stanley & Konstantareas, 2007). In general, the play skills of children with autism have been shown to be of lower frequency, less complexity, and lacking in novelty when compared to children who are typically developing (Rutherford et al., 2007). Since 2000, the importance of pretend play in the diagnosis of autism has become so widely accepted that it has been incorporated into several assessment instruments (Autism Diagnostic Observation Schedule [ADOS]: Lord, Rutter, Di Lavore, & Risi, 1999; Autism Diagnostic Interview [ADI]: Lord, Rutter, & LeCouteur, 1994). Although pretend play differences emerge consistently between children with and without autism, the hypothesized reasons responsible for these differences remain somewhat less understood.

In a recent study by Rutherford and colleagues (2007), seven factors were examined as potential mediators of the play differences in children with autism. Five of these factors argued that play differences are the result of an underlying deficiency in (1) general cognitive maturity and symbolic capacity; (2) executive performance and cognitive flexibility; (3) joint attention and theory of mind; (4) social learning and imitation skills; and (5) spontaneous performance as opposed to actual competence. The remaining two factors contend that differences in pretend play are the result of developmentally deviant patterns, not simply delay, and that this difference is specific to symbolic play not sensorimotor play. Comparisons were made over a 2-year time period between children with autism, children with other developmental disorders, and children who were typically developing on independent and scaffolded sensorimotor and pretend play. Children with autism showed a developmental delay in all play measures as compared to children with developmental delays and those who were typically developing regardless of measurement time. As expected, the mental age of 3 served as an important landmark for the development of symbolic play. Changes in all play skills emerged across this 2-year period. Regression analyses attempted to isolate which factors were responsible for changes in play across the preschool period. Regression analyses were tailored to test competing theoretical explanations, that is, the impact joint attention, executive function, imitation skills, and cognitive development have on functional and symbolic play skills. Diagnosis was a useful predictor for understanding all forms of play, with the addition of joint attention only important for understanding spontaneous symbolic play. The fact that joint attention, not imitation skills, appeared to be the most important added predictor for understanding symbolic play emphasizes Hobson's (2002) contention that social reciprocity and shared affect are essential for the development of symbolic play.

The findings from the Rutherford et al. (2007) study support an "autism-specific deficit" in symbolic play. Furthermore, these findings are indicative of the essential role of play in the assessment process for children with autism. Although the authors failed to examine the role of play in differentially diagnosing children with autism from children with Asperger syndrome, the fact is that play assessments were useful in discriminating children with autism from children with other developmental disabilities. Finally, this research lends credence to the usefulness of play for fine-tuning diagnosis on the autism spectrum and argues convincingly for the need for future research on the importance of play in the diagnostic process for children with developmental disabilities.

Interventions for Children with Autism and Asperger Syndrome

Interest in improving the functional skills of children diagnosed with autism and Asperger syndrome has increased dramatically during the last decade. The earliest formalized general approaches to intervention with these children focused primarily on addressing behavioral deficits (Lovaas, 1987; McEachin, Smith, & Lovaas, 1993), including attention, imitation, language, self-help, and play skills (Greenspan, Wieder, & Simons, 1998; Mesibov, Shea, & Schopler, 2004; Mundy, Sigman, Ungerer, & Sherman, 1987). The most commonly used, empirically supported intervention with young children who have autism is applied behavior analysis (ABA; Lovaas, 1987). ABA originated at the University of California in 1987 and was designed to address the executive function and behavioral deficits that have often been hypothesized to be at the heart of autism. The goal behind many ABA interventions is to teach children to learn by developing the essential skills of attending, imitation, language, preacademics, and self-help through discrete trials training. ABA relies entirely on a trained behavioral therapist who identifies important target behaviors and delivers essential reinforcers/punishers designed to strengthen or diminish the behaviors in question. Behavioral interventions have been quite successful at improving the functional behaviors of children diagnosed with autism and Asperger syndrome, with less known about their impact in improving symbolic play. Additionally, these ABA therapies have been criticized largely over their failure to teach generalizable skills and their lack of ecological validity.

In contrast to the ABA approach wherein the emphasis is on behavioral change, a second commonly used approach is the TEACCH program (Treatment and Education of Autistic and Related Communication Handicapped Children). TEACCH focuses on increasing functional and autonomous skills through enhanced communication abilities. Pioneered by Eric Schopler at the University of North Carolina in the 1970s, the TEACCH program was novel in its use of parents as cotherapists and in its emphasis on visual learning modalities (Schopler, Mesibov, & Hearsey, 1995). Not unlike the ABA approach, Project TEACCH argues for clear structure and predictability in interventions designed to enhance spontaneous communication skills in children diagnosed with autism.

Although the Lovaas and Schopler treatment methods have a place of prominence in the field of autism, other methods have also been discussed including sensory integration, music, script training, peer modeling, and play therapies (Terpstra, Higgins, & Pierce, 2002). One of the most promising new approaches is therapeutic play (e.g., Floor Time; Greenspan et al., 1998). Therapeutic play programs are designed to address the social and communication challenges faced by these children and their families. One such example, Floor Time, adopts a social-pragmatic approach which argues that children with autism can learn in the context of play from the relationships that they have with important people in their lives. This developmental, individualized, and relationship (DIR) model emphasizes "interaction," with adults following the child's lead in an effort to motivate the child to connect with the outside world. According to Greenspan and Wieder (2006), DIR and Floor Time activities are designed to enhance self-regulation, intimacy, two-way communication, and emotional thinking and ideas. This child-centered approach addresses functional skills in an integrated fashion using parents as therapists.

A recent pilot study entitled "Play Project Home Consultation (PPHC) Project" provides important data on the cost-effectiveness of programs based on Greenspan's Floor Time model (Solomon, Necheles, Ferch, & Bruchman, 2007). Parents were instructed to play with their child 15 hours per week. Pre- to post-rating changes on the Functional Emotional Assessment Scale showed significant improvement for the group as a function of the intervention. Individual difference analyses suggested that 45.5% of the children demonstrated "good to very good" developmental improvement. The lack of a control group precludes a definitive statement about whether the PPHC treatment program specifically was responsible for the improved functioning of children. Nonetheless, the provision of one-to-one play opportunities 15 hours a week appeared to enhance the functioning of children with autism and therefore warrants further investigation.

More recently, novel teaching efforts have been directed toward addressing the symbolic play deficits of children with autism. Herrara and colleagues (2008) employed a virtual reality procedure to improve the symbolic play skills of two autistic children. In their case study they convincingly demonstrate the advantages of the virtual reality medium for teaching symbolic play skills in school-age children. After 28 sessions using the "Virtual Supermarket" program, the two subjects demonstrated improvements in both functional and symbolic play, as well as imagination. Although the design costs of this methodology may prove somewhat costly, once developed it can be implemented with a variety of subjects and therefore would be cost-effective.

UNANSWERED QUESTIONS REGARDING PLAY AND DEVELOPMENTAL DISABILITIES

The importance of play in the assessment and treatment of young children with developmental disabilities has been highlighted in this chapter. As an assessment technique, play assessments can provide a useful window into the cognitive and linguistic functioning of young children. Additionally, traditional cognitive and linguistic batteries often require skill sets (e.g., verbal comprehension and production skills, attentional skills, and pointing skills) that young children with developmental disabilities do not possess. Play assessments offer hope for understanding subtle differences among groups of developmentally delayed children.

In a recent pilot investigation by Short and her colleagues (Short, Gorovoy, Russ, & Lewis, 2009), free-play skills were examined in a small sample of preschool children diagnosed with SLI (10), ADHD (10), and Asperger syndrome (4). Using the Affect in Play Scale, Preschool Version, differences in symbolic play, functional play, behavioral factors, and language were examined. Children with ADHD earned higher ratings on the cognitive aspects (i.e., organization, imagination, and comfort) of their play than did children with SLI. Additionally, the children with Asperger syndrome earned the lowest cognitive ratings on their play when compared to either of the other two groups. No differences in negative affect exhibited in play were noted between children with ADHD and those with SLI, whereas more negative affect was noted for the children with Asperger syndrome. Positive affect differences were noted between the three groups, with children with SLI evidencing less positive affect in their play than both of our other groups. Overall affect level in play was lower for the children with SLI than the children with ADHD or Asperger syndrome. Differences in functional play emerged as well, with children with Asperger syndrome exhibiting greater functional play than children with either ADHD or SLI.

Behavioral differences were striking in our groups. As predicted, intrusions were more common on the part of children with ADHD. That is, they did not wait for task instructions to be completed before playing with the toys, their themes were short and not well developed, and their play had considerable momentum. Both children with SLI and children with Asperger syndrome sat patiently, albeit passively, throughout the instructional period. Children with SLI were quiet throughout play, but highly engaged. Children with Asperger syndrome were more inclined to imitate the play instructions rather than to generate novel play patterns, with perseverations evidenced in their play.

In an effort to examine whether language impacted the scoring of play skills for this sample, tapes were rescored with the sound turned off. All children's play scores were lower in the absence of audio information, thus suggesting that the presence of language enhanced the examiners' understanding of the children's play. Another important discovery from this methodological change was the differential impact of sound elimination on the children's performance. The sound manipulation (presence/absence) had the greatest impact on the children with ADHD as compared to our other two groups. That is, children with ADHD were rated as better players when the experimenter could hear what they were saying than when he or she had to rely exclusively on their behavioral enactment of the play.

The present study, although preliminary in nature, offers hope that brief play assessments can provide important information regarding diagnostic differences in children with developmental disabilities. Not only were cognitive differences identified, but so too were affective and behavioral differences identified in this brief play assessment. New research in our lab is being conducted on the effectiveness of play interventions with children diagnosed with ADHD, SLI, and Asperger syndrome. The hope is that the play intervention that capitalizes on parent–child interaction and provides extended practice in symbolic play may differentially enhance the children's skill repertoire. That is, the play intervention may be a contextually supportive medium for children with language disabilities to practice new linguistic skills. For children with ADHD, the hope is that the play medium may be useful for learning increased self-control and sustained attention (i.e., development of longer, more elaborated themes). Finally, for children diagnosed with Asperger syndrome, play may be a useful medium for developing greater symbolic play. By working and reworking on script-like play scenarios, children may broaden their cognitive and emotional skills while still enjoying themselves.

Much work is needed to provide better educational supports for young children with developmental handicaps and their families. Play assessments and interventions appear to be ideally suited to enter the world of a young child and teach him or her to master new skills necessary for daily living. The arena of play provides the child with a nonthreatening place to learn, practice, and refine skills in a variety of domains, while simultaneously providing the parent, clinician, and teacher with an ideal arena in which to perform their evaluation of the child. The APS (Russ, 1987) is ideally suited for use as an assessment device with young children because of its ease of administration, brevity, standarization, and ease of scoring. Children with developmental disabilities need careful and frequent evaluation in order to assure adequate developmental progress. The APS is a useful tool for clinicians in their ongoing evaluation.

REFERENCES

Abikoff, H., Hechtman, L., Klein, R. G., Weiss, G., Fleiss, K., Etcovitch, J., et al. (2004). Social functioning in children with ADHD treated with long-term methylphenidate and multimodal psychosocial treatment. *Journal of the American Academy of Child and Adolescent Psychiatry, 43*(7), 820–829.

Alessandri, S. M. (1992). Attention, play, and social behavior in ADHD preschoolers. *Journal of Abnormal Child Psychology, 20*(3), 289–302.

Alessandri, S. M., & Schramm, K. (1991). Effects of dextroamphetamine on the cognitive and social play of a preschooler with ADHD. *Journal of the American Academy of Child and Adolescent Psychiatry, 30,* 768–772.

Atwood, T. (1998). *Asperger's syndrome: A guide for parents and professionals.* London: Jessica Kingsley.

Bagnato, S. J., & Neisworth, J. T. (1994). A national study of the social and treatment "invalidity" of intelligence testing for early intervention. *School Psychology Quarterly, 9,* 81–102.

Barkley, R. A. (2002). Psychosocial treatments for attention-deficit/hyperactivity disorder in children. *Journal of Clinical Child Psychiatry, 63,* 36–43.

Barkley, R. A. (1990). *Attention-deficit/hyperactivity disorder: A handbook for diagnosis and treatment.* New York: Guilford Press.

Barkley, R. A. (1997). *ADHD and the nature of self control.* New York: Guilford Press.

Barkley, R. A., Cook, E. H., Diamond, A., Zametkin, A., Thapar, A., Teeter, A., et al. (2002). International consensus statement on ADHD. *Clinical Child and Family Psychology Review, 5*, 89–111.

Beilinson, J., & Olswang, L. (2003). Facilitating peer group entry in kindergarteners with deficits in social communication. *Language, Speech, and Hearing Services in Schools, 34*, 154–166.

Bishop, D. V., & Adams, C. (1990). A prospective study of the relationship between specific language impairment, phonological disorders and reading retardation. *Journal of Child Psychology and Psychiatry, 31*, 1027–1050.

Blackman, J. (1999). Attention deficit/ hyperactivity disorder in preschoolers: Does it exist and should we treat it? *Pediatric Clinics of North America, 46*, 1011–1025.

Brinton, B., & Fujika, M. (2006). Social intervention for children with language impairment: Factors affecting efficacy. *Communication Disorders Quarterly, 28*(1), 39–41.

Brown, J., Redmond, A., Bass, K., Liebergott, J., & Swope, S. (1975, November). *Symbolic play in normal and language-impaired children.* Paper presented at the American Speech–Language–Hearing Association annual convention, Washington, DC.

Bucy, J., Smith, T., & Landau, S. (1999). Assessment of preschoolers with developmental disabilities and at-risk conditions. In E. V. Nuttall, I. Romero, & J. Lalesnik (Eds.), *Assessing and screening preschoolers: Psychological and educational dimensions* (pp. 318–339). Boston: Allyn & Bacon.

Campbell, T. F., Dollaghan, C. A., Rockette, H. E., Paradise, J. L., Feldman, H. M., Shriberg, L. D., et al. (2003). Risk factors for speech delay of unknown origin in 3-year-old children. *Child Development, 74*, 346–357.

Campbell, S. B. (1987). Parent-referred problem three-year-olds: Developmental changes in symptoms. *Journal of Child Psychology and Psychiatry, 28*, 835–846.

Casby, M. W. (1997). Symbolic play of children with language impairment: A critical review. *Journal of Speech and Hearing Research, 40*(3), 468–479.

Conners, C. K. (1997). *Conners' Rating Scales—Revised: Technical manual.* Toronto: Multi-Health Systems.

DeKroon, D., Kyte, C. S., & Johnson, C. J. (2002). Partner influences on the social pretend play of children with language impairments. *Language, Speech, and Hearing Services in the Schools, 33,* 253–267.

Faraone, S. V., Short, E. J., Findling, R. L., Manos, M. J., Skolnik, R., & Biederman, J. (2002). Efficacy of adderal and methylphenidate in attention-deficit/ hyperactivity disorder: A drug–placebo and drug–drug response curve analysis of a naturalistic study. *International Journal of Neuropsychopharmacolgy, 5*(2), 121–129.

Fattig, M. (2008). Early indicators: High functioning autism and Asperger syndrome. *Disabled World: A Disability and Seniors Information Community.* Retrieved from *www.disabled-world.com/artman/publish/article_2255. shtml.*

Feurstein, R. (1979). *The dynamic assessment of retarded performers: The learn-*

ing potential assessment device, theory, instruments, and techniques. Baltimore: University Park Press.

Feurstein, R. (1980). *Instrumental enrichment: An intervention for cognitive modifiability.* Baltimore: University Park Press.

Gillon, G. T. (2004). *Phonological awareness: From research to practice.* New York: Guilford Press.

Greenspan, S. L., Wieder, S., & Simons, R. (1998). *The child with special needs: Encouraging intellectual and emotional growth.* Reading, MA: Addison-Wesley.

Haywood, H. C., & Lidz, C. S. (2006). *Dynamic assessment in practice: Clinical and educational applications.* Cambridge, UK: Cambridge University Press.

Herrera, G., Alcantud, F., Jordan, R., Blanquer, A., Labajo, G., & De Pablo, C. (2008). Development of symbolic play through the use of virtual reality tools in children with autistic spectrum disorders: Two case studies. *Autism, 12*(2), 143–157.

Hobson, P. (2002). *The cradle of thought: Exploring origins of thinking.* London: Macmillan.

Holmes, E., & Willoughby, T. (2005). Play behavior of children with autism spectrum disorder. *Journal of Intellectual and Developmental Disability, 30*(3), 156–164.

Johnson, C., Beitchman, J. H., Young, A., Escobar, M., Atkinson, L., Wilson, B., et al. (1999). Fourteen year follow-up of children with and without speech/language impairments: Speech/language stability and outcomes. *Journal of Speech, Language, and Hearing Research, 42,* 744–760.

Johnson-Martin, N. M., Attermeir, S. M., & Hacker, B. J. (2004). *The Carolina curriculum for infants and toddlers with special needs.* Baltimore: Brookes.

Lerner, J., Mardell-Czudnowski, C., & Goldberg, D. (1987). *Special education for the early childhood years* (2nd ed.). Englewood Cliffs, NJ: Prentice Hall.

Lewis, V., Boucher, J., Lupton, L., & Watson, S. (2000). Relationships between symbolic play, functional play, verbal, and non-verbal ability in young children. *International Journal of Language and Communication Disorders, 35*(1), 117–127.

Li, C., Walton, J. R., & Nuttall, E. V. (1999). Preschool evaluation of culturally and linguistically diverse children. In E. V. Nuttall, I. Romero, & J. Lalesnik (Eds.), *Assessing and screening preschoolers: Psychological and educational dimensions* (pp. 296–317). Boston: Allyn & Bacon.

Linder, T. W. (1993). *Transdisciplinary play based intervention.* Tucson, AZ: Therapy Skill Builders.

Linder, T. W., Holm, C. B., & Walsh, K. A. (1999), Transdisciplinary play-based assessment. In E. V. Nuttall, I. Romero, & J. Lalesnik (Eds.), *Assessing and screening preschoolers: Psychological and educational dimensions* (pp. 161–185). Boston: Allyn & Bacon.

Lombardino, L., Stein, J., Kricos, P., & Wolf, M. (1986). Play diversity and structural relationships in the play and language of language-impaired and language-normal preschoolers: Preliminary data. *Journal of Communication Disorders, 19*, 475–489.

Lord, C., Rutter, M., Di Lavore, P. C., & Risi, S. (1999). *Autism Diagnostic Observation Schedule—ADOS*. Los Angeles: Western Psychological Services.

Lord, C., Rutter, M., & LeCouteur, A. (1994). Autism Diagnostic Interview Revised: A revised version of a diagnostic interview for caregivers with possible pervasive developmental disorders. *Journal of Autism and Developmental Disorders, 24*, 659–685.

Lovaas, O. I. (1987). Behavioral treatment and normal educational and intellectual functioning in young autistic children. *Journal of Consulting and Clinical Psychology, 55*, 3–9.

Lovell, K., Hoyle, W., & Siddall, M. (1968). A study of some aspects of the play and language of young children with delayed speech. *Journal of Child Psychology and Psychiatry, 9*, 41–50.

McEachin, J. J., Smith, T., & Lovaas, O. I. (1993). Long-term outcome for children with autism who received early intensive behavioral treatment. *American Journal on Mental Retardation, 97*(4), 359–372.

Mesibov, G. B., Shea, V., & Schopler, E. (2004). *The TEACCH approach to autism spectrum disorders*. New York: Springer-Verlag.

Mundy, P., Sigman, M., Ungerer, J., & Sherman, T. (1987). Nonverbal communication and play correlates of language development in autistic children. *Journal of Autism and Developmental Disorders, 17*(3), 349–364.

Pelham, W. E., & Fabiano, G. A. (2008). Evidence-based psychosocial treatment for ADHD: An update. *Journal of Clinical Child and Adolescent Psychology, 37*, 184–214.

Pelham, W. E., Gnagy, E. M., Greiner, A. R., Hoza B., Hinshaw, S. P. Swanson J. M., et al. (2000). Behavioral versus behavioral and pharmacological treatment in ADHD children attending a summer treatment program. *Journal of Abnormal Child Psychology, 28*, 507–525.

Pelham, W. E., Wheeler, T., & Chronis, A. (1998). Empirically supported psychosocial treatments for attention deficit hyperactivity disorder. *Journal of Clinical Child Psychology, 27*(2), 190–205.

Piaget, J. (1962). *Play, dreams, and imitation in childhood*. New York: Norton.

Rappley, M. D., Mullan, P. B., Alvarez, F. J., Eneli, I. U., Wang, J., & Gardiner, J. C. (1979). Diagnosis of attention-deficit/hyperactivity disorder and use of psychotropic medication in very young children. *Archives of Pediatric Adolescent Medicine, 153*, 1039–1045.

Reilly, N. E., Cunningham, C. E., Richards, J. E., Elbard, H. J., & Mahoney, W. J. (1999). Detecting attention deficit hyperactivity disorder in a communications clinic: Diagnostic utility of the Gordon Diagnostic System. *Journal of Clinical Experimental Neuropsychology, 21*, 685–700.

Rescorla, L., & Goossens, M. (1992). Symbolic play development in toddlers with expressive specific language impairment (SLI-E). *Journal of Speech and Hearing Research, 35*(6), 1290–1302.

Russ, S. (1987). Assessment of cognitive affective interaction in children: Creativity, fantasy and play research. In J. Butcher & C. D. Spielberger (Eds.), *Advances in personality assessment, Vol. 6* (pp. 141–153). Hillsdale, NJ: Erlbaum.

Rutherford, M. D., Young, G. S., Hepburn, S., & Roger, S. J., (2007). A longitudinal study of pretend play in autism. *Journal of Autism and Developmental Disorders, 37,* 1024–1039.

Salvia, J., & Ysseldyke, J. E. (2001). *Assessment.* Boston: Houghton Mifflin.

Sattler, J. M. (2001). *Assessment of children: Behavioral, social, and clinical foundations* (5th ed.). San Diego, CA: Author.

Sattler, J. M., & Hoge, R. D. (2006). *Assessment of children: Cognitive applications* (4th ed.). San Diego, CA: Author.

Schleifer, M., Weiss, G., Cohen, N., Elman, M., Cvejic, H., & Kruger, E. (1975). Hyperactivity in preschoolers and the effect of methylphenidate. *American Journal of Orthopsychiatry, 45,* 38–50.

Schopler, E., Mesibov, G. B., & Hearsey, K. (1995). Structured teaching in the TEACCH system. In E. Schopler & G. Mesibov (Eds.), *Learning and cognition in autism* (pp. 243–267). New York: Kluwer Academic/Plenum.

Short, E. J., Freebairn, L., Hansen, A., & Lewis, B. A. (2008). ADHD symptoms in children with speech and language disorder. *Advances in ADHD, 2*(4), 112–119.

Short, E. J., Gorovoy, S., Russ, S., & Lewis, B. (2008, April). *Assessment of preschoolers with ADHD, language disorders, and Asperger syndrome: Insights from affect in play.* Paper presented at the Society for Research in Child Development annual meeting, Denver, CO.

Short, E. J., Manos, M. J., Findling, R. L., & Schubel, E. (2004). A prospective study of stimulant response in preschoolers. *Journal of the American Academy of Child and Adolescent Psychiatry, 43*(3), 251–259.

Short, E. J., & Miller, D. J. (1981). Metamemory in preschoolers: The 4- and 5-year-olds' sensitivity to memory instructions in a game-like context. *Genetic Psychology Monographs, 103,* 221–241.

Shriberg, L. D., Tomblin, J. B., & McSweeny, J. L. (1999). Prevalence of speech delay in 6-year-old children and comorbidity with language impairment. *Journal of Speech, Language, and Hearing Research, 42,* 1461–1481.

SLI Consortium. (2002). A genomewide scan identifies two novel loci involved in specific language impairment. *American Journal of Human Genetics, 70,* 384–398.

SLI Consortium. (2004). Highly significant linkage to the SLI1 locus in an expanded sample of individuals affected by specific language impairment. *American Journal of Human Genetics, 74,* 1225–1238.

Solomon, R., Necheles, J., Ferch, C., & Bruchman, D. (2007). Pilot study of a parent training program for young children with autism: The Play Project Home Consultation program. *Sage Publications and The National Autistic Society, 11*(3), 205–224. (DOI:10.1177/1362361307076842)

Stanley, G. C., & Konstantareas, M. M. (2007). Symbolic play in children with autism spectrum disorder. *Journal of Autism and Developmental Disorders, 37,* 1215–1223.

Tallal, P., & Gaab, N. (2006). Dynamic auditory processing, musical ability, and language development. *Trends in Neuroscience, 29*(7), 382–390.

Terpstra, J. E., Higgins, K., & Pierce, T. (2002). Can I play?: Classroom-based interventions for teaching play skills to children with autism. *Focus on Autism and Other Developmental Disabilities, 17*(2), 119–128.

Tomblin, J., Records, N., Buckwalter, P., Zhang, X., Smith, E., & O'Brien, M. (1997). Prevalence of specific language impairment in kindergarten children. *Journal of Speech, Language, and Hearing Research, 40*, 1245–1260.

Vygotsky, L. (1986). *Thought and language.* Cambridge, MA: MIT Press.

Wolraich, M. L., Lambert, E. W., Bickman, L., Simmons, T., Doffing, M. A., & Worley, K. A. (2004). Assessing the impact of parent and teacher agreement on diagnosing attention-deficit hyperactivity disorder. *Journal of Developmental and Behavioral Pediatrics, 25*(1), 41–47.

Zito, J. M., Safer, D. J., dosReis, S., Gardner, J. F., Boles, M., & Lynch, F. (2000). Trends in the prescribing of psychotropic medications to preschoolers. *Journal of the American Medical Association, 283*, 1025–1030.

PART IV

Play in Evidence-Based Prevention Programs in School Settings

12

Play and Head Start

Sandra J. Bishop-Josef and Edward F. Zigler

OVERVIEW OF HEAD START

Head Start is the largest and oldest (begun in 1965) early childhood intervention program in the United States. From the beginning, the basic Head Start program has been a center-based preschool serving primarily poor children ages 3–5. Initially just a summer program, Head Start is now typically a half-day, school-year program, although some children attend for 2 years. In addition, Head Start has been making progress in converting many Head Start centers to full-day, full-year programs, allowing them to provide child care as well as preschool education and comprehensive services. Federal guidelines mandate that at least 90% of the children served be from families with incomes below the poverty line; at least 10% of the enrollment must be children with disabilities. Head Start programs receive 80% of their funding from the federal government and the rest (which can be in-kind services) from other, usually local, sources.

In fiscal year 2009, approximately 1,600 Head Start grantees served over 900,000 children and their families. Funding for the program in 2009 was over $7 billion (U.S. Department of Health and Human Services [USDHHS], 2010). Local programs are overseen by policy advisory councils consisting of parents, staff, and community representatives. Head Start embodies a comprehensive approach, providing a broad range of services to children and their families. Each program is required to provide six core components: early childhood education, health screening and referral, mental health services, nutrition education and meals, social services for the child and family, and parent involvement. Although they must adhere to national performance standards in these areas, programs are encouraged to adapt their services in response to local needs and resources. Since its inception, one of the goals of Head Start has been to prepare children for school entry. In the early years of the program, however, the overall mission of Head Start was ambiguous. This ambiguity was eliminated by the 1998 Head Start reauthorization, which mandated that the mission of Head Start is to "promote school readiness by enhancing the social and cognitive development of children through the provision of educational, health, nutritional, social and other services to enrolled children and families" (USDHHS, 2008).

PLAY IN HEAD START

History

As we discuss below, play has a prominent place in Head Start curricula. From its inception in 1965, Head Start has been a comprehensive, whole-child program. The founders of Head Start believed that preparing children who live in poverty for school requires meeting all of their needs, not just focusing on their academic skills. Although Head Start was established before the creation of a strong knowledge base on the potential of intervention programs to promote young children's development, Head Start's founders recognized the importance of social and emotional factors for cognitive development and school readiness. The founders also recognized the importance of play for children's learning.

Despite these beginnings, Head Start fell victim to the excessive focus on cognitive skills and naive environmentalism that became common in the 1960s (Zigler, 1970). This view held that minimal environmental interventions during the preschool years could yield dramatic increases in children's cognitive functioning. A book by Joseph McVicker Hunt, *Intelligence and Experience* (1961), was the bible of this point of view and had an immense effect. Hunt argued that the right environmental input could raise children's IQs by as much as 30–70 points. Given that IQ is among the most stable of all psychological measures, this promise was completely unrealistic.

When researchers began to evaluate Head Start, they were drawn to assessments of cognitive functioning, particularly IQ test scores (Zigler & Trickett, 1978). The researchers ignored the rich, comprehensive nature of the Head Start intervention and focused on one narrow outcome.

Evaluators also became enthralled with the results: relatively minor interventions—even 6–8 weeks of Head Start—seemed to produce large increases in children's IQs. These gains were soon found to be caused by improvements in motivation rather than changes in cognitive functioning (Zigler & Butterfield, 1968). Yet findings such as these did not (and still do not) deter the use of IQ as a primary measure of Head Start's effectiveness (Raver & Zigler, 1991; Zigler & Trickett, 1978). This practice is understandable in that measures of IQ were readily available, easy to administer and score, and deemed reliable and valid, whereas measures of socioemotional constructs were and still are less well developed. Also, IQ was a construct that policymakers and the public could easily understand, and it was known to be related to many other behaviors, particularly school performance.

Soon, researchers lost faith in IQ as a measure of Head Start's success (Raver & Zigler, 1991), when the 1969 Westinghouse Report (Westinghouse Learning Corporation and Ohio University, 1969) found that Head Start children failed to sustain their cognitive advantages once they moved to elementary school. This report nearly proved fatal to Head Start because some critics concluded that this failure to sustain cognitive gains meant that Head Start was ineffective. However, investigators began to understand that Head Start children's rapid IQ gains could be explained by motivational factors (e.g., less fear of the test and the tester), rather than by true improvement in cognitive ability (Zigler & Trickett, 1978). Experts also pointed out the numerous difficulties and biases in using IQ to evaluate comprehensive intervention programs (e.g., Zigler & Trickett, 1978).

In the early 1970s, the Office of Child Development (OCD; now the Administration on Children, Youth, and Families [ACYF]) articulated everyday social competence as the overriding goal of Head Start and encouraged broader evaluations to measure more accurately the program's effectiveness (Raver & Zigler, 1991). However, no accepted definition was available of social competence, much less established measures. Therefore, OCD funded the Measures Project in 1977, a multisite study to develop a battery of measures of the factors making up social competence, including but not limited to appropriate cognitive measures. Zigler and Trickett (1978) also suggested approaches to assessing social competence that included measures of motivational and emotional variables, physical health and well-being, achievement, and formal cognitive ability. This comprehensive definition of social competence was later echoed by the National Educational Goals Panel, a semigovernmental group composed of federal and state policymakers, who officially defined school readiness as consisting of five dimensions: (1) physical well-being and motor development, (2) social and emotional development, (3) approaches to learning, (4) language development, and (5) cognition and general knowledge (Kagan, Moore, & Bredekamp, 1995). Zigler, Gordic, and Styfco (2007) further argued that in young children at the time of school entry, everyday social competence and school readiness are one and the same.

Thus, by the late 1970s to early 1980s, the naive cognitive–environmental view had largely been rejected, and a renewed appreciation of the whole child and the value of play was becoming evident. Books by David Elkind, *The Hurried Child* (1981) and *Miseducation: Preschoolers at Risk* (1987), argued that children were being pushed too hard, too early, especially with respect to intellectual tasks. As a past president of the National Association for the Education of Young Children, Elkind commanded respect, and his books were very popular and important in moving both professionals and the general public toward a view that social and emotional development is a valuable part of child development that strongly affects intellectual growth. There was also a renewed appreciation for the value of play. The "risks" associated with academic activities in preschool can be overstated, however. The pendulum had certainly swung too far when many Head Start teachers refused to even put letters of the alphabet on the walls of Head Start classrooms.

During the 1980s, however, the pendulum had already started to swing back in the opposite direction. In 1982, the Reagan administration cut most of the funding for the Measures Project, supporting only the site that was developing measures of cognitive functioning. During the Reagan and George H. W. Bush years, the Head Start administration was again focusing almost exclusively on cognitive measures to assess the program's effectiveness (Raver & Zigler, 1991). Further, the cognitive measurement system that emanated from the Measures Project (i.e., Head Start Measures Battery) was accompanied by a curriculum, which led to concerns about "teaching to the test" and worries that play would be devalued.

The tide began to shift yet again during the next decade (Zigler, 1994). The 1998 reauthorization of Head Start explicitly stated that the goal of the program is "school readiness," defining *readiness* in terms of physical and mental health, social and emotional development, parental involvement, and preacademic skills (Raver & Zigler, 2004). Finally, a sensible middle ground seemed to have been reached, a consensus that learning is fostered by more than cognitive training. However, the tide turned again shortly thereafter, culminating in the recent attack on play.

In recent years, many preschools and elementary schools have reduced or even eliminated play from their schedules (Bodrova & Leong, 2003; Brandon, 2002; Johnson, 1998; Murline, 2000; Vail, 2003). In some locations, dress-up areas and blocks are being removed from preschool classrooms (Steinhauer, 2005; Vail, 2003). In sum, Bodrova and Leong (2003) described the current situation as "the disappearance of play from early childhood classrooms" (p. 12).

Play is being replaced by lessons focused on cognitive development, particularly literacy and reading (Brandon, 2002; Fromberg, 1990; Johnson, 1998; Steinhauer, 2005; Vail, 2003). One expert stated: "We are not allowing normal, creative, interactive play. We are wanting kids to sit down and write their names at 3 and do rote tasks that are extremely boring at a young age" (Adele Brodkin, quoted in Steinhauer, 2005, p. 4). The lessons addressing cognitive development often involve "children sitting at tables engaged in whole-class activities" (Whitehurst, 2001, p. 16), instead of activities such as making Play-Doh gifts, with the teacher engaging the children in conversations about their work (contrasting example of "child-centered approach" provided by Whitehurst, 2001, p. 9). Some teachers have argued that "the instruction techniques that early childhood education experts say are ideal for learning frequently are derided as 'just play' by administrators and policymakers pushing what they consider to be more academically oriented curricula" (Brandon, 2002, p. 1).

The policy change away from play and toward cognitive development resulted partially from findings showing the poor academic achievement of many American children, in comparison with students from other nations (Elkind, 2001). The change also reflects an attempt to eliminate the well-documented achievement gap between children from low socioeconomic backgrounds and minority families and those from higher income, nonminority backgrounds (Raver & Zigler, 2004).

The George W. Bush administration did much to fuel the current attack on play. The president spoke often about reforming education, including preschool education, by focusing on cognitive development, literacy, and "numeracy." Mrs. Bush, a former librarian, hosted a White House Summit on Early Childhood Cognitive Development—not child development or even the whole of cognitive development. The focus was on literacy, one cognitive skill out of many related to school success. In the 2001 reauthorization, the Elementary and Secondary Education Act (Public Law 89-10), first passed in 1965, was renamed the No Child Left Behind Act (Public Law 107-110). The new law added the president's initiative that all children be able to read by third grade (Bush, 2003). The reading mandate and accompanying testing resulted in further emphasis on literacy training in the early elementary grades.

Parents of young children are also increasingly demanding preschool content that they view as "academic" rather than play (Vail, 2003). For example, one preschool director commented about parents: "They agree in theory that play is important, but they say, 'Could you just throw in the worksheets, so I can see what they are learning?'" (Vail, 2003, p. 16). Another noted: "All parents want now are worksheets, and they want them in their babies' hands as early as possible" (Bodrova & Leong, 2003, p. 12). An article in the National Association for the Education of Young Children's (NAEYC) journal provided guidance for teachers who need to defend play-based preschool environments from attacks by individuals, including parents, who question their value (Stegelin, 2005). As parents are the "customers" of early childhood programs, programs are likely to eventually succumb to parental pressure and change curricula to reflect parental preferences, even if these are ill-advised, such as devaluing play.

The focus on cognition and literacy also found its way into policies and proposals for Head Start. The Bush administration initially wanted to change Head Start from a comprehensive intervention to a literacy program (Raver & Zigler, 2004; Steinberg, 2002; Strauss, 2003; Zigler, 2003). However, changing the law governing Head Start would have required considerable time. To move the program in the desired direction more quickly, the administration imposed new protocols on how the program should be run (decisions that were within its power). For example, a new national reporting system (NRS) was instituted that required standardized testing of all Head Start 4-year-olds, at the beginning and end of the year, to assess their cognitive development (language, preliteracy, and premath skills). The results of the testing (consisting of four brief tests) were to be used to determine whether centers were performing adequately. Critics feared that funding decisions would be based on children's test scores. Another fear was that teachers would "teach to the test," focusing only on the narrow range of skills assessed by the NRS. Data supported the validity of this latter fear: the U.S. Government Accountability Office (GAO, 2005) found that at least 18% of Head Start programs changed their instruction to correspond to the content of the NRS standardized testing. The GAO stated that this could prove detrimental to children if teachers omit other equally important skills from their curricula and called for studies to examine the impact of the changes. Fortunately, as will be detailed below, the recent reauthorization of the Head Start legislation eliminated the NRS.

In addition, as part of his early childhood initiative "Good Start, Grow Smart," President Bush announced a national program to train all Head Start teachers on strategies to promote literacy (USDHHS, 2002). In response, DHHS developed the Strategic Teacher Education Program (STEP), which included training on a literacy curriculum developed by the Center for Improving the Readiness of Children for Learning and Education (CIRCLE). Training was held in June 2002 for 3,000 Head Start teachers and a follow-up training was conducted in November 2002 (Advisory Committee on Head Start Research and Evaluation, 2003). This training was to be followed up by these teachers then training other Head Start teachers, back at their home sites (i.e., a train-the-trainer model). Although the training was supposed to be voluntary, Head Start personnel reported pressure to participate (Strauss, 2002). Some argued that the training essentially established a national curriculum, thereby violating the "local control" tradition that was designed to ensure that Head Start is responsive to the needs identified in each local community.

During 2003, Congress began work to reauthorize Head Start. The reauthorization process typically adjusts program details to keep budgets and services current. This time, however, Congress sought to redesign Head Start. A version of a bill later passed in the House (H.R. 2210) removed language in the law relating to what has always been one focus of Head Start, social and emotional development. Most occurrences of these words were replaced with the word *literacy*. This version also stopped assessments of children's social and emotional functioning in ongoing national evaluations of Head Start (Schumacher, Greenberg, & Mezey, 2003). Instead, representatives wanted assessments of whether children meet specified goals on preliteracy and premath tests. The assessment goal prevailed in the bill that eventually passed the House (by one vote), although the obliteration of language pertaining to social and emotional competence and evaluations did not.

The Senate also introduced a Head Start bill, the Head Start Improvements for School Readiness Act (S. 1940). This bill did not call for drastic changes like those in the House bill (Schumacher & Greenberg, 2004). However, the Senate bill included a detailed list of items that all Head Start children must learn.

Many experts criticized the proposed changes to Head Start policy that overemphasized cognitive development and standardized testing, which they argued are inappropriate (Raver & Zigler, 2004; Steinberg, 2002; Stipek, 2004; Strauss, 2003). David Elkind (2001), in a piece reminiscent of Piaget's constructivist views entitled "Young Einsteins: Much Too Early," argued that young children learn best through direct interaction with their environment. Before a certain age, they simply are not capable of the level of reasoning necessary for formal instruction in reading and mathematics. Elkind believed this fact of development explained why the pioneers of early childhood education developed hands-on models of learning. Elkind's article was accompanied by a counterpoint by Whitehurst (2001), titled "Young Einsteins: Much Too Late." Whitehurst, who was subsequently appointed director of the Institute of Education Sciences at the U.S. Department of Education by President Bush, claimed that "content-centered" approaches (i.e., academically oriented) are more likely to facilitate children's literacy learning. Raver and Zigler (2004) disagreed, criticizing the emphasis on cognitive development and standardized testing as being far too narrow and unsupported by scientific evidence on how children learn. They advocated continued attention to, and assessment of, children's social and emotional development, viewing this domain as synergistic with intellectual development. With regard to the Elkind–Whitehurst debate, the authors of this chapter agree with Stipek (2004) that quality preschool education requires pursuing both hands-on, play-based learning and direct instruction of academic skills simultaneously. Kagan and Lowenstein (2004), in a comprehensive review of the literature on school readiness and play, reached the same conclusion. Without taking sides on whether emotion or cognition should be primary, more than 300 scholars signed a letter protesting the plan to carry out standardized testing in Head Start and questioning the validity of the proposed assessments (Raver & Zigler, 2004; see also Meisels & Atkins-Burnett, 2004). The concerns of these scholars were borne out by the GAO study (2005) that severely criticized the NRS. The GAO found that the reliability and validity of the NRS have not been established, and argued therefore that "results from the first year of the NRS are of limited value for accountability purposes." Critics have also questioned the wisdom of Congress "micromanaging" Head Start, which has always been a program run at the local level and tailored to meet the needs of children and families in each particular locality.

Congress was unable to pass a bill reauthorizing Head Start during the 108th session, so efforts began anew in the 109th Congress. In the 109th Congress, the issue of a focus on literacy/numeracy versus a whole-child approach took a back seat to other matters. For example, the legislation proposed in the House sought to reduce the power of the policy councils, a major attack on one of the key components of Head Start, parent involvement. The Senate bill, however, did not seek to diminish the policy councils. Despite considerable effort, the 109th Congress also failed to pass a Head Start reauthorization bill.

Finally, in fall 2007, Congress passed the Improving Head Start for School Readiness Act (Public Law 110-134) and President Bush signed it into law in December. The legislation has several key positive features. Most relevant to this discussion, the reauthorization makes clear that a new assessment framework, recommended by the National Academy of Sciences (Snow & Van Hemel, 2008), will be used in Head Start. This framework will replace the NRS.

Performance Standards

As discussed previously, from its very inception, Head Start has embodied a focus on the whole child. Included in this comprehensive approach is recognition of the importance of play for child development. Several of the Head Start performance standards for education and early childhood development (USDHHS, 1998; 45 CFR, 1304.21) include a focus on play.

Performance standard 1304.21 (a) (4) describes the various means by which Head Start programs must "provide for the development of each child's cognitive and language skills" (USDHHS, 1998, p. 68). This standard identifies play as one of the primary strategies for promoting children's cognitive and language skills and requires that Head Start programs support "each child's learning, using various strategies, including experimentation, inquiry, observation, play and exploration" (1304.21 [a] [4] [i]; USDHHS, 1998, p. 68). With regard to literacy and numeracy, in particular, this standard requires that programs support "emerging literacy and numeracy development through materials and activities according to the developmental level of each child" (1304.21 [a] [4] [iv]; USDHHS, 1998, p. 70). The guidance section for this standard lists ways adults can support the development of literacy and numeracy, including "games, dramatic play, fingerplays, puzzles, blocks" (p. 71). The standard also mentions play as a means of promoting the development of language skills and urges adults in Head Start to encourage "dramatic play in which children act out familiar activities, such as going to the grocery store or the library, and using the telephone" (1304.21 [a] [4] [iii]; USDHHS, 1998, p. 70). Thus the performance standard regarding cognitive and language development includes several explicit references to how play can be used to support this development.

Play is also mentioned in the Head Start performance standard concerning physical development (1304.21 [a] [5]; USDHSS, 1998). This standard requires Head Start programs to "promote each child's physical development by providing sufficient time, indoor and outdoor space, equipment, materials and adult guidance for active play and movement that support the development of gross motor skills" (p. 71). The standard further states: "A child's gross motor development is important to overall health. As such, that development is important to the achievement of cognitive skills" (p. 71), again linking play and cognitive development.

The Head Start performance standards require that programs implement a curriculum (1304.3 [a] [5]; USDHHS, 1998). *Curriculum* is defined as a written plan that includes:

1. The goals for children's development and learning
2. The experiences through which they will achieve these goals
3. What staff and parents do to help children achieve these goals
4. The materials needed to support the implementation of the curriculum

Any curriculum used in Head Start must meet these definitional criteria. The curriculum also must provide for "the development of cognitive skills by encouraging each child to organize his or her experiences, to understand concepts, and to develop age appropriate literacy, numeracy, reasoning, problem solving and decision making skills which form a foundation for school readiness and later school success" (1304.21 [c] [1] [ii]; USDHHS, 1998, p. 79). The guidance for this standard lists various ways adults in Head Start can support children's cognitive development, including "supporting play as a way for children to organize their experiences and understand concepts" (p. 79). Thus, when discussing the Head Start curriculum, the performance standards again include a focus on play.

Play as Part of the Curriculum

The curricula used in Head Start also demonstrate an understanding of the value of play and its essential role in children's learning. The Head Start performance standards do not prescribe any particular curriculum. Programs are free to write their own curriculum, use a locally developed curriculum, or purchase a published curriculum. A U.S. General Accounting Office (2003) study found that most Head Start programs were compliant in implementing a curriculum. Further, the majority (58%) of Head Start programs used one of two published curricula: either the Creative Curriculum (36%) or the High Scope curriculum (22%).

Creative Curriculum

The Creative Curriculum for Preschool (Dodge, Colker, & Heroman, 2002) focuses on children's active learning through play and stresses the importance of social and emotional development for learning. It is based on research in child development and children's learning. Each classroom has 11 interest areas: blocks, dramatic play, toys and games, art, library, discovery, sand and water, music and movement, cooking, computers, and outdoors. The curriculum has six content areas (literacy, mathematics, science, social studies, the arts, and technology), and learning in each of these content areas occurs in each of the interest areas. For example, literacy activities are infused throughout each of the 11 interest areas, rather than just in the library area or during book-reading activities (Heroman & Jones, 2004). Teachers label toy boxes with drawings of the toys they contain, as well as with the words naming the toys. The cooking area has picture-and-word instructions for activities like washing hands. The daily schedule is posted with both pictures and words outlining the day's activities.

Several of the interest areas include a focus on play (Dodge et al., 2002). For example, the dramatic play area encourages children to engage in imaginative play. This play can be used to promote cognitive development, including literacy and numeracy. For example, vocabulary development is enhanced when the teacher introduces props for the play scenarios and teaches children the props' names (e.g., stethoscope and tongue depressor for playing "doctor's office"). Prewriting skills can be developed through using writing tools and paper of various kinds (e.g., prescription pads). Premath skills can also be developed in the dramatic play area (e.g., providing a height chart and scale for the doctor's office). Play is incorporated into the outdoor interest area and used in the service of cognitive development. For example, to promote preliteracy skills, teachers can ask children to explore outdoors and record on clipboards what plants they observe. Later, in the classroom, children can use resource books to find pictures of what they discovered outside. They can also make charts and graphs to organize their observations, which promotes premath skills.

High Scope Curriculum

The High Scope curriculum (Hohmann & Weikart, 1995) encourages children to pursue their own interests and takes advantage of children's natural desire to communicate what is meaningful to them to others. It was developed in the early 1960s for the High Scope Perry Preschool Project, one of the most studied preschool intervention programs. The curriculum is based on Piaget's theory of cognitive development, particularly his central idea that children actively acquire knowledge through interacting with the physical environment, which includes play. The curriculum includes 58 key experiences for children, grouped into 10 categories: creative representation, language and literacy, initiative and social relations, movement, music, classification, seriation, number, space, and time. As with the Creative Curriculum, the High Scope classroom is divided into various interest areas, including blocks, house, toy, book, sand and water, and outdoors. Also similar to Creative Curriculum, literacy and numeracy learning occurs in all of the interest areas. The High Scope curriculum stresses the need for a daily routine, including a "plan–do–review" sequence. Children plan what activities they want to engage in, engage in these activities during "work" times (or, more accurately, "play" times), and end by recalling and reflecting on what they have done. In each of these phases, there are opportunities for gaining preliteracy skills. For example, children can describe their plans to the teacher or make a drawing of their plans. During the work time, children locate toys by going to bins labeled with both pictures of the toys and their names. In reviewing the activity, children are required to use words to describe what they have done.

Program Vignette

The following vignette comes from a local Head Start program, provided by an education coordinator. It provides an example of how play can function in the context of Head Start.

"I recently observed an example of the importance of play in the case of a 4-year-old boy, who was a serious behavior problem in class. He exhibited extremely aggressive actions which were very disturbing, both to teachers and the other children. No one would play with him and his negative behavior was escalating. One day, outside, the boy had six other boys engaged in a game without any coercion at all. There was no football, but it became obvious that that was what they were playing. The child was using his stocking hat as the football (his idea), explaining the 'rules,' and running around the playground. There was no tackling involved, as they were using tagging to bring the player down. Teachers were very wary and tempted to end the game before anyone got hurt. Fortunately, they held back and allowed the so-called 'problem' child his time to shine. The smile on his face and his obvious pride spoke volumes. His play was the key to helping the boy to cope with his unresolved conflicts and feelings of inadequacy at home. Without play, this may have taken much longer to discover or, sadly, would not have been discovered at all."

In this example, play provided a way for the boy, who had behavior problems, to relate to his peers. The play scenario also allowed the teachers to see another aspect of the boy, beyond his problematic behavior. In the context of the play, the boy could learn skills such as self-regulation, collaboration, and the importance of following rules. The boy's pride likely reflects an increase in his self-confidence, gained through successful play. As we discuss below, such skills, although often considered social or emotional, are essential for learning.

EMPIRICAL SUPPORT

Research on Head Start's Impact

The question of whether Head Start affects children's educational success has been a matter of long-standing debate. This debate may have been fueled, in part, by the fact that Head Start focuses on the whole child, its performance standards demonstrate an appreciation for the key role of play in children's learning, and programs typically employ curricula with a strong emphasis on play. In Head Start children learn through active engagement with people and materials in the very rich classroom environment, including substantial time in both free and structured play (Dodge et al., 2002; Hohmann & Weikart, 1995; Zigler & Styfco, 2001).

The task of assessing Head Start has been further handicapped by the failure of Head Start to have a clear, consistent, and agreed-upon goal.

As described above, the impact of Head Start has often been assessed by examining IQ scores. A consistent finding over the years has been that the IQ is increased as a result of a child experiencing Head Start, but that this result "fades out" over the next few years. Even the 1998 reauthorization, which clearly stated that the goal of Head Start was to improve children's school readiness, did not solve the efficacy issue. The question of just how much improvement in school readiness is necessary to constitute the success of the Head Start program remains unresolved. The Bush administration interpreted this as meaning that to be successful, Head Start graduates should begin school as equally ready as middle-class children. However, this is an unrealistic goal for the Head Start program (Brooks-Gunn, 2003). We must be realistic about what 1 or even 2 years of Head Start can reasonably be expected to achieve for young children living in environments of extreme poverty and subsequently going on to typically inferior elementary schools. To overcome such negative environmental factors, poor children need programs from conception through age 8 or third grade (Zigler & Styfco, 1993).

Barnett (2004) conducted a critical review of the extensive body of research examining Head Start and other preschool programs' effects on children's cognitive development. He concluded: "The weight of the evidence indicates that a wide range of preschool programs including Head Start can increase IQ scores during the early childhood years, improve achievement, and prevent grade retention and special education" (p. 242). Barnett cited many methodological shortcomings in studies to date, however, and called for better research designs in future studies.

One somewhat better designed study has demonstrated positive effects of Head Start on children's literacy development. This study comparing Head Start children to a comparison group found that Head Start children developed preliteracy skills significantly faster than children in the comparison group (Abbott-Shim, Lambert, & McCarty, 2003). For both receptive vocabulary (the Peabody Picture Vocabulary Test) and phonemic awareness (the Early Phonemic Awareness Profile), the comparison group showed only normal maturation from pretest to posttest, whereas Head Start children had rates of growth that were significantly faster than those of the comparison group.

The FACES study (Head Start Family and Child Experiences Survey; Administration for Children and Families, Office of Planning, Research and Evaluation [ACF OPRE], 1997, 2003) also offers evidence of Head Start's effects on school readiness. FACES provides information on outcomes for nationally representative samples of children served by Head Start. There have been three waves of the FACES study, in 1997, 2000, and 2003. Results to date indicate that children show substantial gains on measures of school readiness, particularly vocabulary and early writing skills, over the course of participating in 1 year of Head Start. These children continue to show gains in vocabulary, early writing skills, and early math skills in kindergarten. Further, the gains that children made in Head Start predicted their achievement in kindergarten (ACF OPRE, 2003).

Head Start has also been found to reduce the cost of crime (Garces, Thomas, & Currie, 2002; Fight Crime: Invest in Kids, 2004). Currie and her colleagues' study comparing children who attend Head Start to their siblings led to the conclusion that Head Start has "both short-run and long-run positive impacts on children" (Currie & Neidell, 2007, p. 84). These effects include greater educational achievements and less criminal behavior of young adults. The educational achievements include better test scores and lower grade repetition among former Head Start participants. Consistent with all other studies, this study also noted that Head Start does not bring poor children up to the average achievement level of nonpoor children. A surprising finding of the Currie et al. study was that while blacks showed the same benefits as whites upon leaving Head Start, unlike whites blacks did not maintain the advantage through the early grades of school. Currie et al. attributed this to the poorer schools blacks went to and perhaps family factors as well. The findings of this study also indicated that Hispanic and white children in Head Start were about 19 percentage points more likely to attend college. For blacks, the percentage on schooling attainment was found to be small and not statistically significant. For this group, Head Start as relative to other preschool experiences was found to be associated with a reduction in the chance of being arrested by around 12 percentage points. Currie et al. concluded that schooling effects for whites were quite large, while the crime effects for blacks were also quite large in magnitude.

A study recently published in *Science* demonstrated the positive impact of Head Start on children's cognitive skills, including prereading, prewriting and premath skills. Head Start children improved on all of these skills (although not as much as students in non-Head Start preschool programs) (Gormley, Phillips, & Gayer, 2008).

The most recent assessment of the efficacy of Head Start comes from the National Impact Study, a random-assignment, longitudinal study in which Head Start and control children will be followed through the third grade (ACF OPRE 2000). The National Impact study was mandated by Congress in the 1998 reauthorization of Head Start. First year findings (USDHHS, 2005) and findings through first grade (USDHHS, 2010) have been released to date. At the end of their year of participation in Head Start, positive findings were obtained for attendees across a wide array of measures, although these benefits were in the small to modest range. More positive findings were obtained for 3-year-olds than 4-year-olds. The gap in reading skills for Head Start children compared to the national norm were approximately only half as great as was found for the non-Head Start control group. In addition to cognitive measures, the 3-year-old Head Start children were superior on social–emotional variables such as frequency and severity of problem behaviors. Further, Head Start parents engaged in significantly more behaviors related to enhancing school readiness than did non-Head Start parents (e.g., reading to the child). Head Start parents, as compared to non-Head Start parents, also displayed parenting behaviors more similar to mainstream parents (e.g., less corporal punishment). A better health outcome was also found for Head Start children than for non-Head Start children (e.g., overall child health status and dental care). However, the numeracy skills of Head Start children were not different from the comparison group. Further, by the end of kindergarten and first grade, only a few statistically significant differences remained between Head Start attendees and the comparison group. Although critics of Head Start might use the National Impact Study kindergarten and first-grade findings to argue that Head Start does not work, the second author (Zigler, 2010) has provided a more nuanced interpretation of the results. He concludes that the study holds many insights into what Head Start needs to do better to achieve the desired results and has prompted a quality improvement roadmap. Data from subsequent years of the National Impact study will likely prove similarly useful.

Another recent study, using a regression-discontinuity design, also examined the effects of Head Start (Ludwig & Miller, 2007). Unlike the findings of Currie and her colleagues, Ludwig and Miller found evidence of positive impacts of Head Start for both blacks and whites. A very dramatic finding of the Ludwig and Miller study was reduced mortality rates for children age 5–9 from causes that could be affected by Head Start, but not other causes. Ludwig and Miller also found that Head Start attendance increased educational attainment by about half a year and the likelihood of attending some college increased by about 15%.

Research on Play and Its Impact on Children's Learning

Although Head Start was founded before there was an established knowledge base on the potential of intervention programs to promote young children's development, Head Start's founders recognized the importance of social and emotional factors, as well as cognitive development. Since that time, a body of research has demonstrated the importance of these factors for school readiness (Raver, 2002; Shonkoff & Phillips, 2000). For example, emotional self-regulation has been found to be an especially important component of learning (Raver & Zigler, 1991). Children must be able to focus their attention on the task at hand, filtering out distractions. They must be able to control their emotions when in the classroom, during both individual and group activities. They must be able to organize their behavior and listen to the teacher. All of these are essentially noncognitive factors that foster learning. Further, this type of emotional self-regulation can be developed through play when children take turns, regulate one another's behavior, and learn to cooperate (Bredekamp, 2004).

Play also provides opportunities for acquiring many cognitive skills. Although play is often thought of in terms of "free play," dictated by the child, play can also be educationally focused, directed by the teacher or parent to reach specific educational goals. Through both forms of play, children can learn vocabulary, language skills, concepts, problem solving, perspective taking, representational skills, memory, and creativity (e.g., Davidson, 1998; Newman, 1990; Russ, Robins, & Christiano, 1999; Singer, Singer, Plaskon, & Schweder, 2003). Play has also been found to contribute to early literacy development (Christie, 1998; Owocki, 1999).

In addition, play has been shown to contribute to social development, including social skills such as turn taking, collaboration and following rules, empathy, self-regulation, self-confidence, impulse control, and motivation (e.g., Corsaro, 1988; Klugman & Smilansky, 1990; Krafft & Berk, 1998). These factors have an impact on cognitive development and are just as important in learning to read as the ability to recognize letters or sounds.

The research to date on Head Start's impact on child development has not focused on play per se. However, given that the curricula used in Head Start focus largely on children's learning through play, it is likely that at least some of the impact of Head Start can be attributed to play. Data from studies of the curricula used in Head Start provide further evidence of the importance of play. Preliminary research on the Creative Curriculum has provided some support for the curriculum's effectiveness. One study evaluated the use of the curriculum in the Department of Defense's Sure Start preschool program (Abbott-Shim, 2000). Examining 10 randomly selected classrooms, researchers found that children made significant gains on receptive vocabulary, language production, print awareness, and mathematical problem solving over the course of 1 year of participation in the Sure Start preschool. However, this study did not have a comparison group. The United States Department of Education's preschool curriculum evaluation research grants program funded randomized controlled studies of the Creative Curriculum in two sites (Vanderbilt and the University of North Carolina at Charlotte [UNC]; Preschool Curriculum Evaluation Research Consortium, 2008). At both sites, no impacts on student-level outcomes were found, at either prekindergarten or kindergarten. However, the UNC study found positive impacts at the classroom level on a variety of measures: overall classroom quality, teacher–child relationships, early literacy instruction, and early language instruction.

There is considerable longitudinal evidence available on the High Scope curriculum's effectiveness, given its use in the longitudinal Perry Preschool Project. Low-income 3- and 4-year-olds (N = 123) were randomly assigned to the Perry Preschool Project or to a no-preschool comparison group. Researchers have followed the children over time, assessing them every year from ages 3 to 11, and then at ages 14, 15, 19, 27, and 40. The most recent study at age 40 found that Perry Preschool attendees were more likely to have graduated from high school and have a job, had higher earnings, and had committed fewer crimes than the comparison group (Schweinhart, 2004). Preschool attendees performed better on intellectual and language tests during early childhood, on school achievement tests between ages 9 and 14, and on literacy tests at age 19 and 27. A cost–benefit analysis determined that the project returned $17 for every dollar invested. Schweinhart and colleagues determined that the program cost $15,166 per participant and had an economic return to society of $258,888. The savings to society came in the form of reduced costs for crime, special education, and welfare, as well as increased tax revenue from participants' increased wages.

Marcon (1999) also found evidence for the value of child-initiated curricula and play for later school outcomes. Her study evaluated three approaches to preschool education: child-initiated, academically focused, and a combination. She found that although children who had been in more academically focused preschools were less likely to be held back, by fourth grade they had significantly lower grades than children who had experienced more child-initiated preschool models.

Studies of the "Tools of the Mind" curriculum for preschool and kindergarten classrooms provide further evidence for a play-based approach to learning. The curriculum (Bodrova & Leong, 2001, 2003), based on Vygotsky's theory of cognitive development and the work of his student Elkonin, use sociodramatic play to foster literacy. These classrooms contain dramatic play areas where children spend a substantial amount of time daily, and dramatic play permeates many classroom activities. Teachers support children's play by helping them create imaginary situations, providing props, and expanding possible play roles. Children, with the teacher's assistance, develop written play plans, including the theme, the roles, and the rules that will govern the play. Preliminary evaluations of the Tools of the Mind curriculum supported its effectiveness (Bodrova & Leong, 2001; Bodrova, Leong, Norford, & Paynter, 2003). In one study, children who spent 50–60 minutes of a 2½-hour program engaging in supported sociodramatic play scored higher on literacy skills than did children in control classrooms (Bodrova & Leong, 2001). Thus, play, rather than detracting from academic learning, actually supported it.

More recent research, reported in *Science*, showed positive effects of the curriculum on executive functioning, particularly cognitive control (Diamond, Barnett, Thomas, & Munro, 2007). In this study, 147 5-year-olds in a low-income, urban U.S. school district were randomly assigned to classrooms using either the Tools of the Mind curriculum or a balanced literacy curriculum. Children were then evaluated on two measures of executive functioning. One exercise tested the children's ability to hold abstract rules in the mind. Most children in Tools of the Mind completed the test successfully, compared to fewer than one-third of children in the balanced literacy curriculum. In another exercise designed to test the children's ability to focus attention, ignore distractions, and switch the focus of attention, children in the Tools of the Mind classrooms outperformed children in balanced literacy classrooms on their ability to switch focus.

Other experts have also developed play-based curricula and provided evidence of their beneficial effects on cognitive development. For example, Learninggames (Sparling & Lewis, 2003) offers caregivers (and parents) activities to enhance child development, including cognitive development, from birth to age 5. The Learninggames curriculum was developed in the Carolina Abecedarian Project, which provided an early education program to poor children from infancy through age 5. Longitudinal results indicated that children in the project had higher scores on tests of cognitive ability from preschool to age 21 and higher reading and math achievement from elementary school to age 21, completed more years of education, and were more likely to attend college than children in the control group (Campbell, Ramey, Pungello, Sparling, & Miller-Johnson, 2002).

The Singers' Learning Through Play/Circle of Make-Believe project (Singer & Singer, 2004) uses videotapes and a manual to train parents and caregivers of low-income children to play pretend games involving school readiness concepts with the children. Results from several studies indicate that children who engaged in the pretend games with their parents and caregivers had school readiness scores superior to those of a comparison group.

RECOMMENDATIONS FOR RESEARCH

The research reviewed in the previous section provides clear evidence of the importance of play for children's learning. Play has been found to contribute to development in the domains of social, emotional, and cognitive development, including language, numeracy, and literacy. Play is children's work (Piaget, 1962).

However, more research is needed on the impact of play on learning, particularly in the context of Head Start. As mentioned above, the National Impact Study of Head Start is ongoing. However, discerning the effects of play will remain difficult, as play is only one component of Head Start's comprehensive approach to enhancing participants' school readiness. Thus, it is extremely difficult to disentangle the effects of play from those of Head Start's other components. Further studies of play-based curricula, including those used in Head Start, would shed additional light on the effects of play on learning.

RECOMMENDATIONS FOR PRACTICE AND THE DEVELOPMENT OF PREVENTION PROGRAMS

One of the major lessons learned from over 40 years of Head Start is the need to focus on the whole child. The whole child includes his or her need for play. Unfortunately, as discussed above, there has been a 50-year debate between proponents of a cognitive approach and those who focus on social–emotional aspects of learning. The whole-child approach, embodied in Head Start, reconciles these extreme positions.

Proponents of the whole-child approach do not deny the importance of cognitive skills. However, cognitive development is only one aspect of human development. Cognitive skills are very important, but they are so intertwined with the physical, social, and emotional systems that it is shortsighted, if not futile, to dwell on the intellect and exclude its partners.

Consider what goes into educational achievement. It involves mastery of academic content, for certain. But a prerequisite to achievement is good physical health. The child who is frequently absent from school because of illness or who has vision or hearing problems will have difficulty learning, as will children who suffer emotional problems such as depression or posttraumatic stress disorder. By the same token, a child who begins kindergarten knowing letters and numbers may be cognitively prepared, but if he or she does not understand how to listen, share, take turns, and get along with teachers and classmates, this lack of socialization will hinder further learning (Raver, 2002). In fact, kindergarten teachers, when asked about school readiness, emphasize the importance of socialization factors more than literacy or other cognitive skills (Piotrkowski, Botsko, & Matthews, 2000). To succeed at school, a child must receive appropriate education, of course, but he or she must also be physically and mentally healthy, have reasonable social skills, and have curiosity, confidence, and motivation to succeed. This broader view was endorsed in the authoritative book *From Neurons to Neighborhoods* (Shonkoff & Phillips, 2000), in which the finest child development thinkers in the nation pointed out the importance of emotional and motivational factors in human development and learning.

In the future, in order to optimize children's development and success in school, the whole-child approach must be a balanced approach in which each domain of development receives the same amount of emphasis. Head Start should adopt the accepted view that the subsystems of development are equal in importance and operate synergistically.

A relatively new curriculum that is sensitive to the child's need for play is Ann Epstein's *The Intentional Teacher: Choosing the Best Strategies for Young Children's Learning* (2007) which was published by the premier early childhood education organization, the National Association for the Education of Young Children. Like other early childhood education scholars, Epstein argues that we can intentionally teach preschool literacy and numeracy skills, but should do so in a developmentally appropriate way, incorporating play. This approach is similar to Bodrova and Leong's Tools of the Mind curriculum. Epstein points out that preschool teachers should organize learning experiences for preschoolers that concentrate not only on didactic teaching, but also attempt to recognize a teaching opportunity as it arises and take advantage of these "teachable moments." These practices would not represent a large leap for Head Start teachers. Epstein's guide provides specific teaching strategies for interacting intentionally with children in key subject areas (literacy, mathematics, scientific reasoning, social development and social studies, as well as physical movement and visual art). Epstein is currently continuing to develop the intentional teaching approach under the auspices of the High/Scope Foundation. This curriculum would fit well with Head Start's whole-child approach.

In sum, four decades of research and practice offer unequivocal evidence for the critical importance of play for children's development. Head Start, with its central whole-child approach, recognizing the important role of play, serves as a model for developmentally appropriate early childhood practice.

REFERENCES

Abbott-Shim, M. (2000). *Summary of the Sure Start program evaluation.* Retrieved February 28, 2005, from *www.teachingstrategies.com/pages/document.cfm?pagedocid=86.*

Abbott-Shim, M., Lambert, R., & McCarty, F. (2003). A comparison of school readiness outcomes for children randomly assigned to a Head Start program and the program's wait list. *Journal of Education for Students Placed at Risk, 8,* 191–214.

Administration for Children and Families, Office of Planning, Research and Evaluation. (1997). *Head Start Family and Child Experiences Survey (FACES),* *1997–2008.* Retrieved February 26, 2005, from *www.acf.hhs.gov/programs/* *opre/hs/faces/index.html.*

Administration for Children and Families, Office of Planning, Research and Evaluation. (2000). *Head Start Impact Study 2000–2006.* Retrieved February 26, 2005, from *www.acf.hhs.gov/programs/opre/hs/impact_* *study/index.html.*

Administration for Children & Families, Office of Planning, Research and Evaluation. (2003, April). *Head Start FACES 2000: A whole-child perspective on* *program performance. Executive summary.* Retrieved February 26, 2005, from *www.acf.hhs.gov/programs/opre/hs/faces/reports/executive_summary/* *exe_sum.html.*

Advisory Committee on Head Start Research & Evaluation. (2003). An overview of Head Start literacy, mentor-coaching, and Strategic Teacher Education Program (STEP). Retrieved May 25, 2005, from *www.acf.hhs.gov/* *programs/hsb/research/hsreac/jun2003/jun03_step_overview.htm.*

Barnett, W. S. (2004). Does Head Start have lasting cognitive effects? In E. Zigler & S. Styfco (Eds.), *The Head Start debates* (pp. 221–249). Baltimore: Brookes.

Bodrova, E., & Leong, D. J. (2001). *Tools of the Mind: A case study implementing the Vygotskian approach in American early childhood and primary classrooms.* Geneva, Switzerland: International Bureau of Education.

Bodrova, E., & Leong, D. J. (2003). Chopsticks and counting chips: Do play and foundational skills need to compete for the teacher's attention in an early childhood classroom? *Young Children, 58,* 10–17.

Bodrova, E., Leong, D. J., Norford, J. S., & Paynter, D. E. (2003). It only looks like child's play. *Journal of Staff Development, 24,* 47–51.

Brandon, K. (2002, October 20). Kindergarten less playful as pressure to achieve grows. *Chicago Tribune,* p. 1.

Bredekamp, S. (2004). Play and school readiness. In E. F. Zigler, D. G. Singer, & S. J. Bishop-Josef (Eds.), *Children's play: The roots of reading* (pp. 159–174). Washington, DC: Zero to Three Press.

Brooks-Gunn, J. (2003). Do you believe in magic?: What we can expect from early childhood intervention programs. *Social Policy Reports, 17,* 1.

Bush, G. W. (2003, January 8). *Remarks by the president on the first anniversary* *of the No Child Left Behind Act.* Retrieved September 10, 2003, from *www.* *whitehouse.gov/news/releases/2003/01/20030108-4.html.*

Campbell, F. A., Ramey, C. T., Pungello, E. P., Sparling, J., & Miller-Johnson, S. (2002). Early childhood education: Young adult outcomes from the Abecedarian Project. *Applied Developmental Science, 6,* 42–57.

Christie, J. F. (1998). Play as a medium for literacy development. In E. P. Frombreg & D. Bergen (Eds.), *Play from birth to twelve and beyond: Contexts,* *perspectives, and meaning* (pp. 50–55). New York: Garland.

Corsaro, W. A. (1988). Peer culture in the preschool. *Theory into Practice, 27,* 19–24.

Currie, J., & Neidell, M. (2007). Getting inside the "black box" of Head Start quality: What matters and what doesn't. *Economics of Education Review, 26*, 83-99.

Davidson, J. I. F. (1998). Language and play: Natural partners. In E. P. Fromberg & D. Bergen (Eds.), *Play from birth to twelve and beyond: Contexts, perspectives, and meaning* (pp. 175–183). New York: Garland.

Diamond, A., Barnett, W. S., Thomas, J., & Munro, S. (2007, November 30). Preschool program improves cognitive control. *Science, 318*(5855), 1387–1388.

Dodge, D. T., Colker, L., & Heroman, C. (2002). *The creative curriculum for preschool* (4th ed.). Washington, DC: Teaching Strategies.

Elementary and Secondary Education Act of 1965, Public Law 89-10, 64 Stat 1100 20 USC 6301.

Elkind, D. (1981). *The hurried child: Growing up too fast, too soon.* Reading, MA: Addison-Wesley.

Elkind, D. (1987). *Miseducation: Preschoolers at risk.* New York: Knopf.

Elkind, D. (2001). Young Einsteins: Much too early. *Education Matters, 1*(2), 9–15.

Epstein, A. S. (2006). *The intentional teacher: Choosing the best strategies for children's learning.* Washington, DC: National Association for the Education of Young Children.

Fight Crime: Invest In Kids. (2004). *Quality pre-kindergarten: Key to crime prevention and school success.* Accessed on October 9, 2008, from *www.fightcrime.org/issue_earlyed.php.*

Fromberg, D. P. (1990). An agenda for research on play in early childhood education. In E. Klugman & S. Smilanksy (Eds.), *Children's play and learning: Perspectives and policy implications* (pp. 235–249). New York: Teachers College Press.

Garces, E., Thomas, D., & Currie, J. (2002). Longer-term effects of Head Start. *American Economic Review, 92*, 999-1012.

Gormley, W. T., Phillips, D. A., & Gayer, T. (2008, 27 June). Preschool programs can boost school readiness. *Science, 320*, 1723–1724.

Head Start Act of 1998. Public Law 105-285.

Heroman, C., & Jones, C. (2004). *Literacy: The Creative Curriculum approach.* Washington, DC: Teaching Strategies.

Hohmann, M., & Weikart, D. P. (1995). *Educating young children: Active learning practices for preschool and child care programs* (2nd ed.). Ypsilanti, MI: High/Scope.

Hunt, J. M. (1961). *Intelligence and experience.* New York: Ronald Press.

Improving Head Start for School Readiness Act of 2007, Public Law 110-134, 121 Stat. 1363.

Johnson, D. (1998, April 7). Many schools putting an end to child's play. *New York Times*, pp. A1, A16.

Kagan, S. L., & Lowenstein, A. E. (2004). School readiness and children's play: Contemporary oxymoron or compatible option? In E. F. Zigler, D. G. Singer, & S. J. Bishop-Josef (Eds.), *Children's play: The roots of reading* (pp. 59–76). Washington, DC: Zero to Three Press.

Kagan, S. L., Moore, E., & Bredekamp, S. (Eds.). (1995). *Reconsidering chil-*

dren's early development and learning: Toward common views and vocabulary (GPO 1995-396-664). National Education Goals Panel, Goal 1 Technical Planning Group. Washington, DC: U.S. Government Printing Office.

Klugman, E., & Smilansky, S. (1990). *Children's play and learning: Perspectives and policy implications.* New York: Teachers College Press.

Krafft, K. C., & Berk, L. E. (1998). Private speech in two preschools: Significance of open-ended activities and make-believe play for verbal self-regulation. *Early Childhood Research Quarterly, 13,* 637–658.

Ludwig, J., & Miller, D. L. (2007). Does Head Start improve children's life chances?: Evidence from a regression-discontinuity design. *Quarterly Journal of Economics, 122,* 159–208.

Marcon, R. (1999). Differential impact of preschool models on development and early learning of inner-city children: A three cohort study. *Developmental Psychology, 35,* 358–375.

Meisels, S. J., & Atkins-Burnett, S. (2004). Public policy viewpoint: The Head Start national reporting system: A critique. *Young Children, 59,* 64–66.

Murline, A. (2000, May 1). What's your favorite class?: Most kids would say recess. Yet many schools are cutting back on unstructured schoolyard play. *U.S. News and World Report,* 50–52.

Newman, L. S. (1990). Intentional and unintentional memory in young children: Remembering vs. playing. *Journal of Experimental Child Psychology, 50,* 243–258.

No Child Left Behind Act of 2001. Public Law 107-110, 115 Stat 1535, 20 USC 6361, Part B, Subpart 1, Sec. 1201.

Owocki, G. (1999). *Literacy through play.* Portsmouth, NH: Heinemann.

Piaget, J. (1962). *Play, dreams, and imitation in childhood.* New York: Norton.

Piotrkowski, C. S., Botsko, M. B., & Matthews, E. (2000). Parents' and teachers' beliefs about children's school readiness in a high-need community. *Early Childhood Research Quarterly, 15,* 537-558.

Preschool Curriculum Evaluation Research Consortium. (2008). *Effects of preschool curriculum programs on school readiness* (NCER 2008–2009). Washington, DC: National Center for Education Research, Institute of Education Sciences, U.S. Department of Education. Washington, DC: U.S. Government Printing Office. Retrieved July 30, 2010, from *ies.ed.gov/ncer/pubs/20082009/pdf120082009 _rev.pdf.*

Raver, C. C. (2002). Emotions matter: Making the case for the role of young children's emotional development for early school readiness. *Social Policy Report, 16*(3).

Raver, C. C., & Zigler, E. F. (1991). Three steps forward, two steps back: Head Start and the measurement of social competence. *Young Children, 46,* 3–8.

Raver, C. C., & Zigler, E. F. (2004). Public policy viewpoint: Another step back?: Assessing readiness in Head Start. *Young Children, 59,* 58–63.

Russ, S. W., Robins, A. L., & Christiano, B. A. (1999). Pretend play: Longitudinal prediction of creativity and affect in fantasy in children. *Creativity Research Journal, 12,* 129–139.

Schumacher, R., & Greenberg, M. (2004, January 23). *Head Start reauthoriza-*

tion: A section-by-section analysis of the Senate HELP Committee bill (S. 1940). Washington, DC: Center for Law and Social Policy.

Schumacher, R., Greenberg, M., & Mezey, J. (2003, June 2). *Head Start reauthorization: A preliminary analysis of H.R. 2210, the "School Readiness Act of 2003."* Washington, DC: Center for Law and Social Policy.

Schweinhart, L. J. (2004). *The High Scope Perry Preschool Study through age 40: Summary, conclusions, and frequently asked questions.* Retrieved February 27, 2005, from *www.highscope.org/Research/PerryProject/PerryAge-40SumWeb.pdf.*

Shonkoff, J. P., & Phillips, D. A. (Eds.). (2000). *From neurons to neighborhoods: The science of early childhood development.* Washington, DC: National Academy Press.

Singer, D. G., & Singer, J. L. (2004). Encouraging school readiness through guided pretend games. In E. F. Zigler, D. G. Singer, & S. J. Bishop-Josef (Eds.), *Children's play: The roots of reading* (pp. 175–187). Washington, DC: Zero to Three Press.

Singer, D. G., Singer, J. L., Plaskon, S. L., & Schweder, A. E. (2003). A role for play in the preschool curriculum. In S. Olfman (Ed.), *All work and no play: How educational reforms are harming our preschoolers* (pp. 59–101). Westport, CT: Greenwood Press.

Snow, C. E., & Van Hemel, S. B. (Eds.). (2008). *Early childhood assessment: Why, what, and how.* Washington, DC: National Academies Press.

Sparling, J., & Lewis, I. (2003). *Learninggames: The Abecedarian curriculum 36 to 48 months.* Chapel Hill, NC: MindNurture.

Stegelin, D. A. (2005). Making the case for play policy: Research-based reasons to support play-based environments. *Young Children, 60,* 76–85.

Steinberg, J. (2002, December 4). For Head Start children, taking a turn at testing. *New York Times,* p. B10.

Steinhauer, J. (2005, May 22). Maybe preschool is the problem. *New York Times,* section 4, pp. 1, 4.

Stipek, D. (2004, May 5). Commentary: Head Start: Can't we have our cake and eat it too? *Education Week,* pp. 43, 52.

Strauss, V. (2003, January 17). U.S. to review Head Start program: Bush plan to assess 4-year-olds' progress stirs criticism. *Washington Post,* p. A1.

U.S. Department of Health and Human Services. (1998). *Head Start program performance standards and other regulations.* Title 45 of the Code of Federal Regulations, Parts 1301–1308. Washington, DC: Author.

U.S. Department of Health and Human Services. (2002). *HHS fact sheet. Head Start: Promoting early childhood development.* Retrieved May 25, 2005, from *fatherhood.hhs.gov/factsheets/fact20020426b.htm.*

U.S. Department of Health and Human Services, Administration for Children and Families. (2005). *Head Start Impact Study First year findings.* Retrieved October 23, 2008, from www.acf.hhs.gov/programs/opre/hs/impact_study/reports/first_yr_finds/first_yr_finds.pdf.

U.S. Department of Health and Human Services, Administration for Children and Families. (2010). *Head Start Impact Study, final report.* Retrieved July

19, 2010, from *www.acf.hhs.gov/programs/opre/hs/impact_study/reports/ impact_study/hs_impact_study_final.pdf.*

U.S. Department of Health and Human Services, Administration for Children and Families, Office of Head Start. (2008). *About the Office of Head Start.* Retrieved October 23, 2008, from *www.acf.hhs.gov/programs/ohs/about/ index.html#factsheet.*

U.S. Department of Health and Human Services, Administration for Children and Families, Office of Head Start (2010). *Head Start Program fact sheet.* Retrieved July 17, 2010, from *www.acf.hhs.gov/programs/ohs/about/ fy2010.html.*

U.S. General Accounting Office. (2003). *Head Start curriculum use and individual child assessment in cognitive and language development* (GAO-03-1049). Washington, DC: Author.

U.S. Government Accountability Office. (2005, May). *Head Start further development could allow results of new test to be used for decision making* (GAO-05-343). Retrieved May 23, 2005, from *www.gao.gov/new.items/ d05343.pdf.*

Vail, K. (2003, November). Ready to learn. What the Head Start debate about early academics means for your schools. *American School Board Journal, 190.* Retrieved May 25, 2005, from *www.asbj.com/2003/11/1103coverstory.html.*

Westinghouse Learning Corporation and Ohio University. (1969). *The impact of Head Start: An evaluation of the effects of Head Start on children's cognitive and affective development* (Vols. 1 and 2). Report to the Office of Economic Opportunity. Athens, OH: Author.

Whitehurst, G. J. (2001). Young Einsteins: Much too late. *Education Matters, 1*(2), 9, 16–19.

Zigler, E. F. (1970). The environmental mystique: Training the intellect versus development of the child. *Childhood Education, 46,* 402–412.

Zigler, E. F. (1994). Foreword. In M. Hyson, *The emotional development of young children: Building an emotion-centered curriculum* (pp. ix–x). New York: Teachers College Press.

Zigler, E. F. (2003). Foreword. In M. Hyson, *The emotional development of young children: Building an emotion-centered curriculum* (2nd ed., pp. x–xi). New York: Teachers College Press.

Zigler, E., & Butterfield, E. C. (1968). Motivational aspects of changes in IQ test performance of culturally deprived nursery school children. *Child Development, 39,* 1–14.

Zigler, E., Gordic, B., & Styfco, S. J. (2007). What is th goal of Head Start?: Four decades of confusion and debate. *NHSA Dialog, 10,* 83–97,

Zigler, E., & Styfco, S. J. (Eds.). (1993). *Head Start and beyond: A national plan for extended childhood intervention.* New Haven, CT: Yale University Press.

Zigler, E., & Styfco, S. J. (2001). More than the three Rs: The Head Start approach to school readiness. *Education Matters, 1*(2), 12.

Zigler, E., & Trickett, P. (1978). IQ, social competence, and evaluation of early childhood intervention programs. *American Psychologist, 33,* 789–798.

13

Play Intervention and Prevention Programs in School Settings

Sandra W. Russ and Beth L. Pearson

Research on play intervention and prevention programs is a very young field. Even though a large body of research supports the relationship between pretend play and adaptive functioning in children (as reviewed in Chapter 1), there have not been large-scale research programs in developing play interventions that then become widely used. There are a number of reasons for this state of affairs. The recognition of the importance of play in childhood goes in and out of fashion in the culture. Also, it is difficult to carry out studies that are rigorous and can build on one another in different research labs and with different research teams. Large-scale funding is required. Finally, pretend play ability is best developed naturally, over a number of years, in homes that value and enjoy the child's play and provide time for play to occur. It remains to be determined how much progress can be made in time-limited interventions with children who do not have good play skills.

This chapter presents some of the individual studies and programs that do exist and that provide some empirical support for interventions that facilitate play skills and improve functioning in other areas of child development.

FACILITATING PLAY SKILLS

Pretend play relates to important areas of adaptive functioning in children and is a frequently used technique in child psychotherapy (Russ, 2004; Singer & Singer, 1990). Although a large body of research supports the importance of play in child development, there is little research on how to improve play skills that would be relevant to the use of play in therapy. Specifically, we need to learn what techniques influence cognitive and affective processes expressed in play and, in turn, which processes influence important areas of functioning in children.

Pretend play has an important role in child development, as reviewed in Chapters 1 and 2. Pretend play involves pretending, the use of fantasy and make-believe, and the use of symbolism. Fein (1987) defined *pretend play* as a symbolic behavior in which "one thing is playfully treated as if it were something else" (p. 287). Fein also stated that pretense is charged with feelings and emotional intensity, so that affect is intertwined with pretend play. Singer and Singer (1990) viewed play as involving the interaction of cognitive and affective processes. Russ (2004) articulated specific types of cognitive processes and affective processes in play. *Cognitive processes* include the ability to organize a story, to generate a number of different ideas, to use fantasy, and to use symbolism and transformation of objects. *Affective processes* include the expression of emotion and the expression of affect-laden themes, as well as emotion regulation. In therapy, play has been seen as a vehicle for emotional expression (Landreth, 1991). Integration of emotion into a meaningful narrative for the child could also be important in therapy.

An important question is "Can play skills be taught and pretend play ability be developed?" And, if we can teach children to be better players, will the improved skills affect their real-life functioning and behavior?

There have been efforts to improve children's play skills. Many of these play-training studies have been in an academic context rather than in a therapeutic context. Smilansky's (1968) study was one of the first to demonstrate that teachers could teach play skills. She worked with kindergarten children from low socioeconomic backgrounds in Israel for 90 minutes a day, 5 days a week, for 9 weeks. The children who engaged in sociodramatic play, with help from their teachers, showed significant cognitive improvement when compared with children in other groups. The teachers helped the children develop their play by commenting, making suggestions, and giving demonstrations.

Play training has been found to be effective with developmentally disabled populations (Hallendoorn, 1994; Kim, Lombardino, Rothman, & Vinson, 1989). Additionally, Hartmann and Rollett (1994) reported positive results with elementary schoolchildren in Austria, where teachers instructed children from low socioeconomic backgrounds in play 4 hours per week. When compared with a comparable control class, the play intervention group had better divergent thinking and were happier in school.

One of the methodological problems with many studies in the play facilitation area is the lack of adequate control groups. Smith (1988, 1994) has consistently raised this issue in reviewing the play intervention literature. Smith stressed that adequate research design requires the inclusion of a control group that involves experimenter–child interaction in a form other than pretend play. He concluded that when this kind of control group is included, usually both the play group and the control group improve. Dansky (1999) reached a different conclusion after reviewing the play-training literature. He found that many studies did have adequate control groups that controlled for involvement of the experimenter (Dansky, 1980; Shmukler, 1984–1985; Udwin, 1983). Dansky concluded that there were consistently positive results in studies with adequate control groups that demonstrated that play tutoring, over a period of time, did result in increased imaginativeness in play and increased creativity on measures other than play.

Barton and Wolery (2008), in a review of the literature on play with children with disabilities, concluded that there is a consistent relation between pretense behaviors in the child and adult prompting and modeling. However, there were many methodological problems with the studies. Few studies had information about procedure fidelity or generalization across settings, people, or toys. Barton and Wolery did think that teachers could prompt pretend play in the classroom, but they argued that for generalization to occur, multiple exemplars of materials and multiple trainers should be used.

Kasari, Freeman, and Paparella (2006), in a randomized controlled study with children with autism, found that a play intervention did result in increased symbolic play. This was a very rigorous study that began the intervention at the child's current developmental level of play. The training involved modeling and prompting. Children in the play group, compared with children in the joint attention and control groups, had increased symbolic play that generalized to play with mothers. This study was reviewed in detail in Chapter 8 and will not be reviewed again here. It is an important study because it is so well done and is a randomized controlled study that increased play ability.

A Pilot Study with School-Based Children

It is important to study specific techniques that improve play skills. It is also important to identify processes and mechanisms that account for the increase in specific play skills or changes in other areas of functioning. Improvements in cognitive and affective play processes need to be differentiated. In order to accomplish this, the field needs measures of play that can differentiate these processes.

Russ (1987, 1993) developed the Affect in Play Scale (APS) to measure cognitive and affective processes in play. Since the development of this instrument, we have been able to measure specific processes in play. It is important to be able to identify and measure specific cognitive and affective processes so that we can investigate which specific processes relate to adaptive functioning such as creativity and also investigate specific change processes in child psychotherapy (Shirk & Russell, 1996). In the play area, the APS enables us to investigate the effect of specific interventions on specific processes in play.

In a pilot study by Russ, Moore, and Pearson (2004, 2007), we developed a play intervention that attempted to facilitate specific cognitive and affective processes in pretend play. We investigated whether cognitive and affective processes could be differentially affected by different types of play intervention techniques. The pilot study included a control group that controlled for time and interaction with an interested adult. This study also developed a play intervention protocol that could be replicated in other studies and be used as a manual in play therapy. In developing the play intervention, we followed guidelines from previous studies.

In this study, specific play intervention techniques were clearly spelled out and were based upon common techniques used by play therapists. Russ (1998) outlined a number of techniques used by play therapists, such as labeling and reflection of feelings, empathy, and articulation of cause and effect (e.g., she is feeling sad because she lost her toy). These techniques were the foundation of the intervention. Previous play interventions have used such techniques as modeling (Knell, 1993), positive reinforcement (Knell, 1993; Bodiford-McNeil, Hembree-Kigen, & Eyberg, 1996), reflection, and imitation (Bodiford-McNeil et al., 1996). Our study utilized these methods as well, through the use of standardized prompts.

The pilot study investigated the effectiveness of two different play interventions on play skills in comparison with a control group in a school-based population. One play intervention script focused on improving imagination and organization of the narrative. The other play intervention script focused on increasing affective expression in play. In addition, outcome measures of creativity, coping, life satisfaction, and classroom behavior were administered to explore the association of play with adaptive functioning. It was hypothesized that both play interventions would result in improvements on all play skills when compared with the control group. Of particular interest was whether or not affect expression techniques would be effective with the affect play skills and imagination expression techniques would be effective with imagination in play. In addition, it was expected that both play intervention groups would have higher scores on the outcome measures of adaptive functioning than the control group.

Fifty children participated in the study, ranging from 6 to 8 years of age in the first and second grades at an urban midwestern elementary school. The children were all in mainstream classrooms. The ethnic-minority composition of the school is 99% African American. The school reports that 92% of the families are at or below poverty level.

An initial pilot phase was conducted with 12 children to develop the intervention protocol. The participants for the pilot phase were drawn from the school that was the setting for the larger study. This enabled investigators to test instructions, scripts, and prompts to determine if they were effective at eliciting affect in play, imagination in play, and/or organization in play in this particular sample. Investigators also used the pilot phase as an opportunity to ensure that the scripts were age-appropriate and to explore the effects of using different toys. We also piloted the puzzles and coloring sheets used with the control group to make sure they were age-appropriate and interesting.

In the main study, children received a baseline measure of affect and fantasy expressed in play, the APS. The administrator of the APS was not involved in the intervention for that child. Next, children were randomly assigned to one of three groups: imagination play intervention, affect play intervention, or control. There were 19 children in the imagination group, 17 children in the affect group, and 14 children in the control group. Each child participated in five, 30-minute individual sessions which usually occurred over a period of 3–5 weeks. Specific instructions and stories were used for each group, and the toys, story lines, and prompts were standardized. In all cases the same play trainer carried out all five sessions with the child. There were four play trainers in the study. The trainers instructed each child to play out approximately four stories per session, and the children were instructed to make up their own story one time each session. The trainers attempted to limit discussion that did not follow the standardized prompts during the sessions. All trainers filled out session checklists at the end of each session indicating stories used, prompts used, and the child's reactions to the stories and prompts. Within 3 weeks of completing the intervention, outcome measures were given in order to assess a variety of cognitive and affective outcomes. Measures were given by a different investigator than the one who conducted the five sessions with the participant and who was blind to group assignment. First, the child again received the APS. In addition, each child received, in the following order, measures of divergent thinking, self-report coping, and life satisfaction.

Intervention Groups

IMAGINATION GROUP

Children in the imagination group were presented with a set of toys including human-like dolls, blocks, plastic animals, Legos, and cars. They were asked to play out stories with high fantasy content (e.g., someone who lives on the moon) and high story organization (e.g., what someone needs to do to get ready for school). Children were encouraged to explore alternate endings for their stories and they were reinforced for being creative and engaging in object transformations. During the 30-minute sessions, the trainer was active with standardized prompts to have a beginning, middle, and end; show details; have the characters talk; pretend something is there (e.g., use a Lego to be a milk bottle); make up different endings; ask what happens next. The trainer used reinforcement, modeling, and praise.

AFFECT GROUP

Children in the affect group played with the same toys as children in the imagination group. The instructions, stories, and prompts were different from the imagination play group. Instead of focusing on fantasy and organization, children were encouraged to express feelings and were asked to play out stories with affective content. For example, a child might have played out a story about someone who was happy because she was going to a birthday party or sad because he had lost his favorite toy. The examiners used modeling, reinforcement, and reflection of feeling states to encourage affective experimentation. Standardized prompts were reflect/label feelings; ask how the dolls are feeling; have the dolls talk to each other about how they are feeling; state they are feeling this way because ... ; and ask what happens next.

Control Group

Children in the control group spent their sessions putting together puzzles and coloring on coloring sheets. The puzzles and coloring sheets were of neutral scenes such as a farm puzzle and pictures of flowers and butterflies. Experimenter interaction was controlled for by using standardized prompts and encouragement unrelated to affect or imagination. For example, children putting a puzzle together might have been asked about the colors in the picture, the content of the picture, or how many puzzle pieces there were. Toy choice (i.e., being able to pick what toys to use, as in the intervention groups) was controlled for by allowing the child to choose whether he or she wanted to start by doing a puzzle or by coloring. The child had the option of changing activities at his or her discretion.

The prompts were to ask what is in the picture; what piece is that; what color is that; how many pieces are there. Examiners were also active in praising children for their effort and helping them with the puzzles.

Fidelity was difficult to establish in this particular sample because of limitations set forth by the school. We were able to videotape the baseline and outcome play measures, but not the five intervention sessions. However, the stories and prompts were standardized and a session checklist was developed to monitor the stories and prompts used in each session. The affect play group had a different set of instructions and prompts used by the trainer than the imagination play group. Also, a totally different set of stories was used for the affect play group than for the imagination play group. Each trainer followed a script for the particular intervention group. An evaluation of the checklists for the intervention groups revealed that 86% of the time the prompt guideline was followed and 89% of the time the story/feeling guideline was followed. No significant differences were found on the number of prompts given by the play trainers across the groups. As an additional exploration of intervention fidelity, mean differences between play trainers on the APS were investigated and no significant differences were found on children's play scores.

The major result of this study was that the play interventions were effective in improving play skills. The affect play condition was most effective in that, after baseline play was controlled for, the affect play group had significantly higher play scores on all play processes. These children had more affect in their play (both positive affect and negative affect), a greater variety of affect content, and better imagination and organization of the story than did the control group. The imagination play group also had significantly more positive affect and variety of affect than the control group. Although most of these individual group comparisons were no longer significant when the Bonferroni correction was applied to correct for chance findings, the effect sizes were medium or, for frequency of affect, large. Another major finding was that, on outcome measures of adaptive functioning, there were significant effects for group. Although the individual contrast comparisons did not reach significance, inspection of the profile plots indicate that the play groups (usually the affect play group) had higher scores on most of the measures of divergent thinking, coping, and life satisfaction. The one exception was the teacher rating of classroom functioning in which the control group had higher scores than the imagination group.

The affect play intervention was the most effective intervention in improving play skills. By having children play out stories involving emotion, both positive and negative, we were able to improve play skills as measured by the APS. It is worth noting that the APS play measure was quite different from the play intervention situation in that there were only a few props (two puppets and a few blocks), whereas the intervention used a variety of toys. Also, the instructions for the APS are very unstructured ("play any way you like"), whereas the play intervention was quite structured and the child was directed to make up stories with specific themes. Thus, the finding that play changed on the unstructured outcome play measure suggests that the effect of the play intervention would generalize to a natural play situation. Future research should investigate this question.

The finding that the affect play group increased both affective expression in play and cognitive abilities of imagination and organization of the story suggests that involvement of affect also influences processes of imagination and fantasy. In order to express emotion, the child called on storytelling and imagination. Developing a narrative around the emotion may be a powerful process for children. The imagination play group was significantly better than the control group in frequency of positive affect and variety of affect. That the imagination play group improved positive affect and had a wider range of affect expression suggests that using one's imagination involves positive affect. This finding is consistent with results from the creativity research in which positive affect facilitates creativity and imagination (Isen, Daubman, & Nowicki, 1987). Another possible explanation for the overall greater improvement in the affect play group is that the instructions and prompts we used in the affect play group were better in facilitating affect in play than the instructions and prompts in the imagination group were in facilitating fantasy and imagination. Perhaps if we had used other techniques or stories, they would have been more effective. Future research should explore this possibility.

The finding that both play groups increased the positive affect in play is important. Pretend play is fun for most children and may stimulate positive affect themes such as stories about having fun, being happy, and caring about others. This result could have implications for mood regulation in children.

There were significant effects for group on all outcome measures. Although the individual group comparisons did not reach significance, the profile plots indicate that the play groups had higher scores on these variables, with the exception of classroom behavior. Because no baseline measures were given, we cannot say that the play intervention resulted in improvement in these areas. However, because this study utilized a randomized design and the results are in the direction of the hypotheses, we have every reason to expect that we would find this effect in a replication that included baseline measures. Future research should include baseline measures for all outcome measures.

The results suggest that improving play skills could improve creative thinking and coping ability. These results are consistent with previous research (Dansky, 1980; Russ, Robins, & Christiano, 1999) and would be a fruitful area of future research. Both the creativity measure and the coping measure used in this study involved generating a variety of solutions to a problem. The play interventions did not directly train for this ability. Rather, the play interventions had the children make up stories and express emotions. One prompt in the imagination group asked the children to think of different endings. Nevertheless, the creativity and coping tasks were sufficiently different from the play interventions to conclude that they were not being taught the specific task. The finding that play groups had higher scores on the life satisfaction measure is important. The affect expression or use of fantasy could improve the mood of children. The increase of positive affect expression in both groups could account for the difference in subjective well-being and should be explored in future research.

There are a number of limitations to this study. First, the play trainers were not blind to the hypotheses of the study and we had no ratings of videotapes of the interventions by observers to assess fidelity.

Second, there was no way to determine which specific instructions and prompts were most effective. We are currently carrying out several play intervention studies that are videotaping the play so we can asses fidelity of the researchers and investigate which specific techniques are most effective.

Finally, the sample was small. A larger sample would provide more power for the statistical analyses.

In a follow-up study of these children by Moore and Russ (2008) 4–8 months later, the imagination group had improved play skills over time. The affect group did not maintain the play changes over this period. It may be that an increase in affect expression from a play intervention is temporary whereas focus on imagination and pretend in play could be longer lasting. Much more research needs to be done with this protocol.

Implications

These findings have important implications for child therapy in which play is used. The affect play intervention had a large effect on the amount of affect expressed on the outcome play measure. This result suggests that we can increase the expression of affect in play with a play intervention. The expression of emotions in play therapy could be increased by a structured play technique such as the one used in this study. This is especially important for affect-constricted children or children with posttraumatic stress disorder, where expression of affect in a safe setting can be therapeutic. By having children make up various stories and directing them to express affect, with modeling and reinforcement by the therapist, children could increase affect expression quickly. The play intervention scripts and prompts developed for this study could be used by therapists at various points in therapy. This protocol could be used in short-term interventions, where it is important to "get to" uncomfortable thoughts and emotions quickly. By first helping the child to express affect in general, he or she might then be able to express emotions that were relevant to his or her life. The development of manuals for the use of play in therapy is essential in order to build an empirical base for the use of play in therapy.

The protocols developed for this study could also be used in play prevention intervention programs. Teachers, parents, and teacher aides could use these protocols to improve play skills, which in turn may increase creative problem solving and coping ability. The play interventions are easy to follow and carry out. Children in our study enjoyed them. They could be incorporated into home and school settings.

PLAY INTERVENTIONS
AND FUNCTIONING IN SCHOOL

One of the few studies to utilize play in a school-based mental health intervention with at-risk students was conducted by Nafpaktitis and Perlmutter (1998). They investigated the effect of this program on school adjustment of first to fourth grade at-risk children, using a wait-control design. Children participated in individual play sessions with trained and supervised nonprofessional child aides. This study was part of the Primary Intervention Program (PIP) in California public schools based on Cowen, Hightower, Johnson, Sarno, and Weissberg's (1989) prevention programs. After screening, at-risk children for mild to moderate school adjustment difficulties were referred for this early intervention program. The children were randomly assigned to one of two groups, the intervention group or the wait-control group. The intervention group participated once a week for 12 weeks in 30-minute individual play sessions. Child aides, who were carefully trained, conducted play sessions according to a nondirective play model. The child aide made verbal observations about the child's activities and expression of feelings. The adult participated in the play if the child wanted him or her to. If not, he or she engaged in a parallel activity.

The major finding of this study was that children at risk for school adjustment significantly improved in school adjustment after they participated in individual play sessions with a trained paraprofessional. The outcome variable was teachers' ratings of school adjustment. The play intervention was most effective in helping children to become more outgoing and confident, to get along better with peers, and to improve learning and task orientation. The intervention did not decrease acting out or improve frustration tolerance. Children were rated again 12 weeks after the last play session. Ratings declined from postintervention to follow-up but were still better than at baseline. The authors present the possibility that booster sessions may be needed to maintain the improvement. Theoretically, it was assumed that a relationship with a caring adult and the use of play accounted for the change. Ideally, there would have been a comparison group controlling for time spent with an adult. Nevertheless, this was a carefully done study with promising results.

There are also some play interventions that target specific kinds of behavioral or cognitive outcomes in children. Several of these are discussed below.

A study by Baumer, Ferholt, and Lecusay (2005) focused on the role of pretense in narrative development in young children. They examined the effects of the playworld educational practice on the development of narrative competence in 5- to 7-year-old children. The playworld educational practice, derived from play pedagogy developed in Scandinavia, consists of joint adult–child pretense based on a work of children's literature, discussion, free play, and art production. They described playworld as a form of guided pretense in which children are supported by adults. Their study was a pre- and post-quasi-experimental intervention. One experimental and one control classroom were chosen because those teachers were willing to commit to a yearlong study. The two interventions were matched in number of sessions, number of adults and children, and use of the same text (C. S. Lewis's *The Lion, the Witch, and the Wardrobe*) so that the effects of play and dramatization could be isolated. In the playworld group, which lasted for 2 hours for 14 sessions, children enacted the text and then discussed the text. Children could then draw or engage in free play with the props. Pre- and postintervention, children received a measure of narrative competence. Results were that children in the playworld condition showed significant improvements in narrative length, coherence, and comprehension, but not in linquistic complexity, when compared with the control condition. Baumer et al. concluded that the results of this study support the importance of play in promoting narrative competence, a literacy skill that is predictive of academic success. Given findings such as these, play and art should be kept in the elementary school curricula.

Bellin and Singer (2006) also found, in a nationally tested study, that pretend play improved literacy skills in preschool children. They used a video-based program for parents and other caregivers that uses make-believe play, "My Magic Story Car." Children watch pretend play games on the video and then play the games. Key literacy skills improved after the program was utilized. In addition, the majority of children continued to play the make-believe games on their own without adult intervention and teach the games to other children.

Ogan and Berk (2009) recently reported on a play intervention study that targeted self-regulation with preschool children. In this study, children in a nondirected play condition over a period of weeks showed a significant increase in self-regulation. In a study reported in a dissertation by Ogan (2005), 38 4- and 5-year-olds enrolled in Head Start whose pretense was high in antisocial themes were given a battery of self-regulation measures. The children were then randomly assigned to one of two conditions in which they received eight weekly individual play-training sessions. One group was adult-directed with much coaching and correction of inappropriate play themes. The adult-supported play group joined at the invitation of the child. Results were that adult direction constricted the play. The adult-supported group showed greater improvement on measures of self-regulation.

In her dissertation Beth Pearson (2008) focused on hope and school adjustment in a preschool population. Pearson developed a cognitive-behavioral play (CBP) intervention based on Knell's (1993) cognitive-behavioral play therapy (described in Chapter 10, this volume). Forty-eight children were randomly assigned to one of three conditions: a CBP intervention, a free-play condition, and a puzzles/coloring control condition. In the CBP intervention, the research drew on several cognitive-behavioral play strategies. These strategies included teaching children that stressors can be coped with, modeling a problem-solving approach, modeling the use of positive self-statements such as "If I practice, this will get easier," encouraging the children to generate multiple solutions to problems and to use positive self-statements, and praising them for engaging in play activities. In the free-play condition, the children heard the same stories, but play was unguided. Pre- and postintervention measures were administered. This study used an independent assessor for the assessment measures and a fidelity rater who was blind to the hypotheses who rated 19% of the intervention sessions. The major findings were that the CBP intervention play group had significantly higher hope and social competence and less anxiety than the control group, on teacher report measures. This study was the first to provide empirical support for cognitive-behavioral play strategies.

Several studies have used focused play interventions to reduce anxiety in children. These studies were reviewed in Chapter 1. Brief play interventions have reduced anxiety around hospital fears (Cassell, 1965; Johnson & Stockdale, 1975; Rae, Worchel, Upchurch, Sanner, & Dainiel, 1989) and reduced separation anxiety (Barnett, 1984; Milos & Reiss, 1982). The results of these studies suggest that play helps children deal with fears and reduce anxiety and that something about the play itself serves as a vehicle for change. The involvement of fantasy and make-believe is involved in the reduction of anxiety. The studies controlled for the variable of an attentive adult. Results also suggest that children who can already use fantasy and make-believe are more able to use play to resolve problems when the opportunity arises. Teaching children good play skills would provide children with a resource for future coping with fears and anxiety.

FUTURE DIRECTIONS

The promising results of the play intervention studies just reviewed are beginning to build an empirical base for the use of play interventions to bring about change in a variety of areas. The important cause–effect relationship between play and adaptive functioning is being supported. The implications of these studies for practice is that brief play interventions that target specific behaviors and cognitive and affective processes can be developed. They need to be refined and investigated in future research.

Empirically supported play modules that focus on specific issues could become a part of interventions for children. Russ first proposed this concept in 1995. Recent research is making this a more realistic possibility. This is consistent with Kazdin's (1993) idea of having various modules in psychotherapy, especially for children with multiple problems. If we can develop specific play interventions that target areas such as school anxiety, literacy, coping strategies, self-regulation, imagination, and affect expression, then these time-limited play intervention modules could be adapted for use in therapy or for large-scale prevention intervention programs.

For play intervention in therapy, research studies should:

- Focus on play interventions that target anxiety. Research to date suggests that pretend play is especially helpful in processing anxiety and fears. Investigating the effectiveness of play with anxiety disorders and posttraumatic stress disorder is a logical next step.

Also, investigating the use of play with specific types of anxiety-producing situations such as medical situations, starting school, or natural disasters could benefit large number of children.

- Identify specific play techniques and develop manuals. When is modeling and prompting by an adult helpful and when is a free-play situation with little adult intervention most helpful?
- Investigate mechanisms of change. Why does play help reduce anxiety? Is it because of slow exposure to the fear and desensitization? Is the narrative that is developed the more important variable? These important questions about therapy process need to be explored.
- Investigate the use of play intervention modules with specific problems and populations. Is it useful to teach play skills to high-risk groups? Will increased play skills benefit them in other ways?

Ideally, there would be play centers in schools. In addition to recess, there would be pretend play breaks where children could participate in guided pretend play sessions. This kind of center is consistent with Gardner's (1991) call for a restructuring of the school experience. He described Project Spectrum, an early childhood education program, as having different physical areas for different learning domains. A center for pretend play would fit with this model. Teachers and teacher aides could guide pretend play. It is essential that different types of play interventions receive empirical support. As these interventions are developed, the play intervention scripts can be made available to parents and teachers. We are just at the beginning of developing empirically tested play interventions that are helpful to children. Results of the play intervention studies that have been carried out are promising. Play is a resource that our society needs to invest in for the welfare of our children and our society.

REFERENCES

Barnett, I. (1984). Research note: Young children's resolution of distress through play. *Journal of Child Psychology and Psychiatry, 25,* 477–483.

Barton, E., & Wolery, M. (2008). Teaching pretend play to children with disabilities: A review of the literature. *Topics in Early Childhood Special Education, 28,* 109–128.

Baumer, S., Ferholt, S., & Lecusay, R. (2005). Promoting narrative competence through adult-joint pretense: Lessons from the Scandinavian educational practice of playworld. *Cognitive Development, 20,* 576–590.

Bellin, H., & Singer, D. (2006). "My Magic Story Car": Video-based play intervention to strengthen emergent literacy of at-risk preschoolers. In D. Singer, R. Golinkoff, & K. Hirsh-Pasek (Eds.), *Play = learning: How play moti-*

vates and enhances children's cognitive and social-emotional growth (pp. 101–123). New York: Oxford University Press.

Berk, L., Mann, T., & Ogman, A. (2006). Make-believe play: Wellspring for development of self-regulation. In D. Singer, R. Golinkoff, & K. Hirsh-Pasek (Eds.), *Play = learning: How play motivates and enhances children's cognitive and social-emotional growth* (pp. 74– 100). New York: Oxford University Press.

Bodiford-McNeil, C., Hembree-Kigin, T. L., & Eyberg, S. (1996). *Short-term play therapy for disruptive children.* King of Prussia, PA: Center for Applied Psychology.

Cassell, S. (1965). Effect of brief puppet therapy upon the emotional response of children undergoing cardiac catheterization. *Journal of Consulting Psychology, 29,* 1–8.

Cowen, E., Hightower, A. D., Johnson, D., Sarno, M., & Weissberg, R. (1989). State-level dissemination of a program for early detection and prevention of school maladjustment. *Professional Psychology: Research and Practice, 20,* 309–314.

Dansky, J. (1980). Make-believe: A mediator of the relationship between play and associative fluency. *Child Development, 51,* 576–579.

Dansky, J. (1999). Play. In M. Runco & S. Pritzker (Eds.), *Encyclopedia of creativity* (pp. 393–408). San Diego, CA: Academic Press.

Fein, G. (1987). Pretend play: Creativity and consciousness. In P. Gorlitz & J. Wohlwill (Eds.), *Curiosity, imagination, and play* (pp. 281–304). Hillsdale, NJ: Erlbaum.

Gardner, H. (1991). *The unschooled mind.* New York: Basic Books.

Hartmann, W., & Rollett, B. (1994). Play: Positive intervention in the elementary school curriculum. In J. Hellendoorn, R. van der Kooij, & B. Sutton-Smith (Eds.), *Play and intervention* (pp. 195–202). Albany: State University of New York Press.

Hellendoorn, V. (1994). Imaginative play training for severely retarded children. In V. Hellendoorn, R. van der Kooij, & B. Sutton-Smith (Eds.), *Play and intervention* (pp. 113–122). Albany: State University of New York Press.

Isen, A., Daubman, K., & Nowicki, G. (1987). Positive affect facilitates creative problem solving. *Journal of Personality and Social Psychology, 52,* 1122–1131.

Johnson, P., & Stockdale, D. (1975). Effects of puppet therapy on Palmar sweating of hospitalized children. *Johns Hopkins Medical Journal, 137,* 1–5.

Kasari, C., Freeman, S., & Paparella, T. (2006). Joint attention and symbolic play in young children with autism: A randomized controlled intervention study. *Journal of Child Psychology and Psychiatry, 47,* 611–620.

Kazdin, A. (1993, August). *Child and adolescent psychotherapy: Models for identifying and developing effective treatments.* Symposium presented at the annual meeting of the American Psychological Association, Toronto.

Kim, Y. T., Lombardino, L. J., Rothman, H., & Vinson, B. (1989). Effects of symbolic play intervention with children who have mental retardation. *Mental Retardation, 27,* 159–165.

Knell, S. (1993). *Cognitive-behavioral play therapy.* Northvale, NJ: Aronson.

Landreth, G. (1991). *Play therapy: The art of the relationship.* Bristol, PA: Accelerated Development.

Milos, M., & Reiss, S. (1982). Effects of three play conditions on separation anxiety in young children. *Journal of Consulting and Clinical Psychology, 50,* 389–395.

Moore, M.., & Russ, S. (2008). Follow-up of a pretend play intervention: Effects on play, creativity, and emotional processes in children. *Creativity Research Journal, 20,* 427–436.

Nafpaktitis, M., & Perlmutter, B. (1998). School-based early mental health intervention with at-risk students. *School Psychology Review, 27,* 420–432.

Ogan, A. (2005). *An investigation of the effects of make-believe play training on the development of self-regulation in Head Start children.* Unpublished doctoral dissertation, Illinois State University, Normal.

Ogan, A., & Berk, L. (2009, April). *Effects of two approaches to make-believe play training on development of self-regulation in Head Start children.* Paper presented at the Society for Research in Child Development, Denver, CO.

Pearson, B. (2008). *Effects of a cognitive behavioral play intervention on children's hope and school adjustment.* Unpublished dissertation, Case Western Reserve University, Cleveland, OH.

Rae, W., Worchel, R., Upchurch, J., Sanner, J., & Dainiel, C. (1989). The psychosocial impact of play on hospitalized children. *Journal of Pediatric Psychology, 14,* 617–627.

Russ, S. (1987). Assessment of cognitive affective interaction in children: Creativity, fantasy, and play research. In J. Butcher & C. Spielberger (Eds.), *Advances in personality assessment* (Vol. 6, pp. 141–155). Hillsdale, NJ: Erlbaum.

Russ, S. (1993). *Affect and creativity: The role of affect and play in the creative process.* Hillsdale, NJ: Erlbaum.

Russ, S. (1998). Play therapy. In T. Ollendick (Ed.), *Children and adolescents: Clinical formulation and treatment* (pp. 221–243). Oxford, UK: Elsevier Science.

Russ, S. (2004). *Play in child development and psychotherapy: Toward empirically supported practice.* Mahwah, NJ: Erlbaum.

Russ, S., Moore, M., & Farber, B. (2004, July). *Effects of play training on play, creativity, and emotional processing.* Poster presented at the American Psychological Association meeting, Honolulu.

Russ, S., Moore, M. E., & Pearson, B. L. (2007). *Effects of play intervention on play skill and adaptive functioning: A pilot study.* Manuscript submitted for publication.

Russ, S. W., Robins, D., & Christiano, B. (1999). Pretend play: Longitudinal prediction of creativity and affect in fantasy in children. *Creativity Research Journal, 12,* 129–139.

Shirk, S. R., & Russell, R. (1996). *Change processes in child psychotherapy: Revitalizing treatment and research.* New York: Guilford Press.

Shmukler, D. (1984–1985). Structured vs. unstructured play training with economically disadvantaged preschoolers. *Imagination, Cognition, & Personality, 4,* 293–304.

Singer, D. G., & Singer, J. L. (1990). *The house of make-believe: Children's play and the developing imagination.* Cambridge, MA: Harvard University Press.

Smilansky, S. (1968). *The effects of sociodramatic play on disadvantaged preschool children.* New York: Wiley.

Smith, P. (1988). Children's play and its role in early development: A re-evaluation of the "play ethos." In A. Pellegrini (Ed.), *Psychological bases for early education* (pp. 207–226). Chichester, UK: Wiley.

Smith, P. (1994). Play training: An overview. In J. Hellendoorn, R. van der Kooij, & B. Sutton-Smith (Eds.), *Play and intervention* (pp. 185–192). Albany: State University of New York Press.

Udwin, O. (1983). Imaginative play training as an intervention method with institutionalized preschool children. *British Journal of Educational Psychology, 53,* 32–39.

14

Conclusions and Implications for the Use of Play in Intervention and Prevention Programs

Sandra W. Russ and Larissa N. Niec

What can we conclude about the state of empirical support for the use of pretend play in intervention and prevention programs for children? The impressive work by the authors of the chapters in this book suggest that real progress is being made in both measuring play and in developing interventions strategies that are effectively reducing emotional problems and increasing adaptive processes in children.

Looking first at the child development research on play, pretend play has definitely been established as important in both reflecting cognitive, affective, and interpersonal processes and in facilitating the development of some of those processes. Russ, Fiorelli, and Spannagel (Chapter 1) reviewed the research on cognitive and affective processes in play and concluded that pretend play relates to and facilitates various kinds of problem-solving ability such as divergent thinking (the ability to generate a variety of ideas and solutions), coping strategies, and insight ability. These problem-solving abilities are adaptive in everyday functioning and adjustment. Play also relates to dimensions of adjustment in children, such as emotion regulation and the processing of emotions. Well-conducted play intervention studies have shown that play reduces anxiety and fears in children. Although the mechanisms by which this change occurs remain to be determined, research suggests that the fantasy component is important. Access to emotion in play probably contributes as well and is an important variable to isolate in future research.

Play also relates to many areas of interpersonal functioning, as reviewed by Jent, Niec, and Baker (Chapter 2). They concluded that although play has been associated with such interpersonal processes as perspective taking and empathy, not enough longitudinal and experimental research exists to clearly delineate causal relationships. Jent and colleagues propose four important issues to be considered when evaluating the value of play for use within an intervention: the goals of the intervention program, the ages of the children for whom the intervention is designed, the mechanisms likely to bring about change, and the empirical links among those mechanisms and play.

We are reminded by Jent and colleagues that play should not be interpreted without also considering the influence of culture. Although the structure of children's pretend play appears similar across cultures, the frequency and content of play varies widely.

PLAY AND EVIDENCE-BASED ASSESSMENT

In order to study play, we need to be able to measure play. The chapters in the assessment section reviewed a number of play measures with various degrees of empirical support that can be used in investigating children's functioning. As Kaugars (Chapter 3) concludes, for all of these measures more research is needed with larger, more diverse populations and different research teams. Interestingly, most of the measures described assess specific dimensions of the play itself or of the parent–child play interaction. The Dyadic Parent–Child Interaction Coding System described by Knight and Salamone (Chapter 4) is specific and uniquely suited to assessing therapeutic change during parenting interventions such as parent–child interaction therapy (PCIT). Kernberg's Children's Play Therapy Instrument (Kernberg, Chazan, & Normandin, 1998) measures variables of particular interest to psychodynamic therapists. Russ's Affect in Play Scale was originally designed with a main focus on affect expression in fantasy and range of affect expression, with a secondary focus on imagination (Russ, 1993, 2004). Designing measures to assess specific processes in play is consistent with increasingly refined intervention studies that need to focus on specific processes and mechanisms of change in psychotherapy.

Tharinger, Christopher, and Matson (Chapter 5) effectively demonstrate how well play assessment fits with therapeutic assessment. Play assessment is a natural assessment method that lends itself to the collaboration and short-term intervention that defines therapeutic assessment. Short and colleagues (Chapter 11) speak to the utility of play-based assessment for many populations of at-risk children. For children with language disabilities or attention-deficit/hyperactivity disorder (ADHD) and for very young children, a play assessment approach that is developmentally sensitive can be flexible enough to engage these children.

PLAY AND EVIDENCE-BASED INTERVENTIONS

A number of evidence-based interventions integrate play into therapy. What emerges in several of these chapters is that although the intervention has been supported in a number of studies, the play element has not been isolated and evaluated as a component of treatment. For example, Briggs, Runyon, and Deblinger (Chapter 7) present a thorough discussion of how play is used in trauma-focused cognitive-behavioral therapy. They describe play as a crucial ingredient in this intervention that is used in a number of phases of the intervention depending upon the needs of the child. For instance, play can be used to help the child imagine scenes for relaxation and to reenact traumatic experiences. Briggs and colleagues give numerous, innovative examples of how play is used in this well-supported approach. Future research needs to focus on the role of play in the effectiveness of the intervention.

Pincus and colleagues (Chapter 9) make the same point when discussing the use of play in cognitive-behavioral therapy with anxious children. Again, play is a part of empirically supported treatment packages for anxious children which have been empirically validated. However, the relative impact of the play component has not been investigated. One important point made by Briggs and colleagues (Chapter 7) is that a therapist who is play-oriented and playful can model for children the importance of reengaging with the positive aspects of life. Although this kind of playfulness could be an important quality that brings about change, it may be difficult to measure and document as a mechanism of change.

Knell and Dasari (Chapter 10) provide a sophisticated description of cognitive-behavioral play therapy. Play is the major component of this approach that is based on principles of cognitive-behavioral therapy. Little direct empirical support exists for this approach. Knell and Dasari describe two studies that use principles of cognitive-behavioral play therapy in interventions there were found to be effective. The authors call for more research to support the intervention.

Two chapters looked at play interventions for children with developmental disabilities and ADHD. Short and colleagues (Chapter 11) describe the potential of play intervention for children with ADHD, language problems, and Asperger syndrome. Kasari, Huynh, and Gulsrud (Chapter 8) describe the one randomized controlled intervention study with children with autism that focused on symbolic play. Because they had three groups and the methodology was rigorous, they were able to conclude that symbolic play improved because of the play intervention. This study is a model for play intervention studies with clinical populations. Kasari and colleagues also stress that the play intervention was targeted at the developmental level of the child.

PCIT is an evidence-based behavioral intervention for the treatment of childhood conduct problems that uses play very differently from other interventions discussed in this volume. That is, play is a mechanism to enhance the parent–child relationship and focuses on both parents' and children's behaviors. Rather than facilitating children's pretend play, PCIT fosters parent–child dyadic play, through which parents gain active practice in child-centered skills and behavior management techniques.

As other authors in this volume have noted, Niec, Gering, and Abbenante (Chapter 6) point out that analyses of the mechanisms of change in PCIT are still needed. Identifying the components of PCIT that are critical to its effectiveness is important as pressure increases to disseminate and implement evidence-based interventions faster and more cheaply.

Niec and colleagues also observe that a number of system-, treatment-, and family-level barriers must be addressed so that a greater portion of the children suffering from behavior disorders are able to access evidence-based treatments. Play may be one vehicle for enhancing the parent–child relationship.

PLAY AND EVIDENCE-BASED PREVENTION

Bishop-Josef and Zigler's (Chapter 12) review of Head Start and other preschool play-based curricula like Tools of the Mind emphasize the importance of play-based learning in early child development. They convincingly argue that play-based learning should occur simultaneously with direct instruction of academic skills. Curricula that are play-based have been empirically supported in the development of language skills, literacy, and cognitive and socioemotional abilities. Head Start includes both free-play and structured play activities. Play has not been isolated in the research to investigate the specific impact of the play on outcomes. Bishop-Josef and Zigler also state that evaluating play within the curriculum would be difficult to do. However, they conclude that it is likely that the impact of Head Start is partly due to play, since it is such a large part of the curriculum. One important study that they reviewed is the study by Zigler and Styfko (1993) that concluded that, especially for children with low socioeconomic backgrounds, play-based curricula should be used through the third grade. Children continue to engage in various kinds of play until they are 9 or 10 and research has shown that play interventions can be effective with this older age group.

Russ and Pearson (Chapter 13) describe other play intervention studies with school-based populations. They conclude that there is great potential for using focused, brief, standardized interventions in school settings to effect a variety of areas in child development. The studies emerging from the Russ research lab suggest that play abilities can be facilitated and have the potential to influence creativity, coping, and life satisfaction. Methodologically rigorous studies from different researchers have found that play interventions could reduce anxiety in the school situation. The protocol developed by Pearson (2008), based on cognitive-behavioral play therapy, was effective in reducing anxiety in preschoolers. This intervention protocol should be refined and further developed. The Nafpaktitis and Perlmutter (1998) study found that play sessions improved school adjustment. Classroom aides carried out the play intervention. This study demonstrates that paraprofessionals can be trained to effectively carry out play intervention protocols. Teachers' aides and other paraprofessionals in elementary schools and preschool programs could be trained in empirically supported play intervention protocols.

INTEGRATING PLAY INTERVENTIONS INTO PSYCHOTHERAPY

As focused play interventions are developed, they can be integrated into different psychotherapy approaches. Play intervention modules would be one way of integrating play interventions. Jent, Niec, and Baker (Chapter 2) propose a set of four important guidelines to consider when integrating play into a psychotherapeutic intervention. These guidelines might be applied to a variety of methods of integration. For example, when implementing a play module approach, various play techniques could be implemented in a series of sessions or within a session. For a child with constricted affect, for instance, the five 20-minute play sessions that Russ, Moore, and Pearson developed could be used early in therapy to facilitate expression of emotions (Moore & Russ, 2008). Preliminary research found that the intervention increased affect expression in children from low socioeconomic backgrounds. For the disorganized child, using a play module to develop narratives might bring more coherence to the child's thinking.

Before such a module approach is implemented, it is necessary to better understand the mechanisms through which play facilitates change. The work in this volume raises a number of questions about play: When is modeling a situation through play more effective than just reflecting what is occurring in the moment? When is praise helpful and when is it inhibiting? Research investigating specific play techniques must be carried out in the laboratory before being transferred to clinical settings.

In some forms of therapy, it would be useful to initially assess whether a child can utilize play in treatment. Many children in need of treatment cannot pretend or use fantasy to imagine scenarios. In interventions such as trauma-focused cognitive-behavioral therapy, for example, children must be able to use imagination to create the trauma narrative. A play assessment could determine the abilities of the child to pretend and use fantasy and to express affect in play. If the child could use play, then play could be utilized in the therapy. If not, the therapist would need to decide whether to try to improve the child's play ability in addition to focusing on other issues. For children with constricted affect who can still pretend, using play to access emotion could be effective rather quickly. On the other hand, for children who have major difficulties pretending, using play in a short-term therapy approach would not be a good use of the limited time available. The age of the child would influence decisions about using play as well.

Many traditional play therapy interventions lack support regarding their efficacy to enhance children's functioning. However, as Russ and colleagues (Chapter 1) and Jent and colleagues (Chapter 2) have argued, developmental research demonstrates a robust relationship between play and children's cognitive, affective, and interpersonal processes. In addition, play is a natural mode of communication and interaction for children. It is not surprising, then, that so many evidence-based interventions include play in some form. These psychotherapeutic approaches represent the next generation of play interventions. By integrating play with principles from orientations with strong empirical support, such as cognitive-behavioral therapy, researchers have created developmentally sensitive, efficacious treatments that recognize play as an important aspect of children's behavioral and emotional health.

In conclusion, the field has made significant progress in building an empirical base for play approaches in intervention and prevention programs. A growing number of play assessment instruments exist that have validity studies to support them. Empirically supported interventions are using play as a major component of the treatment package. The play component needs to be isolated to determine the impact of the play.

Although a number of areas exist where play interventions could be further refined, focused studies are finding that play intervention facilitates change and growth in a variety of domains.

Historically, a gap has existed between the basic, developmental research on play and the treatment efficacy research. This volume has brought together the two literatures in hopes that (1) developmental scientists will be stimulated by the intervention research to ask new questions about children's emotional and behavioral processes, and (2) researchers and clinicians developing interventions will consider the data regarding play and child development when creating new treatment approaches.

The field of play research will benefit from increased communication and collaboration among researchers. Increased partnerships between research laboratories and clinical settings will also aid in the development and dissemination of evidence-based play assessment and intervention. As play is rediscovered as an important vehicle for change and growth in children, new research will teach us about how we can help children through play.

REFERENCES

Kernberg, P., Chazan, S., & Normandin, L. (1998). The children's play therapy incident (CPTI): Description, development, and reliability studies. *Journal of Psychotherapy Practice and Research, 7*, 196–207.

Moore, M., & Russ, S. (2008). Follow-up of a pretend play intervention: Effects on play, creativity, and emotional processes in children. *Creativity Research Journal, 20*, 427–436.

Nafpaktitus, M., & Perlmutter, B. (1998) School-based early mental health intervention with at-risk students. *School Psychology Review, 27*, 420–432.

Pearson, B. (2008). *Effects of a cognitive behavioral play intervention on children's hope and school adjustment.* Unpublished dissertation, Case Western Reserve University, Cleveland, OH.

Russ, S. (1993). *Affect and creativity: The role of affect and play in the creative process.* Hillsdale, NJ: Erlbaum.

Russ, S. (2004). *Play in child development and psychotherapy: Toward empirically supported practice.* Mahwah, NJ: Erlbaum.

Zigler, E., & Styfco, S. (Eds.). (1993). *Head Start and beyond: A national plan for extended childhood intervention.* New Haven, CT: Yale University Press.

Index

Page numbers followed by an *f* or *t* indicate figures or tables.